Adverse Reactions
to Drug
Formulation Agents

CLINICAL PHARMACOLOGY

Series Editor

MURRAY WEINER

Division of Clinical Pharmacology and Toxicology
University of Cincinnati
College of Medicine
Cincinnati, Ohio

Volume 1 Nicotinic Acid: Nutrient-Cofactor-Drug, *by Murray Weiner and Jan van Eys*

Volume 2 Drugs in Central Nervous System Disorders, *edited by David C. Horwell*

Volume 3 Clinical Application of Interferons and Their Inducers, Second Edition, *edited by Dale A. Stringfellow*

Volume 4 Beta-Lactam Antibiotics for Clinical Use, *edited by Sherry F. Queener, J. Alan Webber, and Stephen W. Queener*

Volume 5 Receptor Binding in Drug Research, *edited by Robert A. O'Brien*

Volume 6 Drug Therapy in Hypertension, *edited by Jan I. M. Drayer, David T. Lowenthal, and Michael A. Weber*

Volume 7 Adverse Reactions to Muscle Relaxants, *edited by Isaac Azar*

Volume 8 Clinical Pharmacology in the Elderly, *edited by Cameron G. Swift*

Volume 9 Anti-Inflammatory Compounds, *edited by W. R. Nigel Williamson*

Volume 10 Nonsteroidal Anti-Inflammatory Drugs: Mechanisms and Clinical Use, *edited by Alan J. Lewis and Daniel E. Furst*

Volume 11 Drug Stereochemistry: Analytical Methods and Pharmacology, *edited by Irving W. Wainer and Dennis E. Drayer*

Volume 12 Drug Interaction Compendium, *by Murray Weiner*

Volume 13 Receptor Pharmacology and Function, *edited by Michael Williams, Richard A. Glennon, and Pieter B. M. W. M. Timmermans*

Volume 14 Adverse Reactions to Drug Formulation Agents: A Handbook of Excipients, *by Murray Weiner and I. Leonard Bernstein*

Volume 15 Cardiovascular Function of Peripheral Dopamine Receptors, *edited by J. Paul Hieble*

Additional Volumes in Preparation

Drug Therapy in Disease States, *edited by Roger L. Williams, Craig Brater, and Joyce Mordenti*

Adverse Reactions to Drug Formulation Agents

A Handbook of Excipients

Murray Weiner / I. Leonard Bernstein

College of Medicine
University of Cincinnati
Cincinnati, Ohio

MARCEL DEKKER, INC.   New York and Basel

Dedicated by
Dr. Bernstein to his wife, Miriam,
his partner in all of life's endeavors,
and by
Dr. Weiner to the memory of his late wife, Marilyn,
whose love, fidelity, and support remain an inspiration for his
continuing productivity

Library of Congress Cataloging-in-Publication Data

Weiner, Murray
    Adverse reactions to drug formulations: a handbook of excipients.

    (Clinical pharmacology ; v. 14)
    Includes index.
    I. Excipients--Side effects.   2. Drugs--Side effects.
I. Bernstein, I. Leonard.   II. Title.
III. Series. [DNLM: 1. Excipients--adverse effects.
W1 CL764H v. 14 / QV 800 W423a]
RS201.E87W45   1989   615'.7042   89-12041
ISBN 0-8247-7944-4 (alk. paper)

This book is printed on acid-free paper.

MARCEL DEKKER, INC.
270 Madison Avenue, New York, New York 10016

Current printing (last digit):
10 9 8 7 6 5 4 3 2 1

PRINTED IN THE UNITED STATES OF AMERICA

Series Introduction

This is Volume 14 of the Marcel Dekker "Clinical Pharmacology" series that I have been privileged to edit over the past five years. While most of the other works were prepared by numerous chapter authors under the guidance of a volume editor, this entire volume has been personally written by my coauthor and me. It meant a lot of work for us, but it was a labor of love, and we hope we have achieved a unity of style and flow of thought that makes the effort worthwhile.

The decision to write a book about side effects to excipients was the result of an uneasy feeling that the complex role of excipients is generally not well appreciated and often ignored. On the other hand, the perception of undesired consequences attributed to excipients occasionally reaches far beyond reality.

The formulators who decide on excipients are generally experts in physicochemical phenomena, pharmaceutical machinery, and manufacturing procedures rather than clinical medicine. Physicians and patients generally accept the available formulations on the basis of faith in a government-regulated industry. We decided to approach the subject with an outline and review of modern concepts and scientific advances relevant to an understanding of the purposes and potential effects of excipients. Only then could a rational review of individual excipients and classes of excipients according to logical categories be undertaken. Since allergic and nonallergic reactions need to be distinguished and understood, these two categories of side effects are separately described and evaluated. The book includes a section on reactions to materials used in devices and a listing of thousands of excipients in products currently marketed in the United States, as compiled by the FDA.

The process of writing this book was in itself a real learning experience. We hope the fruits of this experience will now be shared with readers in many disciplines who have an interest in understanding the consequences of the use of excipients.

Murray Weiner, M.D.

Foreword

It is paradoxical that science in general pays so much attention to the "active chemicals" in medicinal formulations and so little to the so-called "inactive" ingredients used to provide bulk or coating to a capsule or tablet, to add color, to prevent chemical change, to mask unpleasant taste, or to solubilize the active materials.

Scientists who specialize in biopharmaceutical problems know how complex they can be and also realize how "active" some of these excipients can be on occasion. There are, for example, dramatic adverse reactions to the coloring material, tartrazine, particularly among individuals who are also intolerant of aspirin. A broad spectrum of other reactions to excipients, more subtle and as yet less well documented, is coming to light and beginning to get the attention it deserves.

Testing for bioequivalency of generic products in healthy volunteers places great importance on the need for pharmacokinetic identity of brand and competitor versions but ignores the possibility of misadventure from the presence of different excipients in a proposed generic product.

The present volume is a welcome addition to the scientific literature and is long overdue. It not only brings together a great deal of information not otherwise readily available, but serves as a reminder of the importance of excipients in medicinal products.

Louis Lasagna, M.D.
Center for the Study of Drug Development
Tufts University
Boston, Massachusetts

Preface

Medical attention to adverse reactions induced by excipients in drug formulations is of relatively recent origin. Two major initiatives during the food and drug regulatory process in the United States accelerated this recognition during the last half-century. Both of these evolved from concerns about possible side effects from colorants in foods and drugs. Enactment of the Federal Food, Drug and Cosmetic Act of 1938 was the landmark excipient legislation; it prohibited the use of any *uncertified* coal-tar-derived color in foods and drugs. Certification of drug colorants thereupon became mandatory. The second important event was passage of the Delaney Clause of the Color Additive Amendments of 1960, which specifically banned use of color additives with *any* carcinogenic potential in man and animals. As a result of this regulation, the most commonly used FD&C colorant, amaranth (FD&C Red #2), was delisted in the mid 1970s. Thus up to that time, the major impact of drug safety legislation had been primarily overt toxicity and the carcinogenic potential of drug-based excipients.

Undoubtedly, these new laws also catalyzed heightened awareness about the occurrence of less-well-defined forms of adverse responses, including allergic and pseudoallergic reactions. Beginning in 1959 with the first report of acute symptoms induced by tartrazine in drug consumers, the number of documented morbid reactions to colorants and other excipients has increased in exponential fashion. Although previously noted for many years, the role of excipients in the induction of contact dermatitis also received greater emphasis during this period. Recently, fatal and near-fatal anaphylactic episodes involving sulfite analogs and the sterilizing gas, ethylene oxide, have further raised the level of concern about excipients among federal scientists and legislators. Unfortunately, the widely publicized notoriety given these severe reactions has sparked an increased number of speculative and anecdotal reports concerning suspected excipient-induced adverse reactions that cannot be objectively substantiated. To the uninitiated, who may wish to be informed about possible excipient problems surfacing in the current spate of critical and noncritical literature, it is often difficult to distinguish fact from fiction.

The purpose, content, and format of this book were conceptualized in response to the confusing and scattered body of knowledge about adverse reactions currently attributed to excipients. Major texts of pharmacology and allergy refer only to selected prototypes of abnormal responses elicited by excipients. It was evident that a more detailed reference source about the side effects of drug additives was needed. It was also essential that a text devoted to additive substances should encompass significant factual data about most of the materials currently being used in drug formulations. Finally, it was decided that a simplified organization of the text into nonallergic and allergic categories would best satisfy the clinical backgrounds and needs of most readers. Allergic hypersensitivity was further defined according to the numerical classification of Gell and Coombs. Descriptive accounts of both allergic and nonallergic reactions were subdivided according to predominant anatomical manifestations—symptoms and signs. A designation of pseudoallergy was included to characterize the immunologically nonspecific nature of many reactions caused by excipients. Finally, a special chapter on medical devices was included in this review because of the increasing number of "inactive" additives being incorporated into these materials.

The primary goal of this text is to provide convenient access to and reliable information about excipient-associated adverse reactions. By compiling this ready reference, we hope that practitioners and pharmaceutical scientists will be alerted to the possibility that some apparently drug-related clinical side effects may be caused by nontherapeutic components of drug formulations.

Murray Weiner
I. Leonard Bernstein

Contents

Series Introduction (*Murray Weiner*)   iii
Foreword (*Louis Lasagna*)   v
Preface   vii

Introduction   1

Part I Assessment of Adverse Reactions to Excipients
  1 General Considerations   13
  2 Classification of Adverse Reactions   17
  3 Allergic Reactions   23
  4 Immunopathogenesis of Human Hypersensitivity   39
  5 Diagnostic Procedures for Human Hypersensitivity Diseases and
     Pseudoallergic Reactions   59

Part II Nonallergic Adverse Effects of Excipients by Class of Excipient
  6 Adverse Effects: Bulk Materials   89
  7 Adverse Effects: Coatings   121
  8 Adverse Effects: Flavoring Agents   133
  9 Adverse Effects: Coloring Agents   159
  10 Adverse Effects: Other Addition Products   167

Part III Allergic and Pseudoallergic Reactions by Class of Excipient
  11 Allergic Reactions: Bulk Materials   201
  12 Allergic Reactions: Coatings   223
  13 Allergic Reactions: Flavoring Agents   231
  14 Allergic Reactions: Coloring Agents   253
  15 Allergic Reactions: Other Addition Products   283

Part IV Device Materials
  16 Reactions to Materials Used in the Construction of Devices   343

Part V Appendix
Tabulation of Inactive Ingredients   359

Index   449

Introduction

The formulation of drugs has long been known to be a significant element in the action of medicaments. In earlier times, medications were essentially either extracts of biological material, usually plants, or relatively crude mineral products. The nature of the final product as a powder or a solution or suspension in modified aqueous solvents such as elixirs was intimately related to the steps necessary for the extraction and preservation of the active ingredients. All components of an active medication were considered an integral part of the action of the medicine. Medicinal products were frequently combinations prepared with the expectation that the final effect would not be a simple summation of the action known for each component. It required the skill of a professional pharmacist to combine these ingredients properly so as to achieve the desired final product. Differentiating between active and inactive components was not seriously considered.

With advances in medicine, pharmacology, and the pharmaceutical sciences, few medicines are accepted in scientific circles unless they are well-characterized, individual, biologically active chemical entities, specifically formulated with presumably inert ingredients to accomplish a technical purpose. The addition of inactive components may be necessary for a wide variety of reasons, ranging from flow characteristics required by large-scale machinery to the need for acceptable product uniformity, stability, convenience of use, handling, or pattern of bioavailability. Oral medication, formerly predominantly in liquid form, is now more convenient and generally more stable in economical tablets or capsules. Often the bulk of the desired dose is so small that a "filler" must be added just for practical handling. Control of taste and appearance may motivate additions to the bulk or the coating of a dosage form that make no direct contribution to the medicinal action of the product.

This volume gives medical scientists and practitioners a resource to evaluate problems in therapy that may involve excipients in medications. Recent developments have improved the availability of information identifying the excipients included in commonly prescribed drug preparations, but there is still an information gap concerning the effects and biological mechanisms by which these excipients may cause undesired responses, and the types of clinically observed

1

phenomena that may be due to or influenced by them. This volume is intended to help fill that gap.

Webster's 7th New Collegiate Dictionary defines an "excipient" as "an inert substance added to a prescription in order to confer a suitable consistency or form to the drug; a vehicle." These definitions can be taken to mean that only bulk carriers or solvents of active agents are excipients. For the purposes of this volume, the term "excipient" is more broadly applied to include all agents in a medicinal preparation regardless of their nature, purpose, or quantities employed, other than the components intended as the active ingredients. Impurities of active components that are inadvertently a part of the final medicinal preparation are not considered to be "additives" and are beyond the scope of this review. However, some harmful impurities or breakdown products that are known to reach the final product via an excipient will be discussed. Some important incidentally coadministered agents, such as propellants, sterilizing gases, and potentially harmful materials leached from containers will also be reviewed. However, deliberate adulteration of preparations to achieve a hidden purpose will not be reviewed as a problem of excipients. Incidents such as the undocumented addition of a steroid to the base of a topical cream, or the oriental practice of formulating modern medications in traditional concoctions to achieve one or another presumed advantage, are not reviewed here.

At times the contribution of an excipient to the medicinal effects of the preparation may be critical to the point of being as important to the action of the drug as the recognized active components themselves. While such contributions of excipients to activity are discussed in places, the major emphasis in this volume is on the intrinsic actions of the excipients per se that may be clinically significant, rather than their intended influence on the action of the active component of medication.

In order to develop reasonable attitudes and opinions about excipients with potential harmful effects or with suspected but unproved adverse effects, it is essential to know something about the function the excipient serves, and the risks associated with alternative excipients. This text therefore includes in Parts II and III brief comments about the utility of each excipient, classified and reviewed in accordance with its function in medicinal formulations.

Materials used as excipients are sometimes described as being "natural" or "artificial." Such characterization commonly carries with it strong inferences of "good" and "bad." Natural flavors, for example, are assumed to be directly derived from accepted foods and, therefore, safe, while artificial flavors carry not only the stigma of inferiority but also an implied danger of potential harm. This attitude is understandable since any natural substance that has survived millennia of human experience deserves a degree of confidence that is unavailable to synthesized materials that have been with us for only a few decades or less.

On the other hand, the ancients knew that even many natural substances are highly toxic. Socrates knew the consequences of hemlock and the Borgias knew many natural poisons. Until relatively recent times, tomatoes were considered poisonous, indicating that ancient judgments were not always correct. Tobacco was smoked for hundreds of years and cigarettes used for decades before the carcinogenic potential of this "natural" product was recognized. One of the most potent carcinogens known, aflatoxin, is a natural substance formed by a fungus growing on stored foods such as beans and peanuts. A single dose of 1 mg orally to a rat consistently results in multiple malignancies in a month or two. Using an "artificial" antifungal agent might block the development of this "natural" but harmful agent.

Since there is a wide variety and fairly high incidence of food sensitivities and allergies, it is to be expected that excipients prepared from foodlike natural products may also produce such reactions. Nature can be cruel, and the fact that a substance is of natural origin is not fully reassuring as to its safety.

Another "buzzword" that conjures up implications that may not be justified is the descriptive term "pure." To a chemist, a pure substance is a single agent uncontaminated by other entities. With foods or excipients such as cornstarch or powdered milk, purity is a question of the absence of contaminants or additives. Making some natural excipients more pure in the chemical sense may interfere with their desirable properties as excipients. Natural biological products, even when purified, can have stability problems, particularly the type of instability associated with the capacity to support the growth of microorganisms. In some instances "contaminants" are deliberately left in or added to help preserve the desirable aspects of the excipient. Thus an "impurity" may be useful, and some "impurities" may be deliberately added to prevent development of a more harmful impurity.

Statements indicating that an excipient is natural rather than artificial, or pure rather than commercial or unrefined, can be helpful in describing the nature of the excipient and possible consequences of its use, but should not be allowed to prejudice judgments about the probability that it may cause clinical problems.

Many excipients are available in several forms to serve a variety of purposes. Many of these forms are defined by official or semiofficial bodies such as the United States Pharmacopeia (USP). For example, lactose can be obtained as lactose hydrous USP, lactose anhydrous USP, and lactose spray-dried USP. While these different forms are of critical interest to formulation specialists, they rarely differ in their significance to practitioners concerned with undesired reactions to excipients. Consequently, the different forms will be reviewed separately only when the differences are of known relevance to undesired clinical effects. In some instances, such as with starch, a dozen or more chemically derived forms can have important formulation consequences with essentially no toxic or other clinically significant differences.

In evaluating excipients, as with foods or active drug agents, there is a legal need to declare that an agent is "safe" if it is to be used. However, safety is rarely all-or-none, and a great deal of harm to the public interest can be done by merely raising questions about the lack of absolute safety when the question could only be answered by proving the unprovable, that is, that nothing harmful could ever possibly occur.

In the real world, no activity has zero risk, including inaction. When a given excipient is presented for use, the realistic safety question should not be "what is the risk of using this agent" but rather "what is the risk of using this agent as compared to the risk of *not* using the agent." In other words, if the agent is not to be used, what *will* be used instead, or if nothing is used, what risks accompany *that* decision? Lack of a proper excipient can be accompanied by significant dosage and other quality control problems.

For medications to be made available, they must be formulated. Dozens of considerations ranging from the physical aspects of uniformity, purity, and stability to the attitude of the consuming patient enter into the equation. It is not so much a question of whether excipients are safe, but whether they are as safe as possible, given the formulation requirements of the particular medication. In the last analysis, the physician must make a benefit–risk judgment about each patient for the drug *as formulated*. Some knowledge about the nature, purposes, and consequences of excipients is bound to be helpful.

The spectrum of adverse effects that may result from excipients is much the same as that of drugs, foods, or other materials to which we are exposed. It is common to classify adverse effects into either "toxic" or "sensitivity" reactions. If a reaction is seen more or less uniformly in all individuals, particularly if it is dose-dependent, it is likely to be called a toxic effect. If it occurs only in an occasional individual, even after use of a small dose, the "blame" is put on the individual for being "sensitive" rather than on the agent. This empirical method of classification sometimes conflicts with the mechanistic concept that "toxic" is a direct injurious effect on living cells or tissues that occurs in all individuals, while "sensitivity" implies an immune or "allergic" reaction involving the development of antibodies only in sensitive individuals in response to a foreign agent or allergen with the adverse reaction being a consequence of antigen–antibody interactions. Topically the distinction is made between "primary irritants" and "sensitizing agents."

The problem is considerably more complicated. Some allergic (i.e., antibody-antigen based) reactions are almost universal. A highly antigenic substance such as egg albumin injected into mammals at appropriate intervals is uniformly harmful (causing anaphylaxis) and therefore might be labeled "toxic." Conversely, subjects with an uncommon metabolic enzyme disturbance may create or fail to neutralize a highly and directly toxic metabolite produced from a substance that is harmlessly handled by most people. Such subjects may be uniquely "sensitive" in developing a harmful response that does not involve the immune system. The problem is reviewed in more detail in Part I.

Given the complexities of the body's handling of materials to which it is exposed, and individual differences in response to similar exposures, it can be difficult to classify reactions to excipients dogmatically as toxic or allergic, though in many instances the mechanism is clear.

A prime problem in considering the potential contribution of an excipient to an observed reaction to a medication is the availability of information indicating what excipients were used in that particular preparation. Until relatively recent times, excipients were seldom identified on the label and might be changed without notice to the consuming public. The United States Food and Drug Administration (FDA) currently requires the listing of excipients in preparations "other than oral" ones and must be informed about all components of prescription drugs. However, official knowledge of the inactive ingredients in over-the-counter (OTC) drugs is not required, even though the tragic event that led to the important Food and Drug Act of 1937 involved a toxic excipient used to make an oral liquid formulation of sulfanilamide.

Legal conflicts between "proprietary rights" and availability of government-held data to the public under "freedom of information" laws are being resolved to handle the dilemma of the legitimate need to protect trade secrets and the right of the public to know, both of which are in the public interest.

In May of 1984 the Proprietary Association (PA), an organization whose members are responsible for a major fraction of OTC products in the United States, recommended to its membership that they voluntarily list the inactive ingredients in their products. Effective September 1985, packaging labels list such ingredients alphabetically but not quantitatively. The listing need not include flavors, fragrances, or "certain other ingredients."

In December of 1984 the Pharmaceutical Manufacturers Association (PMA), whose members manufacture a large majority of prescription drugs sold in the United States, agreed to follow the PA recommendations in principle, except that the excipient information is in the package insert rather than on the label. The FDA Drug Bulletin of December, 1985 briefly summarizes the PMA and PA voluntary guidelines.

In late 1986, the USP proposed that the existing requirement for the listing of inactive ingredients on the labels of topical and parenteral preparations be extended to all doseage forms (8). Their proposal differs from the PA and PMA guidelines in that it would not exempt ingredients whose identity are considered a trade secret and that the label requirement would be mandatory rather than voluntary. While flavors and fragrances would not have to be individually listed, the requirements, if put into force, would require lists that run into hundreds of substances for some products. The exclusion of flavors and fragrances is an obviously rational necessity. For example, analysis of the composition of chocolate has identified hundreds of distinct chemical entities (1) in this one natural flavoring agent. The perfume used in one topical steroid product is known to contain 28 ingredients (2), many of which are known to be capable of sensitization.

In spite of these formidable problems, recent progress in labeling rules represent a considerable improvement in the ability of the public and the profession to take into account potential consequences of excipients. It also leads to a greater need for professionals to enhance their knowledge and understanding about excipients. Recognition of this need has led organizations such as the American Academy of Pediatrics to publish excipient commentaries for its members. Periodical publications list the trade names of products that do or do not contain excipients of concern (3,4).

Pharmacopoeal monographs on excipients primarily describe tests and standards for identity, purity, and assay but are generally deficient in tests for physical properties (e.g., particle size, bulk density, flow rate, moisture sorption), tests for function (e.g., cohesiveness, lubricant effect), and information concerning patient acceptability and potential side effects. During the past two decades a large number of excipients have been used frequently in the formulation of dosage forms without being incorporated into pharmacopoeal monographs.

Since the 1960s medical scientists have become increasingly aware of the possible influence of presumably inert excipients on the bioavailability of active ingredients. The rate and completeness of absorption can be significantly altered by a variety of mechanisms involving "inactive" components of formulated drugs. Excipients might even influence the pathway of absorption and hence the pharmacological consequences. If an absorbed steroid makes its way into the systemic circulation via the lymphatics rather than the portal vein, its pharmacologic consequences might be quite different, since the lymphatic route avoids the first pass through the liver. The excipients used might make the difference (5). Beyond the problem of interactions that influence the biological consequences of the active components, there is now increasing concern that ingredients generally regarded as inert may have significant actions in some individuals and under certain circumstances.

A Report on Bioequivalence by the Office of Technology Assessment criticized compendial standards for the lack of information regarding potential influence on bioavailability and the absence of many important excipients from the compendia. The relative magnitude of the problem has expanded with the growth of interest and activity in bioavailability and bioequivalence.

Extensive investigation into the characterization of pharmaceutical excipients has been carried out by industrial and government laboratories, the health services, and academic institutions. Considerable duplication and some wasteful effort have no doubt been expended in this direction. As early as 1963 a

Swiss pharmaceutical educator suggested that a Codex of Auxiliary Substances that are not described in Pharmacopeia would be of great value. Nine years later the major Swiss pharmaceutical companies initiated a collaborative project that led to the publication in German of an Excipient Catalogue in 1974. This loose-leaf book contains monographs for almost 100 official and nonofficial excipients, and includes general descriptive information, names of suppliers, tests and specifications for various parameters obtained from the literature or specifically measured in the laboratories of the collaborating companies, and the intended role of each of the excipients in pharmaceutical dosage forms. The selection of excipients for the Swiss catalogue and some of the information included in the monographs were based to a large extent on the needs of the companies and on documentation available from suppliers such as manufacturers' technical data sheets. At the April 1976, meeting of the Academy of Pharmaceutical Sciences, a project for a Codex in English was approved and implementation was assigned to the Industrial Pharmaceutical Technology Section. The Council of the Pharmaceutical Society of Great Britain approved the request of its Industrial Practice Sub-Committee to collaborate with the Academy of Pharmaceutical Sciences in the preparation of a Codex of Pharmaceutical Excipients. The framework of an organization has been developed in the United States and for the United Kingdom, and there now exists a *Handbook of Pharmaceutical Excipients* with 145 monographs (6). Although these efforts help considerably in better identifying and describing the nature and possible consequences of excipients on bioavailability, the formidable problem of cataloguing clinical reactions that may relate to excipients remains unresolved.

This volume is intended as a scientific treatise based on modern concepts of medicine and pharmaceutical chemistry that call for both rational and empirical conclusions based on objective documented data. The authors recognize, however, that there are fashions in science as in every other area of human endeavor, and it is sometimes necessary to realize that there may be fruitful approaches to a problem that differ from the currently fashionable approach in western science. The way we now attack our problem may not be the sole or even necessarily the best of all possible approaches. Thus, for example, the logic of identifying and dealing with pure ingredients is self-evident. Nevertheless, there are examples in which adverse reactions to a clearly identified agent do not occur if that agent is coadministered with something else (see Part II, chapter 8, Part III, Chapter 13). Thus careful study of pure, isolated material may give dependable, reproducible results, but these results may possibly have only limited relevance to the action of the more complex preparations in which the active material is administered.

In traditional Chinese medicine the effect of a preparation is rarely perceived as being due to one of its active components. Traditional Asian practitioners do not expect the action of a mixture of ingredients to be a mere sum of the action of each component. They do not understand the Western preoccupation with distinctions between active and inactive or excipient components of a medication. A traditional Chinese pharmacist will readily describe the purpose or action of a seven-ingredient prescription. Yet if one asks the reason that a particular ingredient is included, one is likely to be met with a blank stare. The full prescription is perceived as working as a unit, as confirmed by centuries of real world experience rather than resulting from a rigid test in an environment of dubious relevance.

Modern Western scientific medicine tends to dismiss fundamental Asian concepts of nature as a balance between day and night, sun and moon, male and female, yin and yang, with disease being the consequence of a disturbance in nature's balance. Yet Western science does accept the concept of homeostasis, and the need to restore homeostasis when it is disturbed by disease. Traditional Chinese medicine teaches that both kidney and liver disease can cause edema, presumably by an imbalance that may be due to too much yin in one case and not enough yang in another. A Chinese discussion of yin-yang imbalance may sound less strange to the western scientific ear if one substitutes the pairs estrogen/androgen, sodium/potassium, magnesium/calcium, or AMP/GMP for yin/yang. There is need for tolerance and even some humility in examining medicinals from our current, particular vantage point.

Another area of concern is the current preoccupation with "steady-state" blood levels as a goal of formulation and pattern of drug administration. In spite of the almost axiomatic assumption that "steady-state" blood levels are a fundamental goal of drug administration, there are precious few examples where it has been proven that "steady state" is a preferred or even a desirable drug level pattern for achieving a desired therapeutic purpose. In fact there are some instances where "pulse" therapy (i.e., intervals of low levels between "spikes" of high blood levels) is clearly preferable, and many instances where readily achieved periods of peaks and troughs of blood levels are as effective as "steady state" levels that are difficult to achieve. Concepts of numerically precise concentrations that are "therapeutic" or "toxic" are also often fictitious, being more of a scientific aura than a reality (7). Since excipients in formulations are often involved in such fashions, experts in the field need to reexamine not only how they achieve certain formulation goals but also the soundness of the goals they seek to achieve in a particular situation.

This volume is intended to summarize the "state of the art" concerning both minutiae and broad principles that influence the potential for adverse effects from excipients, as seen from the vantage point of long clinical experience in drug development, clinical toxicology, and allergy.

Part I reviews types of adverse reactions that may result from excipients, and is organized in accordance with the nature of the observed biologically significant responses to these agents. Part II reviews excipients classified in accordance with their purpose. It identifies the uses and describes relevant characteristics of commonly used excipients, with emphasis on reported toxic adverse effects attributable to individual or related groups of agents. It does not go into detail about allergic and pseudoallergic reactions, which are reviewed by class of excipient in Part III. Part III follows essentially the same chapter headings and classifications of excipients as Part II, but with emphasis on immunologically related side effects. The introductory comments for each group of excipients are oriented accordingly and are followed by relevant information in the following sequence for each of the individual substances discussed: immunologic reactivity classified by types I, II, III, or IV as defined and discussed in Part I; anatomical sites of hypersensitivity reactions; and pseudoallergic reactions. Par IV deals with side effects of materials in medical devices. The last part of the book is an alphabetical listing of currently used excipients. A standard index identifies where each excipient or type of excipient is discussed. (The alphabetical listing is, of course, not indexed.)

The Introduction and Part I can be read as a study or teaching text. The work as a whole, and particularly Parts II and III, is intended as a reference source to help a reader determine what is generally known about a suspected excipient or whether an observed reaction is likely to be due to an excipient.

There are serious gaps in knowledge and in the availability of information on reactions to excipients. This very problem was a major stimulus for the authors to prepare this volume. Some reports that are poorly documented or of doubtful significance are nevertheless included when this assists in the evaluation of the problem or the identification of possibilities that need to be considered, even if only to be discarded. However, by design, not every report about every excipient known to the authors is automatically reviewed. It is inevitable that some significant reports about specific excipients will escape inclusion. However, the experience and interests of the authors and their associates should keep such instances to a minimum. Thus, if a reader finds very little information in this volume about reactions to a particular excipient, it is highly likely that very little about it has appeared in the available literature, suggesting that adverse effects attributable to that agent have not been reported.

REFERENCES

1. Furia, T.D. and Bellanca, N. *In* Fenaroli's Handbook of Flavor Ingredients. Second Ed., Vol. 2, CRC Press, Cleveland.
2. Fisher, A.A. Perfume dermatitis, Part III: The search for non-sensitizing perfumes. Cutis 27:13 (1981).
3. Aldridge, R.D., Main, R.A. and Smith, M.E. Dyes and preservatives in oral antihistamines. Br. J. Dermatol. 102:545–549 (1980).
4. Aldridge, R.D., Smith, M.E. and Main, R.A. Dyes and preservatives in oral antihistamines. Br. J. Dermatol. 110:351–355 (1984).

5. Giannina, T., Steinetz, B.G. and Meli, A. Pathway of absorption of orally administered ethynylestradiol-3-cyclopentyl ether in the rat as influenced by vehicle of administration. Proc. Soc. Exp. Biol. Med. 121:11175–1179 (1966).

6. American Pharmaceutical Association. Handbook of Pharmaceutical Excipients. Washington, D.C. (1987).

7. Weiner, M. Clinical evaluation of the significance of data generated in Phase I study of new drug. *In* Klinische Pharmakologie, 5th Ed. (Kuemmerle, Hitzenberger, and Spitzy, eds.). Ecomed, Munich, pp. 1–11 (1986).

8. U.S.P.D.I. Update. Proposed labeling of inactive ingredients. No 6, p. 105 (1986).

Part I
Assessment of Adverse Reactions to Excipients

Chapter 1   General Considerations   13

Chapter 2   Classifications of Adverse Reactions   17

Chapter 3   Allergic Reactions   23

Chapter 4   Immunopathogenesis of Human Hypersensitivity   39

Chapter 5   Diagnostic Procedures for Human Hypersensitivity Diseases and Pseudoallergic Reactions   59

1

General Considerations

The assessment of toxic potential has a great impact on the task of determining if and how particular excipients may be a health hazard. At times it is essential to make black and white decisions about grey areas. When these decisions have to be made, it is important to have a clear light in which to judge the depth of the shade of grey. To review adverse responses to excipients intelligently it will be helpful to review these more general issues concerning toxic potential.

The first and perhaps most important debate in this area concerns evaluating the significance of results in animal studies to the clinical situation in humans. As a rule, poisons that kill animals can also kill humans. While large doses may cause severe and obvious effects, the response to smaller doses may be less severe but nevertheless real, or may not become apparent until multiple doses have been administered for a long time. Consequently, animal studies with large doses can yield results that are indicators of potential responses to more moderate doses in humans. Thus, one school of thought advocates that no agent should be used in humans if it causes a serious effect, such as cancer, when used in any dose in animals.

On the other hand, any number of natural and even vital constituents of the body, such as the sex hormones, are clearly carcinogenic when administered in excessive doses in animals. Even ordinary food as a source of calories must be called a "cocarcinogen" by some definitions, since some tumors grow more quickly and kill their hosts more rapidly if the animal is well fed, compared to nutritionally or calorically deprived "controls."

A fundamental question is whether the dose–response curve is more or less linear into the zero-zero point (Fig. 1, left), so that there is no such thing as a "no-effect" dose; or whether some meaningful dose must be exceeded before there is any effect at all, that is, there is an identifiable minimal effective dose (Fig. 1, right). If the facts are as shown in Figure 1, left, no dose of the agent can be considered harmless. On the other hand, if Figure 1, right reflects the true state of affairs, there is no point in prohibiting low doses because only high doses are harmful. If the low-dose end of Figure 1, left could be magnified, some experts consider that there would in every instance be a dose so small as to be totally inactive (see inset). On the other hand, the lower end of Figure 1, right, if adequately magnified, might show that the effect of even the smallest dose is not zero, though it may approach zero asymptotically.

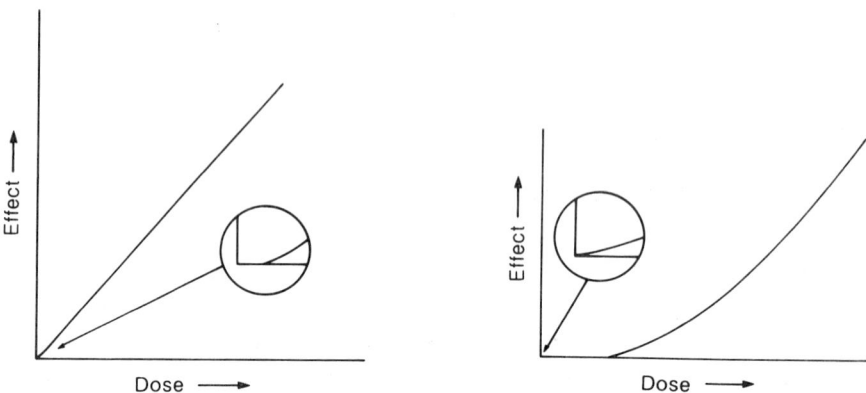

Figure 1 Two hypothetical dose–response curves.

There is good reason to believe that the response of biological systems in the real world is overwhelmingly to require a minimal effective dose: Almost every biological test system shows a need to exceed a certain critical concentration in order to trigger a reaction that results in an observable effect. Many biochemical systems involve the presence of neutralizing mechanisms whose capacity must be exceeded before a foreign substance can interact with a system that causes an adverse effect. For example, studies to explain biochemical species differences (1) indicate that the amount of hepatic thionucleophils available preferentially to bind and neutralize reactive metabolites resulting from drug treatment can determine the dose necessary for a toxic response.

Thus, there is frequently objection to a blanket prohibition of clinically useful agents because chronic massive doses are carcinogenic in animals. In some instances the benefits of the agent are clear, while the presumed risk is theoretical and perhaps nil. The "benefit–risk ratio" of short-term therapy with a "carcinogen" may favor its use.

While this concept of "benefit–risk ratio" is a prime consideration with drugs that can be life-saving or otherwise important, the concept is rarely invoked regarding excipients, since these are generally considered ingredients of convenience rather than necessity. A wide choice of excipients is assumed to be available for any legitimate formulation purpose. Nevertheless, dosage of excipients cannot be ignored. For example, the battles raging over the use of cyclamate or saccharin as sweetening agents in foods are fueled largely by the fact that hundreds of milligrams per day are ingested for years by a large portion of the population. In this context the amount of sweetener required in a teaspoon of medication used for an acute illness is not likely to have any adverse action. Yet it may be argued that sweetness is not an essential characteristic of an effective medication. But if compliance with the doctor's orders is significantly improved, is it not worth adding?

In considering the magnitude of excipient doses that may cause side effects, it is often essential to think of trace impurities or breakdown products with a toxic potential. The detection of such impurities and other materials that may be present in a formulation is dependent on the sensitivity of available analytic methods. Analytic sensitivity has no relevance to the dose of the agent required to cause an adverse effect. Thus unmeasurable amounts of some very potent agents may be capable of distinct pharmacologic action (2), while other agents may be accurately detected at levels orders of magnitude lower than that having any clinical significance. As the state of the analytic art advances, residua of more and more substances are being found in components of medications. Such detection capability can be very important in dealing with potent toxins and particularly with allergens in sensitized subjects. But the rules of dose–response relations apply regardless of analytic capabilities. The fact that a new trace material not previously detected is found anew in a well-established medication is not an appropriate basis for challenging the use of the medication.

Also among the major current problems are the serious but questionable concerns raised by very thorough testing with models of uncertain significance. When an agent with a long history of presumably uneventful use is subjected to such "state of the art" testing, and the results lead to its prohibition, other agents that have not undergone such severe testing may replace it. The potential for harm from these other agents is sometimes less well known and less well studied than that of the agent they replace. Their use may entail a real but unknown risk that is greater than the insignificant but well-documented risk of the former agent.

The next chapter will discuss the classification of adverse reactions, followed by a detailed review of relevant aspects of modern immunologic concepts.

REFERENCES

1. Gillette, J.R. The phenomena of species variation: problems and opportunities. *In* Drug Metabolism from Microbe to Man. (D.V. Parker and R.L. Smith, eds.), Taylor & Frances, London, p. 147 (1976).
2. Paltzer, R., Galeazzi, R.L., Niederberger, W. and Rosenthaler, J. Simultaneous modeling of gopindolol kinetics and dynamics. Clin. Pharmacol. Ther. 36:5 (1984).

2

Classification of Adverse Reactions

I. Direct toxicity   17
II. Immunotoxicology   18
III. Hypersensitivity and allergy   18
IV. Intolerance and idiosyncrasy   19
V. Pseudoallergic reactions   20
    References   21

I. DIRECT TOXICITY

Classic toxicology is concerned primarily with the direct adverse effects of a substance on the normal physiology and morphology of the organism. A broad spectrum of mechanisms may mediate the toxic effect, and it is often of practical as well as theoretical interest to know the basis of the observed effects. Among the direct effects of both natural and xenobiotic excipients are influences on enzymes, receptors, membranes, and intracellular structures. The biochemical phenomena involved include metal chelation, phosphorylation, oxidative and reductive processes, intercalation, free radical formation, and others. In the last analysis, however, empirical observations of toxic effects are the prime basis for toxicologic evaluation.

The traditional view of toxicology is of a scientific method that studies the specific biochemical and pathologic lesions induced by xenobiotics and attempts to elucidate mechanisms of biological processes (1). The principles involved in evaluating this more or less direct type of toxicity were briefly discussed in the introduction and the preceding chapter. In applying these principles, toxicologists are often concerned with damage to target organs because of receptor injury, enzyme defects, prolonged localization or peculiarities of metabolism in certain tissues.

The toxicology of excipients will be reviewed according to precedents established in evaluating drug-related toxic reactions. This approach is appropriate since excipient materials are essential components of clinical drug formulations. Toxic reactions to excipients may be influenced by many variables, including protein-binding effects, membrane changes, chelation, interference with intestinal absorption, or unusually high retention of the material in body tissues if the substance is administered on a chronic basis.

The multiple and complex mechanisms responsible for toxicity in general are the subject of innumerable volumes with a range of subject matter from sophisticated complex biochemical theories concerning genetic nucleotides and double helix intercalation to statistical probit analysis of empirical dose–mortality rate data. These are obviously beyond the scope of this text. Even a general discussion of metabolic toxification and detoxification mechanisms, pharmacokinetics, and pharmacodynamics are outside the practical capacity of this volume. However,these mechanisms will be discussed when they are relevant to the side effects of specific excipients in Part II.

On the other hand, immunological phenomena and methodology as they apply to the problem of reactions to excipients will be reviewed in some detail in the remaining chapters of this part. The review is designed to enhance the understanding of Part III, which deals primarily with allergic reactions to specific excipients. Part II discusses primarily nonimmunological reactions to specific excipients.

II. IMMUNOTOXICOLOGY

The subspecialty of immunotoxicology as a valid approach to investigation of nonpharmacological adverse reactions is still viewed ambivalently by toxicologists and pharmacologists. While it is clearly established that immune mechanisms play a cardinal role in many important drug reactions (e.g., penicillin, quinidine), there is as yet no currently accepted way of predicting immune reactions with the use of in vivo or in vitro models. Since the toxicologist is understandably concerned with animal models in which potential risks can be quantified, the skeptical attitude toward the budding discipline of immunotoxicology will not be entirely dispelled until more precise methodology for determining prospective risk is devised. Current progress in immunologic research and biotechnology in this area will be reviewed in Chapter 4.

III. HYPERSENSITIVITY AND ALLERGY

Immune responses by exogenous agents such as excipients are usually manifested by mechanisms involved in human hypersensitivity and allergy. The most practical classification of human hypersensitivity has been proposed by Gell and Coombs (Table 1) (2). The clinical manifestations of types I, II, and III hypersensitivity are due to humoral antibodies, while type IV reactivity consists only of those reactions mediated by cellular immune mechanisms. Type I reactions are referred to as immediate hypersensitivity and are mediated by a specific

Table 1 Classification of Human Hypersensitivity as Suggested by Gell and Coombs

Type	Antibody(ies)	Immunocyte
I	Reagin (IgE, IgG$_4$)	B
II	Cytotoxic (IgG)	B
III	Immune complex (IgM, IgG)	B
IV	Delayed (cell-mediated)	T

immunoglobulin class known as IgE. Under unusual circumstances, the IgG$_4$ subclass of IgG may also be involved in type I reactions. Type II responses are generally referred to as cytotoxic and may involve either IgM or IgG immunoglobulin isotypes. Type III reactions are due to immune complex reactions and, for the most part, are caused by toxic aggregates of antigen and corresponding IgG antibody. Toxic reactions are more likely observed when these aggregates are presented to body tissues in slight antigen excess. Type IV reactions are exclusively mediated by cellular immunity and include localized cutaneous reactivity (contact dermatitis) or a systemic form of cellular sensitization (tuberculinlike), the sequelae of which may include widespread granulomata and fibrogenesis of vulnerable organs. Although it is often difficult, the ultimate aim of the immunotoxicologist is to define an immunological adverse reaction on the basis of one or several mechanisms known to be involved in one of these models of human hypersensitivity.

IV. INTOLERANCE AND IDIOSYNCRASY

Immunologically mediated reactions may also be confused with or mistaken for an effect that mimics the usual criteria for an immune reaction. Because neither antibody nor cell-mediated immunity can be demonstrated in such conditions, a variety of terms have been used to describe such reactions. For example, an enhanced response to a chemical agent without underlying abnormalities of metabolism, excretion, or bioavailability is called intolerance or the state of a lowered threshold to the normal pharmacological action of that particular agent. Scientific reasons for such exaggerated responses have not been established but it is possible that upregulation of membrane receptors or delayed inactivation of drugs at the drug–receptor interaction level could be responsible. In a sense, intolerance is the converse of tolerance (subsensitivity), which is the state of diminished efficacy after repeated exposure to a drug.

The term "idiosyncrasy" refers to an unusual physical response to an agent occurring in a small number of susceptible individuals (3). This reaction appears after subtherapeutic doses of the material, is unrelated to the expected pharmacological action of the agent, and may occur for the first time without prior contact. The fact that relatively few individuals experience such reactions often is confused with the possibility of an unusual immunological reaction. The small eliciting dose is also compatible with an immune response. However, the important prerequisite of a sensitization or incubation period cannot be demonstrated in such instances and immune reactions cannot be detected by objective techniques. At times it is difficult to differentiate intolerance or idiosyncratic reactions from cumulative toxicity, especially in view of the fact that chronic exposure to chemicals and drugs may induce changes in the body that cannot be equated with acute pharmacological or immunological effects. For example, chronic administration of antibiotics may lead to permanent changes in intestinal flora that could ultimately cause gastrointestinal intolerance symptoms and could be confused with food intolerance or allergy.

V. PSEUDOALLERGIC REACTIONS

A group of reactions known as pseudoallergic or anaphylactoid reactions must also be differentiated from immune-mediated syndromes. These are mediated by agents such as colloid volume expanders (e.g., dextran and gelatin), basic polypeptide agents (polymyxin B, 48/80, ACTH), radiocontrast media, and excipients. A partial list of excipients that cause anaphylactoid reactions is shown in Table 2. Acute reactions to these substances are caused by direct release of mediators from mast cells and basophils, resulting in the classic end-organ effects that these mediators exert. Direct mediator release occurs without evidence of a prior sensitization period, specific IgE antibodies, or antigen–antibody bridging on the mast cell/basophil cell membrane. It has been suggested that this occurs due to activation of a "second" non-IgE receptor on mast cell membranes (4).

Table 2   Representative Additives Causing Pseudoallergic Anaphylactoid Reactions

Class	Example
Colorants	FD&C Yellow Dye #5
Emulsifiers	Cremophor-El
Biocidals	Paraben
Alcohols	Benzyl alcohol
Antioxidants	Sulfites

The nonimmune reaction is immediate, often severe and is therefore referred to as anaphylactoid. Because it is nonimmunological, it may occur the first time that the host is exposed to respective agents. These reactions are of further interest because they can also be elicited by small doses of the offending substance. It has been proposed that some of these reactions could be based in part upon nonimmunological release of anaphylatoxins (C3a, C5a) through activation of the alternative complement pathway. Although this is an attractive hypothesis, substantive evidence for the occurrence of these events after stimulation by the above agents has not been demonstrated in most instances. Neuropeptides such as substance P and endorphins may also activate and induce mediator release from mast cells (5). Osmotic alterations may lead to nonspecific mediator release, but such physical effects are more likely to occur at local tissue sites such as the nose or bronchi.

REFERENCES

1. G.G. Gibson, R. Hubbard, and D.V. Parke, (eds.) Immunotoxicity—Outline of Major Problems in Immunotoxicology. Academic Press, Inc., London, pp. 1–3, (1983).
2. Gell, P.G.H., Coombs, R.R.A., and Lachman, R., eds. Clinical Aspects of Immunology, 3rd Ed. Blackwell Scientific Publications, Oxford (1975).
3. Fingl, E., and Woodbury, D.M. General Principles in the Pharmaceutical Basis of Therapeutics 5th Ed., (L.S. Goodman and A. Gilman, eds.), Macmillan Publishing Co., Inc., New York (1975).
4. Stanworth, D.R. The role of non-antigen receptors in mast cell signalling processes. Mol Immunol 21:1183 (1984).
5. Wasserman, S.I. The regulation of inflammatory mediator production by cell products. Am Rev Respir Dis 135:S46–S48 (1987).

3

Allergic Reactions

I. General principles of immune responses   23
     A. Background   23
     B. Antigens   24
     C. Antibodies   25
     D. Cells of the immune system   26
     E. Complement   32
     F. Idiotypic networks   33
II. Chief categories of human hypersensitivity   34
     A. Immediate hypersensitivity reactions (type I)   35
     B. Cytotoxic hypersensitivity reactions (type II)   35
     C. Immune complex reactions (type III)   35
     D. Delayed hypersensitivity reactions (type IV)   36
     References   36

I. GENERAL PRINCIPLES OF IMMUNE RESPONSES

A. Background

Immunology emerged as a formal discipline in the life sciences at the time that host–parasite relationships were recognized as significant determinants of disease. Although natural resistance and host susceptibility factors were found to be of great importance, interest also focused on immune bodies manufactured by the host. At this time the effects of active immunization by vaccines and passive immunization by heterologous antisera were discovered. In the course of these early investigations, Richet and Portier observed that reinjections of toxins from sea anemones produced toxic and sometimes fatal effects in dogs that had been previously injected with these substances (1). Later, they elaborated on these original observations and called this phenomenon anaphylaxis. This discovery was one of the early building blocks of immunology and paved the way for recognizing human hypersensitivity.

     It is beyond the scope of this book to discuss the principles of immunity and hypersensitiviy in great detail. For such information, the reader should consult recently published texts and reviews on the subject (2-9). However, it is necessary to have a general understanding about how current concepts of immunity and hypersensitivity relate to possible adverse reactions induced by excipient agents.

The immune system is one of the most important barriers to harmful agents in the environment. Two major types of immune responses are recognized. Intrinsic immunity consists of a complicated network of activated proteins and cells that, upon proper stimulation, will migrate to the site of injury, immobilize the offending agent, and phagocytose the agent as a direct clearing mechanism (10). Phagocytes include polymorphonuclear leukocytes, monocytes, and macrophages. Other significant components of innate immunity consist of interferon, the alternate pathway of complement, and acute-phase proteins that increase rapidly during infection. In addition, special lymphocytes known as natural killer (NK) cells recognize cell surface changes on virally infected cells, bind to these sites, and ultimately kill them. Adaptive immunity evolved as a supplementary mechanism of defense when phagocytes were unable to recognize harmful exogenous agents, or the agents could not be immobilized and cleared by complement or acute-phase reactants. Humoral antibodies are protein molecules produced by mature B lymphocytes or plasma cells. The chief functions of antibody are to bind, neutralize, and immobilize a variety of infectious agents prior to phagocytosis and other host clearance mechanisms. Immune defense against viruses, some bacteria, fungi, tumors, and foreign tissues is mediated by T lymphocytes and their secreted polypeptides (lymphokines).

B. Antigens

An antigen is a substance that the host perceives as foreign to itself and that will incite formation of immune bodies in the host. These include immune responses against nonself tissue antigens that are identified by cell surface markers known as human leukocyte antigens (HLA-A, B, C, and D) or major histocompatibility complex class I (corresponding to HLA-A, B, C) and class II (HLA-D, DR, DQ, and DP) antigens. Antigens range in size from simple chemicals to complex proteins and carbohydrates. Whether simple or complex, antigen molecules contain antigenic determinants called epitopes. Epitopes differ from one antigen to another but some antigens consist of a series of repeated epitopes. Epitopes should be considered as molecular configurations with recognition for cells of the adaptive immune system and the antibody products of these cells. Antigens may be considered multivalent or univalent. In multivalent reactions, two or more epitopic determinants are available for cross-linking reactions with circulating antibody or B cell membrane surface immunoglobulin while only one reactive epitopic determinant is required for univalent binding. Univalent antigenicity can also be equated with the haptenic reaction, in which low-molecular-weight chemicals or drugs must first conjugate with endogenous carrier protein before antibody specificity against the ligand (univalent epitope) can be demonstrated (11). Such conjugates will also induce formation of antibodies to the carrier protein and new antigenic determinants formed within the carrier protein by chemical interaction with hapten. If simple chemicals, drugs, or their metabolites lack chemically reactive moieties for successful conjugation to proteins, they are unable to induce synthesis of antibodies and hence are nonimmunogenic. Thus, the distinction between antigenicity and immunogenicity must always be kept in mind, especially in the case of low-molecular-weight compounds. In modern immunologic parlance, it is preferable to relate epitopic density to both antigens and immunogenic properties of an antigen.

C. Antibodies

Antibodies are glycoproteins newly synthesized in response to a specific substance, the antigen. They are synthesized on the endoplasmic reticulum of plasma cells. The unique defensive properties of antibody enable vertebrate animals to produce up to 10^8 different antibody specificities so that antibodies can be synthesized to virtually any natural or synthetic antigen. There are nine different immunoglobulin isotypes (IgM, IgD, IgG_1, IgG_2, IgG_3, IgG_4, IgA_1, IgA_2, and IgE). The basic configuration of immunoglobulin molecules consists of 4 polypeptide chains containing about 1300 amino acids with 2 identical carboxy-terminal heavy chains, and 2 identical N-terminal light chains (either κ or λ) joined by disulfide bridges (Fig. 1) (2,10,12). Both heavy and light chains have constant (C) regions identical in structure for all antibodies of that particular isotypic class. The C region of all immunoglobulin heavy chains is divided into three separate amino acid domains, except IgM and IgE, which have four domains (12). The variable (V) regions make up the N-terminal's 110 or so amino acids of each immunoglobulin chain. Within the V regions of light and heavy chains, there are a total of six hypervariable regions. The amino acid sequences of the various hypervariable regions are folded to form the antigen-combining site. Antibody specificities are determined by a random process of V region gene translocations unique for each different B-cell precursor (13). The translocation process involves the genes coding for both heavy chain and light chain V regions (10,12). C region gene translocations ultimately determine the isotypic class of the immunoglobulin molecule. Upon completion of the translocation process, the various gene clusters are spliced in the sequence of heavy-chain V genes to heavy-chain C genes (VC), and heavy-chain VC genes to light-chain V genes. The net result is that each activated B cell is programmed to secrete a unique variety of isotypic/antigenic specific antibody. Enzymatic cleavage of the immunoglobulin molecule by papain occurs at the hinge region between the first and second domains of the C region of the heavy chain and products Fc, Fab' (monovalent antigen binding) and F(ab')$_2$ (divalent antigen

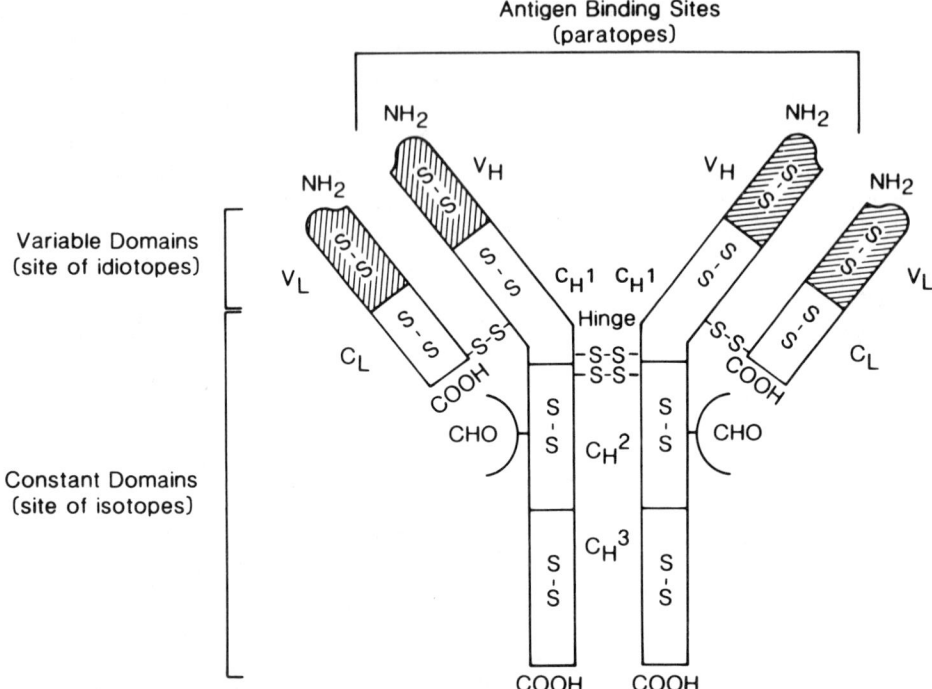

Figure 1 Schematic diagram of a human IgG molecule showing two light (L) and two heavy (H) chains linked by disulfide bonds. Variable regions of light (V_L) and heavy (V_H) chains comprise the antigen combining site (also known as the paratope). There are both light (C_L) and heavy (C_H) constant regions. The constant region of the IgG heavy chain consists of three domains (C_H1, C_H2 and C_H3). IgM and IgE isotypic forms of immunoglobulin molecules have four heavy chain domains (C_H1, C_H2, C_H3 and C_H4). Allotopic or intraspecies determinant sites (not shown) are present chiefly within the heavy chain constant domains.

combining) residues. The specific determinants and physiological properties of the isotypic classes of antibody will be discussed in greater detail below.

D. Cells of the Immune System

Cells of the immune system are derived from bone marrow pleuripotential stem cells and develop through either myeloid or lymphoid differentiation. Some mature cells (neutrophils and macrophages) from both pathways have phagocytic functions. Human leukocytes exhibit morphological heterogeneity that can be demonstrated by monoclonal antibodies directed against cell surface differentiation proteins known as cluster differentiation (CD) antigens, some of which are listed in Table 1. A complete summary of the World Health Organization CD nomenclature has been published elsewhere (14).

Both humoral and cell-mediated immunity are inlcuded in the lymphoid arm of the immune system. Two major types of lymphocytes, T cells and B cells, clearly have different functions, although both subsets mature and become immunocompetent in peripheral lymphoid tissues. This process is thymus-dependent for the T cells. Differentiation of human B cells is not as well understood but probably occurs in both bone marrow and gut-associated lymphoid tissue.

T cells are classified according to both effector and regulatory functions. Effector T cells consist of cytotoxic and delayed hypersensitivity T cells, while the regulatory cells are known as T-helper (T_H) and T-suppressor (T_S) cells. Antigen recognition by T cells occurs through a T-cell receptor that is a molecular complex made up of at least five polypeptide chains (Ti/T3) (15) (Fig. 2). Two of these chains form the idiotypic component of the receptor (Ti), a highly variable heterodimer of two disulfide-linked polypeptide chains (a and β subunits), each of which is encoded by somatic rearrangement from pools of separate gene clusters similar to translocation of immunoglobulin genes. The a and β disulfide-linked chains mediate antigen recognition. They are noncovalently associated with four nonvariable T3 (CD3) polypeptide chains (γ, δ, ϵ, ζ) that mediate signal transduction and inositol turnover after activation by antigen–Ti receptor binding. A small subset of peripheral lymphocytes and thymocytes do not express a and β, but rather γ and δ, Ti chains (16). It has been suggested that expression of the γ/δ heterodimer T-cell receptor may appear early in ontogeny but that productive rearrangements of these gene products only survive in a few T-cell precursors. The function of surviving γ/δ T-cell receptors is not known. In mice, γ/δ protein products have been detected in dendritic epidermal cells and intestinal intraepithelial lymphocytes. The expression of the variable and constant gene regions into a and β gene products occurs in the majority of adult T-cell precursors (17). Simultaneous recognition of the Ti/T3 receptor and class II major histocompatibility complex (MHC) restriction molecules by antigen is suggested by the fact that residues within an immunogenic peptide interact with both MHC and Ti proteins in such a way that the peptide antigen is sandwiched between these two cell surface proteins (18,19). T cells also contain a receptor that mediates sheep-cell rosetting of T cells. This receptor is designated as CD2 or T 11. The T 11 receptor is linked to the Ti/T3 antigen recognition receptor with respect to inositol turnover and IL-2 gene induction. The subsequent secretion of IL-2 acts as an autocrine and augments further proliferation of T cells.

Cytotoxic T cells (T_C) recognize antigens in the context of class I MHC gene products. They are capable of inducing specific lysis of antigen-bearing

Table 1 World Health Organization Classification of Cluster Differentiation Molecules (1986): Partial List

Monoclonal antibodies	CD	Cell distribution and function	Cell specificity
OKT6[a],Leu6[b],T6[c]	1	Cortical T (thymocytes)	
OKT11,Leu5B,T11	2	T activation; erythrocyte rosette	
OKT3,Leu4,T3	3	T receptor (TcR)	
OKT4,Leu3,T4	4	T helper (Th)	T cells
OKT5,Leu1,T,T10[d]	5	T cells/early B	
OKT1,T12	6	B cells; class II MHC receptor	
Leu9	7	$Fc\mu$ R (IgM receptor)	
OKT8,Leu2,T8	8	T suppressor/cytotoxic (Ts/Tc)	
Leu11	16	NK cells, PMN ($Fc\lambda$ RIII)	NK and PMN
Leu12,B4[c]	19	Pre-B cells	
Leu16,B1[c]	20	B cells	
CR2[a],B2[c]	21	B-cell complement receptor 2 (CR2)	
		Epstein-Barr virus receptor	B cells
Leu14	22	Activated B cells	
-	23	Activated B cells/$Fc\epsilon$ R2	
BA-1[d]	24	Pre-B cells	
IL-2 receptor[b]	25	TAC/IL-2 receptor	Mitogen-activated T cells
OKT 10	32	$Fc\gamma$ RII (IgG receptor)	Miscellaneous cells
	35	Complement receptor 1 (CR1)	

[a]Ortho Diagnostics, Inc., Raritan, New Jersey
[b]Becton Dickinson Immunocytometry Systems, Mountain View, California
[c]Coulter Electronics, Inc., Hialeah, Florida
[d]Hybritech, San Diego, California

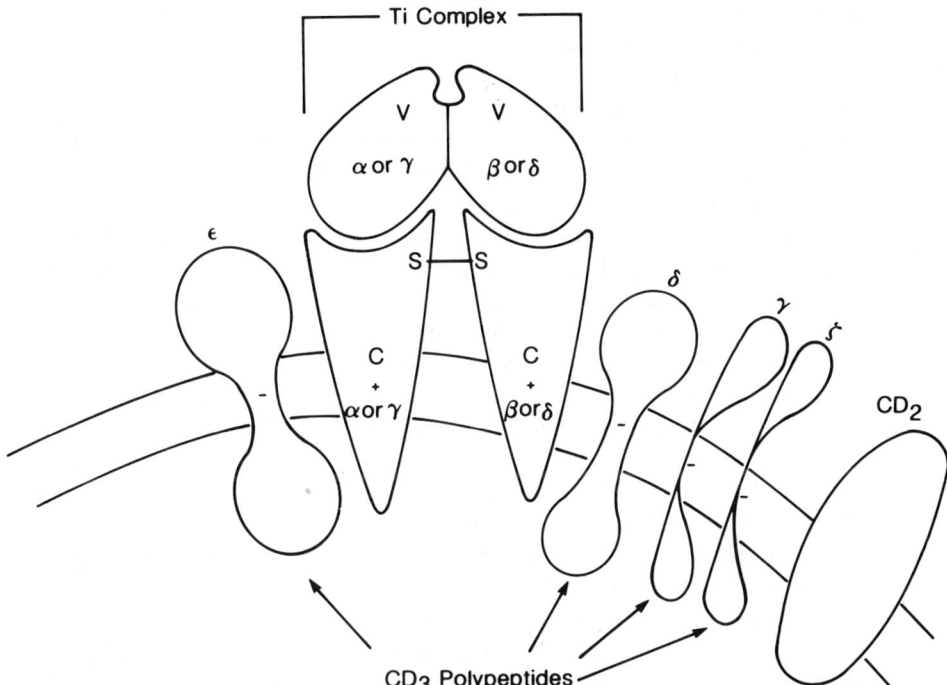

Figure 2 The antigen recognition system of T cells. Each T cell consists of a Ti complex and closely associated polypeptide chains (γ, δ, ϵ and ζ) of membrane CD3 (T3). The Ti complex is a heterodimer of two variable (V) and two constant (C) polypeptide chains. Each of the Ti chains may be either a/β or γ/δ. The CD_2 (T11) transmembrane protein is linked to the Ti/T3 receptor function by providing an intermediary signal for inositol turnover and IL-2 gene induction. Differences of electrical charge between transmembrane components of the Ti C chains and the CD3 polypeptide molecules may facilitate transduction of membrane signals.

target cells that have been modified by virus, hapten, or tumor-associated neo-antigens. They bear the cluster designation of CD8. Delayed-hypersensitivity T cells (T_D) are the effector cells of delayed hypersensitivity reactions. They differ from T_C cells in that they recognize antigens in association with class II MHC molecules and they bear CD4 cell surface antigens.

Cytotoxic effector immune systems are multifaceted. Upon activation by antigen presenting cells (APC), cytotoxic T_C cells are capable of inducing specific lysis of antigen-bearing target cells modified by virus, hapten, or tumor-associated antigens. CD2 or T11 receptor proteins are also present on cytotoxic

T cells and appear to facilitate cell-to-cell contact. Cytotoxic T cells also kill MHC-incompatible (foreign) cells.

The mechanism of T_C cell killing is complex. In addition to a potent lymphokine known as lymphotoxin, T_C cells synthesize a pore-forming protein (perforin) that has been isolated from the granules of these cells. Perforin bears a striking resemblance to the C9 complement protein, a major component of the pore-forming complexes deposited in cell membranes during a complement attack (20,21). Calcium and serine-esterase-independent T_C-mediated lysis has also been reported (22). Recently, activation of T_C by interleukin 2 in vitro has been applied to the adoptive immunotherapy of human cancer (23).

Another killer cell population of lymphoid T cells is designated as the K cell. Membranes of these cells contain IgG Fc_γ receptors that recognize and bind to target cells coded with antibody of this isotypic class, thereby facilitating cell lysis by the K cell. This system is referred to as antibody-dependent cell cytotoxicity.

An antibody-independent mechanism also exists. This is mediated by natural killer cells, which are large granular lymphocytes with the ability to kill directly transformed, virus-infected, or embryonic-derived cells in the absence of antibody. The mechanism of this killing is nonspecific.

Regulatory T cells control the activation, proliferation, and growth of both effector T cells and B cells (24). T-helper cells were first recognized by their ability to interact with and "help" B cells produce specific antibody in response to antigenic stimulation. These cells recognize antigen in the context of MHC class II cell surface components. They contain CD4 surface markers. T-suppressor cells also interact with B cells in the opposite direction of T_H cells, by down-regulating the antibody producing function of B cells in response to antigen. Similar to T_C cells, T_S cells are identified by CD8 differentiation antigens but the MHC restriction system of T_S cells is as yet unknown. While T_C and T_S cells are differentiated primarily by functional in vitro assays, a recent report suggests that T_C cells can be identified by a monoclonal antibody against a surface glycoprotein (S6F1) that is not present on T_S cells (25).

A complex series of cellular interactions is required to initiate the immune response (26). Antigen-presenting cells (macrophages, Langerhans epidermal cells, and B lymphocytes) have the ability to internalize, process, and present protein antigens to T-cell receptors. This processing effect selects those parts or epitopes (usually peptides) of the protein molecule with an affinity for both T-cell receptors and the class II MHC molecules on $T_H CD4^+$ cells. It is thought that $CD4^+$ accessory protein molecules on the surfaces of both APC and T_H cells may stabilize the interaction between APC and T_H, thereby enhancing the antigen recognition process. Macrophage APC cells also secrete a growth-differentiating molecule known as IL-1, which is also required for activation of the T cell at the same time it recognizes the epitopic domain of the peptide antigen.

Antigen presenting cells also process and present virus and tumor antigens that are recognized by class I MHC restriction mechanisms. These APC-processed neoantigens jointly interact with the T-cell receptor and class I MHC surface antigens of $CD8^+$ T_C cells. Similar to antigen recognition by T_H cells, accessory CD8 molecules may also be required to stabilize this interaction. In conjunction with APC-derived IL-1, T_C cells are then activated to pursue their killer functions upon viral or tumor-activated target cells.

The central step in the development of responses to proteins, peptides, and polysaccharides is the activation of T_H $CD4^+$ helper cells, because these cells are essential elements in a complex inducer network of T–T and T–B-cell interactions that directly influence the growth of antigen-specific lymphocyte clones and their differentiation to effector functions. T-helper/inducer cells accomplish this by secreting a variety of polypeptides known as cytokines, which, although nonspecific, potentiate antigen stimulation of B cells. Some of these include γ interferon, interleukin-2 (IL-2 [formerly T cell growth factor]), interleukin-3 (IL-3 [mast cell growth factor]), interleukin-4 (IL-4 [B-cell stimulating factor: BSF-1] mast cell growth factor 2, IgE/IgG_1 enhancing factor), interleukin 5 (IL-5 [B cell growth factor 2, T cell replacing factor, eosinophilic differentiation factor]), interleukin 6 (IL-6 [BSF-2, β_2 interferon, B-cell differentiating factor]) and interleukin 7 (pre-B-cell growth factor) (27–30). The B cell factors (IL-4, IL-5, IL-6, IL-7) stimulate the growth of B cells and their differentiation into plasma cells, thereby enabling antigen-specific clonal expansion of these cells for the purpose of producing cytoplasmic and surface immunoglobulin antibodies directed against specific epitopes of the presenting antigen. The antigen-specific surface immunoglobulin serves as the B cell receptor for future contact with antigen. Excessive production of antibody is regulated by suppressor cytokines secreted by T_S $CD8^+$ lymphocytes. The current model of T-cell "help" in stimulating B-cell humoral antibody production is based on evidence that the B cell internalizes and processes antigen (31). Processed derivatives of the antigen are returned to the B cell surface, where they become associated with class II MHC molecules. T_H lymphocyte bridging with antigen-bearing B cells then occurs because of simultaneous recognition of surface antigen and class II MHC restriction molecules on the B cell surface. Once bridging occurs, T_H lymphocytes supply IL-2 and other B cell factors for ensuing B cell activation, growth, and differentiation (31). Some T cell factors promote a switch in B cell production from IgM and IgD, the first formed classes of antibodies, to other isotypic classes of IgG, IgA, and IgE antibodies (10). Interleukin 4 may have special relevance for IgE-mediated reactions because it augments immunoglobulin class switching to IgE antibodies. Interleukin 4 also induces the expression of low-affinity Fc_ϵ receptors (IgE-binding sites) on B cells, upregulates CD23 antigen expression of B cells, augments IgE production, and enhances the growth of mast cells in vitro (32). In contrast, γ interferon inhibits the production of IgE. Thus the balance between IL-2, γ interferon, and IL-4 may constitute an important determinant of atopic susceptibility.

Immunological effector mechanisms of cellular immunity are dependent on delayed-type hypersensitivity T_D $CD4^+$ cells. These cells respond to T_H cells in T-T interactive mechanisms. The inflammatory response associated with delayed hypersensitivity is mediated and amplified chiefly through production of lymphokines such as IL-2, macrophage activating factor (γ interferon), macrophage inhibitory factor, and others.

E. Complement

Complement is an important amplification system of host defense and consists of a complex group of plasma and cell membrane interactive proteins that are not only directly involved with inflammation and defense against infection but also activated by antigen–antibody reactions (33). There are 15 distinctive proteins in the complement system itself and 10 other control or cofactors for the control of the complement cascade. Several of these proteins (properdin factor B, C2, and C4) are encoded by HLA-linked complement gene loci referred to as MHC class III antigens. The classic or direct pathway of complement activation is antibody dependent, while the alternative pathway of complement activation does not require antibody. Various active and inactive components are generated during activation and progression of the complement cascade and involve a series of enzymatic pathways that convert intermediate protein complexes into active and inactive components. The biological properties of the active components of complement are so potent that several intrinsic inhibitory or control mechanisms are required to limit excessive amounts of complement activation. The pivotal determinant for complement-dependent human adverse reactions is activation of the third component of complement (C3) by both classic and alternate pathways. This ultimately leads to production of bioactive fragments such as anaphylatoxins (C3a and C5a) and neutrophil adherence and chemotactic factor (C5a). Both anaphylatoxins exert spasmogenic effects on vascular smooth muscle in animal models. They not only activate mediator release from mast cells but also cause direct contractile responses of in vitro guinea pig lung strips (34). The C5a anaphylatoxin is more potent than C3a. Recently C4a, a cleavage fragment of C4, has also been identified as an anaphylatoxin (35). The C3b generated as a result of C3 cleavage has the ability to continue the complement cascade. It also opsonizes target cells and serves as an attachment site for phagocytic cells that have specific C3b receptors known as complement receptor 1 (CR1). Because of its high intensity of biological activity, increase of C3b is tightly controlled by two plasma proteins termed factors H and I, which cleave C3b to an inactive form, iC3b. There are cellular complement receptors (CR1, CR2, CR3, CR4, C3e, C5a, C1q, H) for each fragment of C3 metabolism (36).

The CR3 receptor recognizes iC3b and is found on neutrophils, monocytes, and macrophages. The CR2 receptor on B lymphocytes recognizes another degrading fragment of C3. The CR4 receptor that binds C3bi and C3d,g is present on neutrophils and monocytes. The four major complement receptors are thought to play an important role in clearance of immune complexes. After cleavage of C5 into C5a and C5b by C5 convertase, the larger cleavage fragment, C5b, interacts with and is stabilized by C6 and ultimately forms the membrane attack complex, C5b6789. This protein complex has also been described as the pore-forming complex and is deposited in cell membranes during a complement attack (37). These pores prove lethal by disrupting the normal ionic milieu within the cell.

F. Idiotypic Networks

As the complex nature of the immune response became more apparent in the modern era of molecular immunology, another important internal mechanism for regulating the immune response was proposed by Jerne as the idiotypic network hypothesis (Fig. 3). This theory evolved from the prior discovery that the immunoglobulin molecule not only functions as the complementary antibody to an antigen but also itself contains antigenic determinants capable of eliciting specific antibodies called anti-idiotypic antibodies (38–40). By means of these antibody–antibody reactions the immune system internally regulates itself through a complex network of reactions that modulate the normal immune response. Idiotypes refer to epitopes on the hypervariable V regions of antibody molecules. Epitopic determinants in these areas provide the stimuli for production of anti-idiotypic antibodies. Hypervariable epitopes on the latter antibodies can lead to synthesis of antianti-idiotypic antibodies. This network concept of immune regulation emphasizes the potential importance of receptor-specific regulation of the immune system in contrast to instructional (antigen-specific) regulation. Furthermore, the immune system may be perceived as self-determined by the network regulatory system itself, rather than driven by chance contact with foreign immunogens. This is possible because some antianti-idiotypic antibodies are generated by internal images of the antigen that stimulated the original antibody response. Moreover, the effects of antianti-idiotypic antibodies having the internal image of the antigen are functionally similar to classic antibodies generated by foreign antigens. According to the network theory, the states of self-recognition and autoreactivity are also regulated by idiotypic–antiidiotypic interactions. The clinical expression of autoimmune diseases may reflect a pathological dysequilibrium of homeostatic idiotype-anti-idiotype reactions (41). Cogent animal models of this form of dysregulation are myasthenia gravis and Graves' disease induced by anti-idiotypes to acetylcholine receptor and thyrotropin antibody, respectively. Idiotype–anti-idiotypic reactions may

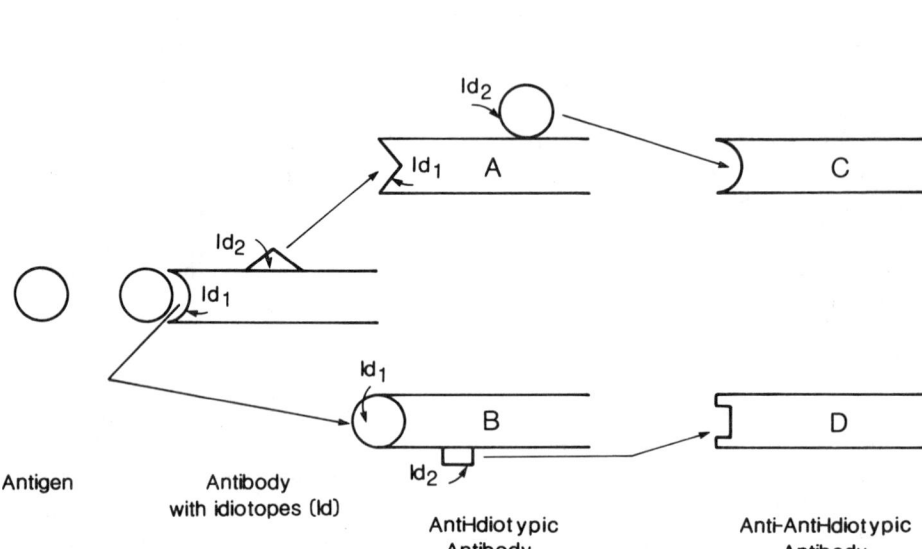

Figure 3 The Jerne network hypothesis: regulation of antibody response by idiotypic-anti-idiotypic networks.

Antibody (Ab1) formed in response to antigen contains multiple idiotopes in its variable region (Id1, Id2 of Ab1). These determinants stimulate the formation of anti-idiotypic antibodies (Ab2; A and B). One species of anti-idiotypic antibody synthesized in response to Id1 of Ab 1 (B in the above diagram) has an internal image of the original antigen and may account for persistence of antibody production without further exposure to the antigen. Other varieties of anti-idiotypic and anti-anti-idiotypic antibodies (Ab3; C and D) regulate production of excess antibody.

also be exploited for preventive and therapeutic interventions in the immune system. Several anti-idiotype monoclonal antibodies are being investigated as vaccines and therapeutic agents.

II. CHIEF CATEGORIES OF HUMAN HYPERSENSITIVITY

It is apparent that humoral and cellular pathways of immunity evolved to protect the host against a multitude of pathogenic insults. However, certain immune responses, both humoral and cellular, have become detrimental to the host and these harmful effects are implied in the term "human hypersensitivity." Inasmuch as excipient agents may be antigenic or allergenic under appropriate circumstances, some of the adverse effects attributed to these agents will necessarily be classified under human hypersensitivity reactions. To characterize and compare allergic responses induced by excipients according to a standardized format, the classification of human hypersensitivity proposed by Gell and Coombs will be used throughout Parts II and III (42).

A. Immediate Hypersensitivity Reactions (Type I)

The term "immediate hypersensitivity" refers to IgE-mediated reactions that are elicited within a few minutes to hours and that may also have a late response component 3–8 hr after the initial reaction. This reaction complex reflects interaction of allergen with its corresponding IgE antibody (either circulating or on the surface of effector mast cells and/or basophils) during the immediate phase and augmentation of the reaction some hours later as a result of recruitment of inflammatory mediators and other effector cells (eosinophils, neutrophils, platelets, and mononuclear cells) with subsequent release of late phase inflammatory mediators (43).

B. Cytotoxic Hypersensitivity Reactions (Type II)

Human hypersensitivity reactions due to cytotoxic antibodies are rare in clinical medicine. In such reactions, the source of antigen is either an epitope(s) of or a new antigenic determinant formed on cell membranes and then perceived by the host as foreign. Specific cytotoxic antibodies (IgM or IgG) formed in response to such neoantigenic membrane epitopes are then redirected to and exert their cytotoxic effects directly upon cell membranes. Two classic examples of this phenomenon are acquired hemolytic anemia (idiopathic or induced by penicillin) and Goodpasture's syndrome, in which cytotoxic antibodies are severely damaging to both pulmonary alveolar and renal glomerular basement membranes.

C. Immune Complex Reactions (Type III)

The toxic effects of immune complexes formed by interaction of antibody with corresponding antigen are thought to play a major pathogenetic role in a variety of human autoimmune diseases including glomerulonephritis, lupus erythematosus, rheumatoid arthritis, vasculitis, and classic serum sickness. If antigen and antibodies combine in the right proportions (usually in slight antigen excess), natural host defense mechanisms are activated. The most important biologically active contributors to this reaction are complement components, leukocytes, and lysosomal enzymes. In both experimental and clinical immune-complex-mediated diseases, deposition of immune complexes in various tissues can be demonstrated by means of direct fluorescent or ferritin conjugated antibody techniques.

D. Delayed Hypersensitivity Reactions (Type IV)

Delayed hypersensitivity or type IV reactions are mediated by T_D CD4$^+$ cells without any evidence of humoral antibody interactions except for K type T cells, which have receptors for the Fc domain of IgG immunoglobulin. Diseases in this category of human hypersensitivity include contact dermatitis, a condition in which the induction and elicitation of the sensitization phenomenon are entirely limited to the skin. Delayed hypersensitivity responses are also systemic and involve lymphoid organs and cells throughout the body. Such involvement evokes the appearance of effector T_D cells that produce proinflammatory lymphokines. These soluble mediators play an important role in the chemotaxis of mononuclear inflammatory cells, the products of which ultimately lead to chronic lymphocytic infiltrates, disseminated granulomata, and fibrosis.

REFERENCES

1. Richet, C. Anaphylaxis, translated by J. Murray Blight. The University Press, Liverpool (1913).
2. Paul, W.E. (ed.). Fundamental Immunology. Raven Press, New York (1984).
3. Samter, M., Talmage, D.W., Rose, B., Sherman, W.B. and Vaughn, J.H. Immunologic Diseases, 3rd Ed. Little, Brown, Boston (1978).
4. Dixon, F.J. and Fisher, D.W. The Biology of Immunologic Disease. Sinauer Associates, Sunderland, Massachusetts (1983).
5. Middleton, E., Jr., Reed, C.E. and Ellis, E.F. Allergy Principles and Practice, 3rd Ed. C.V. Mosby. St. Louis (1988).
6. Kaplan, A.P. (ed.).Allergy. Churchill Livingstone, New York (1985).
7. Patterson, R. Allergic Diseases, 3rd Ed. J.B. Lippincott, Philadelphia (1985).
8. Rose, N.R., Friedman, H. and Fahey, J.L. Manual of Clinical Laboratory Immunology, 3rd Ed. American Society for Microbiology, Washington, D.C. (1986).
9. Stites, D.P., Stobo, J.D. and Wells, J.V. Basic and Clinical Immunology, 6th Ed. Appleton and Lange, Norwalk, Connecticut (1987).
10. Nossal, G.J.V. The basic components of the immune system. N. Engl. J. Med. 316:1320–1325 (1987).
11. Landsteiner, K. The Specificity of Serological Reactions. Dover Publications, New York (1962).
12. Goodman, J.W. Immunoglobulins 1: structure and function. *In* Basic and Clinical Immunology (D.P. Stites, J.D. Stobo and J.V. Wells, eds.) 6th Ed. Appleton and Lange, Norwalk, Connecticut, pp. 27–36 (1987).
13. Korsmeyer, S.J. and Waldmann, T.A. Immunoglobulins II: Gene organization and assembly. *In* Basic and Clinical Immunology (D.P. Stites, J.D. Stobo and J.V. Wells, eds.) 6th Ed. Appleton and Lange, Norwalk, Connecticut, pp. 37–49 (1987).

14. Shaw, S. Characterisation of human leukocyte differentiation antigens. Immunol Today 8:1–3 (1987).
15. Stobo, J.D. Lymphocytes. *In* Basic and Clinical Immunology (D.P. Stites, J.D. Stobo and J.V. Wells, eds.) 6th Ed. Appleton and Lange, Norwalk, Connecticut, pp. 65–81 (1987).
16. Brenner, M.B., McLean, J. Scheft, H. et al. Two forms of the T-cell receptor protein found on peripheral blood cytotoxic T lymphocytes. Nature 325: 689–694 (1987).
17. Pardoll, D.M., Bowlkes, B.J., Bluestone, J.A. et al. Differential expression of two distinct T-cell receptors during thymocyte development. Nature 326:79–81 (1987).
18. Sette, A., Buus, S., Colon, S. et al. Structural characteristics of an antigen required for its interaction with Ia and recognition by T cells. Nature 328: 395–399 (1987).
19. Allen, P.M., Matsueda, G.R., Evans, R.J., Dunbar, J.B. et al. Identification of the T-cell and Ia contact residues of a T-cell antigenic epitope. Nature 327:713–175 (1987).
20. Henkart, P.A. Mechanism of lymphocyte-mediated cytotoxicity. Annu. Rev. Immunol. 3:31 (1985).
21. Podack, E.R. The molecular mechanism of lymphocyte-mediated tumor cell lysis. Immunol Today 6:21 (1985).
22. Ostergaard, H.L., Kane, K.P., Mescher, M.F. and Clark, W.R. Cytotoxic T lymphocyte mediated lysis without release of serine esterase. Nature 330: 71–77 (1987).
23. Rosenberg, S.A., Lotze, M.T., Muul, L.M. et al. A progress report on the treatment of 157 patients with advanced cancer using lymphokine-activated killer cells and inerleukin-2 or high-dose interleukin-2 alone. N. Engl. J. Med. 316:889–905 (1987).
24. Claman, H.N. The biology of the immune response. J.A.M.A. 258:2834–2840 (1987).
25. Morimoto, C., Rudd, C.E., Letvin, N.L. et al. A novel epitope of the LFA-1 antigen which can distinguish killer effector and suppressor cells in human CD8 cells. Nature 330:479–482 (1987).
26. Unanue, E.R. and Allen, P.M. The basis for the immunoregulatory role of macrophages and other accessory cells. Science 236:551–563 (1987).
27. Paul, W.E. and Ohara, J. B-cell stimulatory factor-1/Interleukin 4. Annu. Rev. Immunol. 5:429–459 (1987).
28. Kinashi, T., Harada, N., Severinson, E. et al. Cloning of complementary DNA encoding T-cell replacing factor and identity with B-cell growth factor II. Nature 324:70–76 (1986).
29. Klaus, G.G.B. Unravelling the control of B cells. Nature 324:16–17 (1986).
30. Ross, G.D. and Medof, M.E. Membrane complement receptors specific for bound fragments of C3. Adv. Immunol. 37:217–267 (1985).
31. Lanzavecchia, A. B cell and antigen presentation. Nature 314:537–540 (1987).

32. Snapper, C.M. and Paul, W.E. Interferon-γ and B cell stimulatory factor-1 reciprocally regulate Ig isotype production. Science 236:944–947 (1987).

33. Frank, M.M. Complement in the pathophysiology of human disease. N. Engl. J. Med. 316:1525–1530 (1987).

34. Hugli, T.E., Marceau, F. and Lundberg, C. Effects of complement fragments on pulmonary and vascular smooth muscle. Am. Rev. Respir. Dis. 135:S9–S13 (1987).

35. Frank, M.M. Complement-derived mediators. In Proceedings of the XII International Congress of Allergology and Clinical Immunology, Washington, D.C. (C.E. Reed, ed.), pp. 294–299 (1985).

36. Ross, G.D. and Medof, M.E. Membrane complement receptors specific for bound fragments of C3. Adv Immunol 37:217–267 (1985).

37. Muller-Eberhard, H.J. The membrane attack complex of complement. Annu. Rev. Immunol. 4:503–528 (1986).

38. Jerne, N.K. Towards a network theory of the immune system. Ann. Immunol. (Paris) 125C:373–389 (1955).

39. Kunkel, H.G., Mannick, M. and William, R.C. Individual antigenic specificities of isolated antibodies. Science 140:1218–1219 (1963).

40. Oudin, J. and Michael, M. Une nouvelle forme d'allotypie des immunoglobulines du serum de lapin. C.R. Hebd. Seances Acad. Sci. 257:805–808 (1963).

41. Vaz, N.M., Martinez, A.C. and Coutinho, A. The uniqueness and boundaries of the idiotypic self. In Idiotypy in Biology Medicine (H. Kohler, J. Urbain, and P.A. Cazenave, eds.), Academic Press, Orlando, Florida, pp. 44–59 (1984).

42. Gell, P.G.H., Coombs, R.R.A. and Lachmann, R. (eds.). Clinical Aspects of Immunology, 3rd Ed. Blackwell Scientific Publication, Oxford (1975).

43. Kaliner, M.A. The late phase and its clinical implications. Hosp. Pract. 15:73–83 (1987).

4

Immunopathogenesis of Human Hypersensitivity

I. Type I reactions   39
II. Type II reactions   45
III. Type III reactions   47
IV. Type IV reactions   50
     References   53

I. TYPE I REACTIONS

As early as 1906 the term "allergy," as coined by von Pirquet, was used to characterize reactions that occurred when a host was reexposed to an environmental agent (1). The meaning of altered reactivity implicit in the Greek derivation of the word "allergy" at first was not associated with a specific type of immune response. After Prausnitz and Küstner demonstrated that specific reactivity could be transferred to the skin of a naive recipient by a heat-labile antibody, the terms of "allergy," "allergens," and "allergic antibody (reagin)," subsequently were identified with immediate human hypersensitivity reactions (type I) because skin reactions generally appeared within a short period of time (2). Immune responses leading to type I responses depend upon genetic factors in the host, routes and quantities of exposure, proper conditions for the induction of the immune response, allogeneic and FC_ϵ receptors on effector and regulatory cells, and end-organ responses occurring shortly after the appropriate stimulus.

Although IgE-mediated immune responses confer protective immunity to the parasitized host without causing ill effects, aberrant pathological type I reactions occur in susceptible (atopic) individuals who appear to develop IgE-mediated immune responses because of underlying hereditary factors (3-5). Population studies have demonstrated that infants with increased levels of total IgE are more likely to develop type I clinical sensitivity (5). The inheritance of this trait is postulated to occur by an autosomal recessive mechanism, because an autosomal dominant gene in nonsusceptible (nonatopic) individuals determines the normal total level of serum IgE. This view has been challenged recently as a result of an investigation of 239 members of 40 nuclear and 3 extended families (6). In each extended family, atopy was vertically transmitted and 31 of 47 (66%) offspring of marriages between atopic and unaffected parents were atopic. It was concluded that atopy or the propensity to produce IgE in response to common inhaled allergens is inherited as an autosomal dominant character. Generation of an immune response after exposure to naturally occurring environmental agents also depends upon the presence of immune response genes in susceptible individuals. These have been determined in large human populations by comparing the incidence of skin test reactivity elicted by ultrapurified allergens with the incidence of various human MHC antigens. The most convincing model for the role of immune response genes in type I clinical sensitivity is the significant association between Amb Va (Ra5), a purified component of aqueous short ragweed extract, and a specific (DR2$^+$/Dw2$^+$) class II MHC antigen. More than 95% of Amb Va (Ra5)-positive subjects are Dw2-positive compared to an incidence of 20% Dw2 positivity in Amb Va (Ra5)-negative patients (4). Another interesting immune response association is between HLA-DR3/Dw3 prevalence and sensitivity to purified rye grass allergen (LolpI, LolpII, and LolpIII). General hyperresponsiveness, as determined by multiple skin test responses to a variety of allergens, may also have a genetic basis. Patients with the haplotype of HLA-B8 and HLA-Dw3 are more prone to show general skin test hyperresponsiveness (7). Despite the documented role of immune response and suppressive genes in regulation of specific antibody production to low-molecular-weight chemicals in murine animal models, much less is known about the genetic control of immune responses after exposure to similar agents in humans. In the case of human immune responses induced by chemicals after respiratory exposure, there is as yet no clear evidence that atopic background (as indexed by high total IgE or generalized cutaneous reactivity) is an obligate prerequisite. In fact, the majority of individuals who ultimately develop these immune responses are nonatopic.

The conditions of exposure to an allergen may determine the extent, severity, or duration of immune response to that allergen. The specific sites (respiratory, gastrointestinal, skin, subcutaneous, intramuscular, or intravascular) exhibit somewhat different properties with respect to induction of IgE antibody formation or elicitation of the allergic response itself. Moreover, the route of allergen exposure may determine whether subsequent allergic responses to an allergen are manifested primarily in various organs or as a generalized systemic effect. In general, exposure to small amounts, ranging from nanograms to micrograms, rather than large amounts of naturally occurring allergenic substances, favors the development of specific IgE antibodies in susceptible individuals. For example, it is has been observed that respiratory sensitization to ragweed pollen may occur after as few as three successive seasonal exposures to ragweed pollen. During this period of time, the total amount of inhaled ragweed allergen is probably less than 1 μg/year. Another important exposure determinant of sensitization is the realization that intermittent, in contrast to constant, exposure to small amounts of allergen may greatly enhance the prospects of clinical sensitization to an allergen. This principle of immunization is well documented in animal models, and human correlates also exist. Thus respiratory sensitization to several low-molecular-weight occupational allergens appears to develop more readily in workers exposed to periodic chemical spills rather than those whose exposure is low-level and constant or who are not exposed to accidental spills (8). Another important principle is that symptoms are usually elicited in those end organs originally exposed to the offending allergen, although there are some notable exceptions. Under certain conditions allergens may be absorbed through the skin (chemicals, peptides, or even whole proteins) and elicit remote end-organ or systemic reactions. Generalized reactions may also occur after allergen–antibody reactions in the respiratory, gastrointestinal, or genitourinary systems. Allergens with access to the gastrointestinal system as the primary route of exposure may be subject to different control mechanisms depending on the age of the susceptible host. For example, neonates and toddlers up to the age of 2 are more susceptible to IgE-mediated sensitization by allergens presented to the gastrointestinal tract than older children or adults. Indeed, there is a dramatic shift between gastrointestinal and respiratory sensitization in susceptible children between the ages of 2 and 3. Chronic exposures to either natural or chemical allergens will generally enhance the persistence of clinical sensitivity, except that there tends to be a gradual nonspecific decrease in allergic susceptibility among atopic persons during the latter decades of life. In the case of respiratory sensitization to low-molecular-weight chemicals, specific IgE antibody responses usually disappear within a matter of months, even in workers who have natural atopic susceptibility, provided that further exposure is eliminated. Thus far, one exception to this general rule has been found. Among platinum workers who terminate employment after developing clinical sensitivity, some have been found to maintain a high degree of skin test reactivity to platinum as long as 4 years after discontinuation of employment (9). Why this occurs is not known but it is suspected that certain substances such as platinum may act as nonspecific immunopotentiators (10). Finally, it should be emphasized that atopic individuals have the unusual ability to maintain synthesis of IgE antibodies for years, even though exposure to specific natural allergens is limited to specific seasonal periods of the year. It is postulated that the allergic person's T-cell immune network can be perennially primed by anti-idiotypic antibodies containing allergenlike determinants (i.e., internal allergen images as reflected by idiotypic determinants on the hypervariable segments of IgE heavy and light chains) (4).

Although induction of specific IgE antibodies involves all the previously described cellular interactions between antigen-presenting cells, T_H and T_S cells,

B lymphocytes, MHC recognition factors, and cytokines secreted by macrophages [interleukin (IL-1)] and T cells (IL-2, IL-3, IL-4, IL-5, IL-6, and IL-7), additional regulatory control mechanisms are unique to the synthesis of specific IgE. Several independent investigators have demonstrated a complex group of cytokines elaborated by both T and B cells during synthesis or down-regulation of specific IgE antibodies (11,12). These have been designated as IgE-binding factors. As the names imply, these factors bind to IgE receptors in the membranes of T and B lymphocytes. A group of related IgE-binding factors have been found to potentiate (IgE potentiating factor) the production of IgE antibodies and yet another family of molecules have been demonstrated to downregulate or suppress (IgE suppressor factor) production of these antibodies. Presumably, all individuals regulate the production of IgE antibodies by this complex control network. In the case of atopic individuals, it is postulated that the specific IgE T-suppressor factors may not be functioning properly (12). Alternatively, it is possible that IgE-potentiating factors may exceed proper regulatory controls as is suggested by the marked increase in total and specific IgE in some patients with eczema. The IgE-potentiating and suppressor binding factors share the same structural genes. Their strikingly different functional activities are determined by the degree of posttranslational glycosylation with N-linked oligosaccharides. Two separate nonspecific factors determine whether glycosylation is increased or decreased. Glycosylation-enhancing factor (GEF) is a kallikreinlike protease that enhances the glycosylation process and results in the formation of IgE-potentiating factor by T_H CD4$^+$ cells. Another substance known as glycosylation-inhibitory factor (GIF) (i.e., lipomodulin, a phospholipase inhibitory protein) suppresses the glycosylation process and results in the formation of an IgE suppressor factor. In addition to their profound effects as IgE-binding factors, each of these substances may have other unique properties. Glycosylation-inhibitory factor, for example, not only suppresses IgE but also partially suppresses IgG antibody formation when administered before and after immunization. Glycosylation-enhancing factor not only enhances the production of IgE isotypic antibody but also may directly affect the release of histamine and arachidonic acid metabolites from mast cells. In this way it appears to increase the sensitivity or intrinsic "releasibility" of mast cells and basophils. Thus, GEF appears to have significant dual properties as both a regulator of IgE synthesis and a possible cofactor of mast cell function. Further stimulation of antigen-primed T cells causes the formation of antigen-specific forms of both GEF and GIF (13). The IL-3 lymphokine exhibits mast cell growth factor properties when added to in vitro murine T-cell cultures. However, whether IL-3 lymphokine has similar properties in humans has not been determined. Interleukin-4 also enhances growth of mast cells. In addition, IL-4 plays a major role in the synthesis of IgE by up-regulating the appearance of CD 23$^+$ B cells and the expression of B cell FC$_\epsilon$ receptors (14). IgE-binding factors may also be secreted by Epstein-Barr-virus-infected B cells as well as by nonimmune B cells. It has been determined that IgE-binding factors share homologous epitopes with FC_ϵ receptors on B cells. The functional activity and interaction of B-cell-derived IgE-binding factors with T-cell-derived IgE binding factors has not yet been determined.

Membrane-associate IgE receptors are vital links between the complex cellular interactions that occur during both induction and elicitation of IgE-dependent allergic reactions (15). IgE receptors are transmembrane proteins that consist of one a chain (divided into a 1 and a 2 components) and two β chains joined by a γ chain located at the membrane cytosol interface. Mast cells and basophils contain high affinity receptors (FC_ϵ R_1) while lymphocytes, macrophages, eosinophils, and platelets have low-affinity-type receptors. The low-affinity IgE receptors (FC_ϵ R_2) on macrophages, eosinophils, and platelets have been differentiated from high-affinity FC_ϵ R_1 receptors by CD23 monoclonal antibodies (16), which are specific for the low-affinity-receptor. IgE-induced parasite cytotoxicity is mediated only by macrophages, eosinophils, and platelets. Presumably, the FC_ϵ R_2 receptor is predominant in this system because of its increased affinity for IgE complexes, which are abundant in parasitic infections. Until recently it was thought that only aggregated IgE (dimers or oligomers) bridges could activate the stimulus response signal in the mast cell/basophil membrane. However, recombinant peptides corresponding to a segment of 76 amino acids at the $C_\epsilon 2/C_\epsilon 3$ domain junction of FC_ϵ not only inhibit passive sensitization of human skin mast cells by IgE myeloma protein but also sensitize mast cells to degranulation by anti-IgE in vitro almost as efficiently as myeloma IgE (17). This $C_\epsilon 2/C_\epsilon 3$ amino acid segment is monomeric and folds to generate a cleft between $C_\epsilon 2$ and $C_\epsilon 3$ domains on the surface of the FC_ϵ. It is postulated that justaposition of IgE onto the a chain of FC_ϵ R_1 occurs within this cleft. Once the high-affinity bond between the $C_\epsilon 2$ and $C_\epsilon 3$ domains of the IgE molecule and the corresponding IgE receptor is firmly established, dissociation is a slow process. This accounts for persistence of mast cell/basophil sensitization for long periods of time. After the mast cell/basophil membranes have been sensitized by a sufficient number of specific IgE molecules, subsequent exposure to the specific allergen will result in binding of the allergen to Fab combining sites on two adjacent IgE molecules. This bridging effect is a signal that apparently induces a rapid sequence of biochemical events in the plasma membrane and cytosol of the effector cells. Just after the initial perturbation event, the IgE receptors are apparently immobilized (activated) and internalized. This process provides the signal for a complex interaction between guanosine nucleotide phosphate (GTP) and a GTP-binding regulatory protein, a secretion-signal system that mobilizes both intracellular and extracellular calcium ions required for extracellular release of preformed granule-associated mediators and the generation of new chemical bioactive products from lipid precursors. The biochemical cascade activated by receptor bridging is complex. Among others, membrane-associated enzymes, phosphatidylinositol turnover, inositol triphosphate, diacylglycerol, and protein kinase C play key roles in the activation process (18).

The extent, severity, and duration of allergic reactions in various end organs depend on the number and distribution of mast cells within those organs or the number of basophils, in the case of blood and nasal airways. Such conditions are amply met at respiratory, gastrointestinal, subcutaneous, and intravascular tissue sites. Mast cell mediators consist of vasoactive/spasmogenic compounds, chemotactic agents, enzymes, and proteoglycans (19). The chief performed mediators from mast cell granules are histamine, proteases, proteoglycans, and chemotactic factors. The membrane lipid-derived mediators, which are generated minutes after the allergic reaction occurs, consist of platelet-activating factor (PAF), prostaglandin D_2, and sulfidopeptide leukotrienes (LTC_4, LTD_4, and LTE_4). The generated mediators induce wheal and flare skin responses and smooth muscle contraction including bronchoconstriction both in vitro and in vivo. In addition, PAF induces local platelet and neutrophil aggregation and induces bronchial hyperreactivity. Both preformed neutrophil chemotactic factors of anaphylaxis, eosinophil chemotactic factors, and newly generated leucotriene B_4 chemotactic factors have been identified in mast cells. Chemotactic mediators that attract neutrophils and eosinophils are especially important components of the allergic inflammatory response. These cells are predominant in late phase responses occurring several hours after the initial allergic stimulus. Eosinophils are particularly important because they contain eosinophilic major basic and cationic proteins that are known to be toxic to parasites and various tissues including the lung and skin. Eosinophilic cationic protein induces the formation of functional pores in target cells and in this respect resembles the attack complex of complement and perforin proteins of cytotoxic cells (20). In addition, eosinophils also generate LTC_4, PAF, eosinophil peroxidase and toxic oxygen metabolites in response to a variety of stimuli. Similarly, neutrophils release lysosomal enzymes, toxic oxygen radicals, LTD_4, and PAF in response to activation stimuli. A number of granule-associated proteases and proteoglycans have also been identified in human mast cells. Enzymes that have been identified thus far include tryptase, a chymotryptaselike enzyme, prekallikrein and kininogen. Other lysosomal hydrolases including hexaminidase, arylsulfatase, and glucuronidase also are present in human mast cell granules and are released after IgE-dependent allergen activation in vitro. Human mast cells contain several varieties of polyanionic proteoglycans (21). Heparin-containing mast cells are known as connective tissue mast cells and are present in human skin and lung. Mucosal (gut-associated) mast cells are characterized by their high content of chondroitin sulfate E. Heparin and heparinlike activity may appear in the blood after controlled allergic challenges in humans.

Apart from structural differences of proteoglycans, human mast cells are heterogeneous with respect to chymase enzyme content, distribution in various tissues, and secretory response to compound 48/80, morphine, C5a anaphlyatoxin, and f-met peptides. Thus, mucosal (chymase-negative/tryptase-positive) mast cells are found in greater abundance in lung, alveolar walls, and bowel mucosa than are connective tissue (chymase-positive, tryptase-positive) mast cells. Both types of mast cells are found in nasal submucosa but only mucosal mast cells are present in nasal epithelium. Connective tissue mast cells are the abundant cells in bowel submucosa (22). Connective tissue mast cells exhibit brisk secretory responses to compound 48/80, morphine, C5a anaphylatoxin, and f-met peptides while mucosal mast cells fail to respond to these substances (23,24).

Tissue basophilia of the nose may account for a major proportion of symptoms in patients with allergic rhinitis. These cells are found in nasal secretions during seasonal exacerbations of nasal allergy. Moreover, basophils are the predominant cells of late-phase allergic infiltrates in the nose. Secretory responses of basophils differ from both mucosal and connective tissue mast cells. Basophilic mediator release is stimulated by substance P, C5a anaphylatoxin, and f-met peptides but not by compound 48/80 and morphine. Moreover, both glucocorticosteroids and indomethacin inhibit release of histamine, prostaglandin D_2, and platelet-activating factor from basophils and cutaneous mast cells, while these drugs have little or no inhibitory effects on lung and intestinal mast cells. Basophilic derived kinin and tosyl-L-arginine methyl ester (TAME) esterase as well as histamine, prostaglandin D_2, and leukotriene release has been reported after nasal antigen challenges (25).

Although it has been operationally useful to classify humoral and cellular human hypersensitivity responses as separate entities, it must be emphasized that there are a number of significant regulatory and effector pathogenetic interactions between these two major types of adaptive immunity. Many of the cytokines that regulate production or suppression of IgE are derived from thymus-dependent cells; lymphokines (i.e., IL-3, IL-4) may play a regulatory role in the proliferation and differentiation of mast cells and basophils, as demonstrated in murine T-cell culture systems; IgE-dependent antibody dependent cell cytotoxicity (ADCC) is the primary mechanism of defense against schistosomiasis in humans (3); basophils are the predominant cells of cutaneous basophilia, an animal model of delayed hypersensitivity; and antigen or T-cell mitogens can activate human mononuclear cells to produce several types of histamine-releasing factors, one of which is IgE dependent (26,27).

II. TYPE II REACTIONS

This form of human hypersensitivity is characterized by the development of autoantibodies directed against circulating or fixed tissue components (28). The elicitation phase of the reaction occurs when these autoantibodies bind to specific epitopes in cell membranes. These surface antigen–antibody reactions are in effect local immune complexes that can be visualized by fluorescent-coated antibodies. These membrane-associated antigen–antibody complexes assume a linear appearance when stained by fluorescent antibodies, as contrasted by "lumpy-bumpy deposits" observed at tissue sites affected by type III immune complex disease. Cytotoxic reactions at affected tissues occur subsequent to activation of the classic complement cascade and the formation of the "membrane attack complex" (C5b6789). The membrane attack complex may cause irreparable injury to tissue membranes (e.g., red blood cells) with subsequent osmotic death of the cell. An S protein prevents the attack complex from attaching to target membrane when coupled to C56b-9 (29). Other possible damage mechanisms of type II reactions relate to cleavage of C3 into two major biological fragments, C3a (anaphylatoxin) and C3b by C3 convertase (C4b2a). C3b binds to its receptor (CR1) in target tissues and opsonizes these tissues. C3b is also an essential subunit of two C5 convertases—classic (C4b2a3b) and alternate (C3bBbC3b) pathway types—both of which are capable of binding and cleaving C5 (30). This reaction liberates C5a, a very potent anaphylatoxin and neutrophil chemotactic factor, which attracts neutrophils to the tissue membrane site in great numbers. Although fixed tissues cannot be phagocytized, the activated neutrophils nevertheless release cytotoxic lysosomes.

Some of the classic human diseases with proven type II mechanisms include transfusion reactions, hemolytic disease of the newborn (Rh incompatibility), and autoimmune hemolytic anemias. In some cases, drugs such as penicillin and quinidine may induce cytotoxic antibodies against antigen-altered red blood cell or neutrophil membranes. Antibodies to a glycoprotein of the glomerular basement membrane occur in Goodpasture's syndrome. These antibodies cross-react with a lung basement membrane, the immune consequences of which may result in massive pulmonary hemorrhage. Autoantibodies to acetylcholine receptors in myasthenia gravis, beta$_2$ adrenergic receptors in asthma, and insulin receptors have also been demonstrated. Whether these autoantibodies are actually responsible for cytopathological disorders in these diseases is not certain. The classic explanation for appearance of autoantibodies is cross-reaction between epitopes on exogenous agents (i.e., bacteria and viruses) and tissue autoantigens. Experimental results in autoimmune mice also support the primacy of exogenous inducers rather than abnormalities of Ig germline genes or the genetic elements encoding autoantibodies (31). Another recent hypothesis for the occurrence of membrane and receptor autoantibodies invokes the role of virally encoded membrane proteins and receptors as carriers for enhancing the autoantigenicity of cell surface components (32). This could account for the development of antireceptor hormone antibodies, which in turn could stimulate the formation of anti-idiotypic hormone antibodies.

I. TYPE III REACTIONS

Type III hypersensitivity diseases are mediated by immune complexes, that induce immunopathological damage at various tissue sites. The fact that deposition of immune complexes could be harmful always presented somewhat of a dilemma to immunologists. This is because under ideal homeostatic circumstances, protective antibodies combine with foreign antigens with the ultimate purpose of eliminating these antigens either by phagocytosis or by clearance mechanisms within the reticuloendothelial system. At the same time that clearance is occurring, these circulating immune complexes amplify the humoral adaptive system further by presenting antigen throughout the lymphoid system, thereby making even a stronger antibody response within those tissues (33). The clearance of circulating immune complexes by the reticuloendothelial system occurs primarily in the liver and spleen (34). Cells within the liver are heavily endowed with CR1 receptors, while the spleen clearance mechanism operates by IgG FC_γ receptors. Saturation of the reticuloendothelial system receptors with large doses of immune complexes will result in persistence of circulating immune complexes. Under such circumstances, deposition of immune complexes in other tissues is more likely to occur.

The harmful effects of immune complexes were first proposed by von Pirquet and Schick, who observed that the symptoms of serum sickness could be ascribed to toxic interactions between antigen and antibody (35). Later, Germuth provided direct experimental proof that immune complexes were immunopathogenetic in chronic serum sickness induced in rabbits (30). Similar observations were reported in humans by Lawley et al., who not only confirmed the importance of immune complexes but also showed that complement activation occurred and could be directly associated with the appearance of clinical symptoms (37). These investigators designed a prospective study in patients receiving therapeutic injections with heterologous antithymocyte globulin. The results of this study provided direct evidence that human serum sickness is associated with increased levels of immune complexes and large-scale activation of the complement system.

The pathogenic role of immune complexes depends upon various factors, including the size of the complex, the available combining sites on the respective antigens and antibodies, the characteristics of the antibody component (i.e., affinity and immunoglobulin class) within the complex, the physicochemical nature of the antigen, and the efficiency of complement-dependent opsonification and clearance properties (34). Precipitation of immune complexes occurs because of antigen–antibody lattice formation that is more likely to occur rapidly in states of antibody excess than at equivalence. Apart from the Arthus reaction and IgA immune complexes, precipitation of circulating immune complexes is usually prevented because of several signficant complement interactions with the complex. As soon as antigen and complement-fixing antibody react in body fluids, the classic pathway of complement is activated followed by binding of a large number of C3b molecules to the immune complex (33). Components of the clasic pathway, particularly C1, inhibit lattice formation by interfering with Fc–Fc molecular interactions of IgM and IgG molecules. Even if initial inhibition of immune precipitates does not occur, complement can still lead to their dissolution. This process is dependent upon the alternative pathway of complement. Thus, complement plays a vital homeostatic function by keeping complexes in solution, thereby aiding in the diffusion of antigen–antibody complexes away from their primary sites of formation.

Complement also plays an essential role in the clearance of immune complexes. Opsonized (C3b-coated) immune complexes are recognized by CR1 receptors on the surfaces of various cells. Ninety-five percent of CR1 receptors in the circulation of humans are on the surface of erythrocytes (38). Thus, opsonized immune complexes attach predominantly to CR1 on erythrocytes and are then transported to fixed macrophage systems in the reticuloendothelial system, where the complexes are transferred from erythrocytes to macrophages by as yet unidentified mechanisms, although FC_γ IgG receptors most likely augment this process, particularly in the spleen. Transfer of complexes in the fixed macrophage system ensures safe elimination of immunocomplexes. Large immune complexes are cleared more rapidly than the small ones, probably because of more efficient complement fixation in the former.

Although immunological effects of immune complex interactions reflect the balance between beneficial and detrimental effects upon the host, certain general principles assist in determining whether the balance is tipped one way or the other. A potent antigen induces a strong, high-affinity antibody response. An immune complex formed by these reactants results in brisk complement fixation, optimal antigen elimination, and only transient appearance of immune complexes in body fluids. In contrast, weak antigenic substances are cleared over a much longer period of time. Failure of the normal physiological clearance of immune complexes may occur for a number of reasons: complement deficiencies; failure of several antibody classes or subclasses (i.e., IgA, IgE, IgD, IgG_2, and IgG_4) to fix complement; deficiency or saturation of CR1 receptors on red cells or in the reticuloendothelial system; and diffuse, irreversible disease of the fixed macrophage system (i.e., primary biliary cirrhosis). The deposition of immune complexes in specific tissues depends upon the number of available receptors for C3b and the Fc portions of IgG and IgM molecules, the extent of prior disease within that tissue, and localized increases of vascular permeability induced by chronic, physiological activation of complement.

Immune complexes are commonly found in diseases such as glomerulonephritis, vasculitis, acute infectious diseases (bacterial, viral, and parasitic), and a variety of autoimmune diseases. They are found often in rheumatoid arthritis and systemic lupus erythematosus. Immune complexes are also identified in patients with various malignancies including lymphoproliferative neoplasms, carcinoma of the colon, melanoma, and cancer of the lung. Why some persons develop immune complex disease and others do not is still not understood. Apart from some of the factors mentioned above, genetic factors may play a role in certain diseases. The incidence of immune complex diseases among persons with various deficiencies of complement proteins, particularly the components of the classic pathway, appears to be significantly increased (38,39). Thus, a failure of complement-dependent handling of immune complexes appears to be a plausible explanation for the association between complement deficiencies and disease. Patients with autoimmune diseases frequently have autoimmune antibodies against C3b receptors and/or Fc_γ domains of immunoglobulin molecules. Blocking effects exerted by such antibodies could be responsible for defects in immune complex clearance mechanisms. Immune complexes may initiate the formation of anti-idiotypic antibodies, which form complexes with the specific antibody moiety of the complex. This secondary immune response could account for persistence of chronic circulating immune complexes. However, it should be emphasized that anti-idiotypic-antibody complexes may have important regulatory roles in the homeostatic control of immune responses and the presence of these complexes does not necessarily denote an abnormal disease state. Indeed, physiologically "normal" immune complexes occur in the normal course of infections and metabolism of foods (40).

To summarize, the phlogistic hallmarks of toxic immune complexes include activation of both the classic and alternate pathways of complement, release of biologically active complement components with potent vascular permeability, smooth muscle spasmogenic and chemotactic effects, migration of neutrophils to the site of tissue immune complexes, release of hydrolytic enzymes from these cells, an active attack process on cell membranes, and other complement interactions with coagulation and kininogen pathways. In addition, immune complexes may play a role in modifying antibody-dependent cell-mediated toxicity and in the regulation of antibody production by B cells (34). Furthermore, immune complexes themselves may be regulated by autoanti-idiotypic antibodies. The immunopathogenetic effects of immune complexes may also be enhanced by IgE-dependent release of vasoactive amines that prepare the proper conditions in vessel walls for deposition in tissue sites such as skin or kidney.

Serum sickness is the classic type III mediated disease in both experimental animals and humans (37). Immune complexes can be demonstrated both within the circulation and at various tissue sites including blood vessels, kidney, skin, and joints. "One-shot" serum sickness is a brief and self-limiting disease because most of the immune complexes have been formed for the purpose of essential clearance functions and deposition at tissue sites is transient and nonpersistent. On the other hand, chronic serum sickness may occur in susceptible hosts when there is continuous exposure ("multiple shots") to the antigen and the immune complexes formed are in slight antigen excess, thereby fulfilling the most propitious circumstances for immune-complex-mediated tissue damage. In such cases, immune complexes are most likely to deposit at glomerular basement membrane sites and they can be demonstrated in these locations by fluorescent antibody staining, which delineates a "lumpy-bumpy" pattern of deposition. Another form of localized immune complex disease is the Arthus phenomenon, which, although it can be demonstrated readily in experimental animals, occurs rarely in humans after repeated local injections of a strong antigen at a single subcutaneous site. In this situation, the precipitation and deposition of immune complexes at the site of repeated antigen exposure result in an exaggerated phlogistic response, tissue necrosis, and ulceration.

IV. TYPE IV REACTIONS

Type IV reactions are mediated solely by cellular immune mechanisms, the putative requirements of which are thymic-dependent T lymphocytes. These delayed-hypersensitivity-type cells (T_D) require an intact thymus gland for their development into the mature and active effector cells of cellular immunity. At maturity, they are characterized as $CD4^+$ cells. They recognize antigen in the context of the class II MHC restriction process and they secrete IL-2 and other proinflammatory substances (41). T_D lymphocytes are the essential guardian cells in providing immunity against viral, protozoal, fungal, parasitic, and a number of significant bacterial infections. In addition, cellular immunity plays an important role in protecting against malignancy.

The term "delayed hypersensitivity" was originally used because the time course of these reactions was measured in days or weeks in contrast to the immediate (minutes to hours) reactions observed in types I, II, and III reactions. However, it is now recognized that cellular activation and migration in delayed hypersensitivity occur within a matter of hours, so, in a strict sense, the evolving course of these reactions was not always delayed. Conversely, a major part of the inflammatory response of IgE-mediated immediate reactions may be delayed in time. This constitutes the late phase response, which is thought to be responsible for chronic clinical and pathological abnormalities of type I diseases (42). Delayed hypersensitivity is still referred to as "tuberculinlike hypersensitivity." This term was used for many years because much of the early information about delayed hypersensitivity was derived from the study of the immune response to tuberculin and tubercule bacilli. Tuberculinlike hypersensitivity also implies systemic sensitization of T_D and memory lymphocytes throughout the body.

Contact dermatitis is a special form of delayed hypersensitivity involving the skin and mucous membranes of the body. Although initially localized to the skin site of exposure, it becomes systemic as more memory T_D lymphocytes become activated and migrate to remote areas of skin. There are distinct pathological differences between tuberculinlike hypersensitivity and contact dermatitis (43). Although local tissue swelling is common to both conditions after elicitation by appropriate test antigens, the tissue inflammatory response in contact dermatitis consists of an intense mononuclear cell infiltration, marked edema of the epidermis, and formation of microvesicles that soon become filled with mononuclear cells. As the microvesicles expand, they become visible as skin vesicles. In contrast, the lesion of tuberculinlike hypersensitivity is an indurated swelling with major involvement of the dermis rather than the epidermis. The dermis is infiltrated with mononuclear cells. About 50% of these are lymphocytes and the remainder monocytes. Relatively small numbers of antigen-specific T_D cells are present in local sites elicited by the specific antigen. Since large numbers of mononuclear cells are present in these lesions, it is apparent that the vast majority of lymphocytes found in these delayed hypersensitivity challenge sites are nonspecific inflammatory cells that migrate to the site in response to lymphokine signals. It should be emphasized, however, that antigen-specific T_D lymphocytes are necessary to initiate all such lesions. There is also a tendency for the lymphocytes to assume a perivascular distribution and, as the lesion progresses, there is disruption of collagen within the dermis. If the dose of eliciting antigen is excessive and persists, there may also be progression to a granulomatous reaction, which represents a more advanced type of delayed hypersensitivity. The characteristic cell of granulomatous hypersensitivity is the epithelioid cell, which is a large flattened cell with increased endoplasmic reticulum. As the lesion progresses, multinucleate giant cells also appear in the lesion. Thus, the classic granulomatous lesion of delayed hypersensitivity is composed of a core of epithelioid cells and macrophages (presumably activated) with giant cells dispersed throughout. In active tuberculosis the core area becomes necrotic, with complete destruction of cellular architecture leading to caseation. The central core of these lesions is surrounded by lymphocytes and, as the lesion progresses, there is a proliferation of fibroblasts, increased collagen synthesis, and a fibrotic response throughout the lesion. Granulomatous lesions develop and tend to persist because of persistence of antigen in the lesions. Certain nonimmunological stimuli such as talc may also induce granuloma formation but these can be distinguished from immunologically induced granuloma by the absence of lymphocytes.

Another type of delayed hypersensitivity reaction has unique timing and histopathological features. First described in humans by Jones and Mote, it consisted of a 24 hr "tuberculinlike" skin reaction after repeated intracutaneous injections of small amounts of rabbit serum proteins (44). This "delayed" component was later replaced by an immediate wheal and flare response. Lesions with similar timing have been produced in several experimental animals. This type of immune response has been studied more vigorously in guinea pigs, where it is characterized by a generalized cutaneous, basophilic hypersensitivity response with large sheets of basophils present in the subepidermal layers of the skin (45).

The major factor that differentiates delayed hypersensitivity from the humoral classes of hypersensitivity diseases (types I, II, and III) is the inability of serum to transfer the reaction to naive recipients. In addition, delayed hypersensitivity reactions are independent of complement or complement components. However, transfer of delayed hypersensitivity (tuberculin type or contact) can be readily accomplished in both experimental animals and humans by transferring sensitized lymphocytes to the skin of nonsensitive individuals (46,47). This transfer reaction can only be accomplished with T_D cells. Transfer factor derived from disrupted whole blood leukocytes can also be transferred to nonallergic recipients (41). This material is an antigen-specific, low-molecular-weight, dialyzable material that is resistant to both DNase and pancreatic RNase. Although considerable work has been expended to purify and characterize this substance, its current role in the pathogenesis of delayed hypersensitivity is still not completely determined.

Lymphocytes of the T_D subset also produce and release biologically active, soluble lymphokines (48). The first of these proinflammatory substances to be recognized in delayed hypersensitivity experimental animals was a low-molecular-weight, nonantibody mediator known as macrophage-inhibiting factor. This factor is a potent inhibitor of macrophage migration. Following this discovery, a large number of lymphokines have been isolated from supernatants of in vitro cultures of antigen-stimulated lymphocytes. It is beyond the scope of this chapter to discuss these lymphokines in detail, but the most important ones in the pathophysiology of delayed hypersensitivity are macrophage-activating factor (γ interferon), macrophage-inhibitory factor, lymphocyte-inhibitory factor, leukocyte-inhibitory factor, and lymphocyte-activating factor (48,49). Sensitization of the T_D subset of lymphocytes requires interaction with mononuclear antigen-presenting cells (macrophages) and other regulatory (T_H and T_S) lymphocytes. The antigen presentation to T_D lymphocytes is class II MHC restricted. Concurrent stimulation by macrophage-derived IL-1 further enhances the activation and proliferation of T_D lymphocytes.

Special antigen-presenting cells are involved in contact dermatitis reactions. These cells are known as Langerhans cells and appear to form a continuous network within the epidermis. They are dendritic cells that contain FC_γ and C3b receptors and also express gene-associated Ia (class II MHC) antigens on their cell membranes (50). These surface markers are similar to those present on monocytes and macrophages. They are thought to play essential roles in the induction and elicitation of allergic contact dermatitis and skin graft rejection. Another antigen-presenting population of epidermal dendritic cells with thymic-dependent surface markers (Thy^+) has been discovered in mice (51). The function of these cells is to down-regulate contact sensitization.

Recent experimental work on delayed hypersensitivity in mice suggests that the development of delayed hypersensitivity may be a two-step procedure depending on two separate T-cell responses (52). One T-cell subset produces a mast-cell-dependent factor that stimulates mast cells to release serotonin, a potent vasopermeability factor in mice. This initial preparatory step paves the way for a second set of delayed hypersensitivity T-cells activated by means of classic MHC-restricted antigen stimulation.

Although cellular interactions are similar in cell-mediated immunity and delayed hypersensitivity, the protective effects of cell-mediated immunity are not necessarily synonymous with responses caused by delayed hypersensitivity. Even in some of the classic diseases in which cell-mediated immune mechanisms might offer considerable advantages to the host, there are, nevertheless, situations in which exaggerated responses of delayed hypersensitivity may be deleterious. Exaggerated granulomatous responses leading to fibrosis in tuberculosis, for example, often result in irreversible tissue damage. Massive granulomata in the spleen and liver as a consequence of delayed hypersensitivity reactions to migrating schistosomes are major complications of schistosomiasis. Widespread granulomata and interstitial fibrosis are dreaded delayed hypersensitivity sequelae of hypersensitivity pneumonitis. The progression of such lesions is thought to be due to persistence of antigens that include not only a wide variety of organic dusts but also an increasing number of industrial chemicals (53). Delayed hypersensitivity also causes harmful effects in graft rejection, graft-vs.-host reactions, and autoallergic reactions.

Allergic contact dermatitis may be the most significant type of delayed hypersensitivity with respect to adverse excipient reactions. Contact dermatitis may be induced by a variety of low-molecular-weight chemicals that traverse the skin, combine with dermal proteins to form conjugates, become processed by Langerhans antigen-presenting cells, and ultimately sensitize a subset of effector T_D lymphocytes that are primed for the development of contact dermatitis when the subject is reexposed to the specific antigen.

REFERENCES

1. Von Pirquet, C. Allergie. Munch Med Wochenschr, 53:1457 (1906). Translated from the German original by Carl Prausnitz. *In* Clinical Aspects of Immunology P.G.H. Gell and R.R.A. Coombs, eds.), FA Davis, Philadelphia, (1963).
2. Prausnitz, C. and Küstner, H. Studien uber uberempfindlichkeit, Zentralbl.

Bakteriol. 1 Abt. Orig. 86:160-169 (1921). Translated from the German by Carl Prausnitz. *In* Clinical Aspects of Immunology (P.G.H. Gell and R.R.A. Coombs, eds.), Blackwell Scientific Publications, Oxford, pp. 808-816 (1962).

3. Capron, A., Dessaint, J.P. and Capron, M. Role of IgE in immune defense. *In* Proceedings of the XII International Congress of Allergology and Clinical Immunology (C.E. Reed, ed.), C.V. Mosby, St. Louis pp. 1-5 (1986).

4. Marsh, D.G. Defining human immune response fingerprints toward ultra-pure allergens: immunochemical and genetic aspects of responsiveness toward the Amb V (Ra5) homologues. *In* Proceedings of the XII International Congress of Allergology and Clinical Immunology (C.E. Reed, ed.), C.V. Mosby, St. Louis pp. 242-248 (1986).

5. Kjellman, N.-I.M., Falth-Magnusson, K. and Croner, S. Fetomaternal relationships and predictive value of IgE production. *In* Proceedings of the XII International Congress of Allergology and Clinical Immunology (C.E. Reed, ed.), C.V. Mosby, St. Louis pp. 6-11 (1986).

6. Cookson, W.O.C.M. and Hopkins, J.M. Dominant inheritance of atopic immunoglobulin-E responsiveness. Lancet 1:86-88 (1988).

7. Roitt, I., Brostoff, J. and Male, D. Immunology. Gower Medical Publishing. London, pp. 19.5-19.6 (1985).

8. Bernstein, I.L. Occupational asthma.   In Allergy (A.P. Kaplan, ed.), Churchill Livingstone, New York (1985).

9. Biagini, R.E., Bernstein, I.L., Gallagher, J.S. et al. The diversity of reaginic immune responses to platinum and palladium metallic salts. J. Allergy Clin. Immunol. 76:794-802 (1985).

10. Murdoch, R.D. and Pepys, J. Immunological responses to complex salts of platinum II enhanced IgE antibody responses to ovalbumin with concurrent administration of platinum salts in the rat. Clin. Exp. Immunol. 58:478-85 (1984).

11. Ishizaka, K. Role of IgE-binding factors and glycosylation-modulating factors in the regulation of IgE synthesis. *In* Proceedings of the XII International Congress of Allergology and Clinical Immunology (Reed, C.E., ed.), C.V. Mosby, St. Louis pp. 11-15 (1986).

12. Katz, D.H. Regulation of the IgE system: experimental and clinical aspects. Allergy 39:81-106 (1984).

13. Ishizaka, K. Ige-binding factors and regulation of the IgE antibody response. Annu Rev. Immunol. 6:513-534 (1988).

14. Paul, W.E. and Ohara, J. B-cell stimulatory factor-1/interleukin 4. Annu. Rev. Immunol. 5:429-459 (1987).

15. Metzger, H., Alcaraz, G., Holman, R., Kiner, J.P., Prebluda, V. and Quarto, R. The receptor with high affinity for immunoglobulin E. Annu Rev Immunol 4:419-470 (1986).

16. Capron, A., Dessaint, J.P., Capron, M. et al. From parasites to allergy: a second receptor for IgE. Immunol. Today 7:15-18 (1986).

17. Helm, B., Marsh, P., Vercelli, D. et al. The mast cell binding site on human immunoglobulin E. Nature 331:180-183 (1988).

18. Ishizaka, T. and White, J.R. Triggering mechanisms of basophils and mast cells. *In* Proceedings of the XII International Congress of Allergology and Clinical Immunology (C.E. Reed, ed), C.V. Mostby, St. Louis pp. 159–163 (1986).
19. Wasserman, S.I. The regulation of inflammatory mediator production by mast cell products. Am. Rev. Respir. Dis. 135:S46–S48 (1987).
20. Ding, E., Young, J., Peterson, C.G.B., Venge, P. et al. Mechanism of membrane damage mediated by human eosinophil cationic protein. Nature 321:613–615 (1986).
21. Stracke, M.L. and Metcalfe, D.D. Glycosaminoglycans and proteoglycans in inflammatory cells. *In* Proceedings of the XII International Congress of Allergology and Clinical Immunology, Washington, D.C. (C.E. Reed, ed.), C.V. Mosby, St. Louis, pp. 267–274 (1986).
22. Barrett, K.E. and Metcalfe, D.D. Heterogeneity of mast cells in the tissues of the respiratory tract and other organ systems. Am. Rev. Respir. Dis. 135:1190–1195 (1987).
23. Church, M.K., George J.K.P. and Holgate, S.T. Characterization of histamine secretion from dispersed human lung mast cells: effects of anti-IgE, calcium ionophore A23187, compound 48/80 and basic polypeptides. J. Immunol. 129:2116–2121 (1982).
24. Tharp, M.D., Kagey-Sobotka, A., Fox, C.C. et al. Functional heterogeneity of human mast cells from different anatomic sites. In vitro responses to morphine sulfate. J. Allergy Clin. Immunol. 79:646–653 (1987).
25. Naclerio, R.M., Meier, H.L., Kagey-Sobotka, A. et al. Mediator release after nasal challenge with allergen. Am. Rev. Respir. Dis. 128:597–602 (1983).
26. Thueson, D.O., Speck, L.S., Lett-Brown, M. and Grant, J.A. Histamine release activity (HRA). I. Production by mitogen- or antigen-stimulated human mononuclear cells. J. Immunol. 123:626–632 (1979).
27. Warner, J.A., Pienkowski, M.M., Plaut, M. et al. Identification of histamine releasing factor(s) in the late phase of cutaneous IgE-mediated reactions. J. Immunol. 136:2583–2587 (1986).
28. Roitt, I. Brostoff, J. and Male, D. Immunology. Gower Medical Publishing, London, pp 20.1–20.9 (1985).
29. Podack, E.R. and Müller-Eberhard, H.J. Isolation from human serum of an inhibitor of the membrane attack complex of complement. J. Biol. Chem. 254:9808–9814 (1979).
30. Muller-Eberhart, H.J. The membrane attack complex of complement. Annu. Rev. Immunol. 4:503–528 (1986).
31. Kofler, R., Dixon, F.J. and Theofilopoulos, A.N. The genetic origin of autoantibodies. Immunol. Today 8:374–379 (1987).
32. Cooke, A., Lydyard, P.M. and Roitt, I.M. Autoimmunity and idiotypes. Lancet 2:723–274 (1984).
33. Pepys, M.B. Role of complement in the induction of immunological responses. Transplant. Rev. 32:93–120 (1976).
34. Inman, R.D. and Day, N.K. Immunologic and clinical aspects of immune complex disease. Am. J. Med. 70:1097–1106 (1981).

35. Von Pirquet, C. and Schick, B. Serum Sickness. Williams & Wilkins, Baltimore (1951).
36. Germuth, F.C.Jr. A comparative histologic and immunologic study in rabbits of induced hypersensitivity of the serum sickness type. J. Exp. Med. 97:257–282 (1953).
37. Lawley, T.J., Bielory, L., Gascon, P. et al. A prospective clinical and immunologic analysis of patients with serum sickness. N. Engl. J. Med. 311:1407–1412 (1984).
38. Schifferli, J.A., Ng, Y.C. and Peters, D.K. The role of complement and its receptor in the elimination of immune complexes. N. Engl. J. Med. 315: 488–495 (1986).
39. Frank, M.M. Complement in the pathophysiology of human disease. N. Engl. J. Med. 316:1525–1530 (1987).
40. Husby, S.,Oxelius, V.A., Teisner, B. et al. Humoral immunity to dietary antigens in healthy adults. Occurrence, isotype and IgG subclass distribution of serum antibodies to protein antigens. Int. Arch. Allergy Appl. Immunol. 77:416–422 (1985).
41. Claman, H.N. The biology of the immune response. J.A.M.A. 258:2834–2840 (1987).
42. Kaliner, M.A. The late phase reaction and its clinical implications. Hosp. Pract. 15:73–83 (1987).
43. Fisher, A.A. Contact Dermatitis, 3rd ed. Lea & Febiger, Philadelphia (1986).
44. Jones, T.D. and Mote, J.R. The phases of foreign protein sensitization in human beings. N. Engl. J. Med. 210:120–123 (1934).
45. Richerson, H.B., Dvorak, H.F. and Leskowitz, S. Cutaneous basophil hypersensitivity. I. A new look at the Jones-Mote reaction, general characteristics. J. Exp. Med. 132:564–567 (1970).
46. Chase, M.S. The cellular transfer of cutaneous hypersensitivity to tuberculin. Proc. Soc. Exp. Biol. Med. 59:134–135 (1945).
47. Lawrence, H.S. Transfer factor. In Advances in Immunology, Vol. 11 (F.J. Dixon, Jr. and H.G. Kunkel, eds.), Academic Press, New York, pp. 195–266 (1969).
48. George, M. and Vaughn, M. In vitro cell migration as a model for delayed hypersensitivity. Proc. Soc. Exp. Biol. Med. 111:514–521 (1962).
49. Borish, L., Liu, D., Remold, H. et al. Production and assay of macrophage migration inhibitory factor, leukocyte inhibitory factor and leukocyte adherence inhibitory factor. In Manual of Clinical Laboratory Immunology, 3rd ed. (N. Rose, H. Friedman and J. Fahey, eds.), American Society for Microbiology, Washington, D.C., p. 282 (1986).
50. Stingl, G., Wolff-Schreiner, E. and Pichler, W. et al. Epidermal Langerhans cells bear Fc and C3 receptors. Nature 268:245–246 (1977).
51. Sullivan, S., Bergsrresser, P.R., Tigelaar, R.E. et al. Induction and regulation of contact hypersensitivity by resident, bone marrow-derived dendritic

epidermal cells: Langerhans cells and thy-1 epidermal cells. J. Immunol. 137:2460–2467 (1986).
52. Askenase, P.W. Antigen-specific T cell factors in the delayed-type hypersensitivity cascade. *In* Proceedings of the XII International Congress of Allergology and Clinical Immunology (C.E. Reed, ed.), C.V. Mosby, St. Louis, pp. 146–150 (1986).
53. Fink, J. N. and deShazo R. Immunologic aspects of granulomatous and interstitial lung disease. J.A.M.A. 258:2938–2944 (1987).

5

Diagnostic Procedures for Human Hypersensitivity Diseases and Pseudoallergic Reactions

I. Type I reactions   60
   A. Direct skin tests   60
   B. Indirect skin tests   61
   C. Organ challenge tests   61
   D. Total IgE   62
   E. Radioallergosorbent tests   63
   F. Mediators   64
II. Type II reactions   67
   A. Hemagglutination techniques   67
   B. Complement-dependent cytotoxic antibodies   67
   C. Tissue localization of cytotoxic antibodies   68
III. Type III reactions   68
   A. Immune complexes   68
   B. Interpretation of immune complex tests   72
   C. Autoantibodies   72
IV. Cell-mediated immunity tests   73
   A. Patch tests   73
   B. Tuberculin-like intradermal tests   75
   C. Recall antigens test battery   76
   D. Induction of topical delayed hypersensitivity   77
   E. In vitro correlates of delayed hypersensitivity   77
V. Pseudoallergic reactions   78
   A. Organ challenge tests   78
VI. Immunotoxicological surveys   79
   A. Two-tiered system of immune function testing   80
   B. Experimental contact hypersensitivity   81
   C. Experimental respiratory sensitization   82
   References   82

I. TYPE I REACTIONS

A. Direct Skin Tests

Skin tests (scratch, prick, or intradermal) performed with properly standardized allergens in the appropriate concentrations are the most useful diagnostic techniques in IgE-mediated diseases (1). Skin testing with allergens having a high potential for anaphylactogenicity may be hazardous and should be avoided unless the clinician is fully prepared to treat a potentially lethal systemic reaction (2). However, provided the test conditions are properly controlled, some anaphylactogenic substances may be used with minimal risks for skin testing procedures (e.g., insect venoms, insulin, major and minor penicillin determinants). Acceptable skin testing sites include the ventral surfaces of both lower and upper arms and the dorsolateral areas of the upper arms. Skin tests should not be performed in areas adjacent to the wrists and antecubital fossae. Areas of skin with active inflammation should also be avoided. Generally speaking, the scratch and prick tests are safer than intradermal tests. Scratch tests consist of applying a small drop of concentrated allergen extract (ranging from 1:10 to 1:50) to a small bloodless scratch on the forearm or back. The prick test is performed with individual 25–27 gauge hypodermic needles by an upward pricking motion of the superficial epidermis through a small drop of concentrated allergenic extract (3). Both scratch and prick tests should be performed only if blood is absent from the superficially traumatized site. Negative diluent and positive histamine (equivalent to 1.0 mg/ml histamine base) controls should always be done simultaneously to determine that the skin has normal histamine-reactive properties. A positive skin test is interpreted as a wheal at least 3 mm greater than the saline control accompanied by a flare reaction. This usually appears anywhere from 10 to 20 min after the suspected allergic substance is applied to the skin.

Intracutaneous tests should be performed with a single unitized 0.6 ml hubless syringe with an attached hypodermic needle. The gauge of the attached hypodermic needle may vary from 26 to 30. Detailed information about variability of instruments, technique performance factors, interpretation of skin tests results, reproducibility, sensitivity, specificity, significance and standardization recommendations are available in the recent National Institute of Allergy and Infectious Diseases report, Proceedings of the Task Force on Guidelines for Standardizing Old and New Technologies Used for Diagnosis and Treatment of Allergic Diseases (4). The test consists of a small bleb (varying from 0.01 to 0.05 ml) of the suspected allergen extract at a much more dilute dose (from 1:1,000 or 1:10,000 w/v) injected into the superficial epidermis. This test is read 15 min after application and also consists of a wheal and flare at least 5 mm larger than the diluent control and within the same size range as the positive histamine control (0.01 mg/ml histamine base). When intracutaneous tests at higher concentrations (1:100) are used, late cutaneous responses are likely to occur 4-6 hr after the application of the test (5). These late cutaneous reactions have been shown to be IgE-dependent and are thought to be due to secondary inflammatory infiltration of the area with eosinophils, neutrophils, and subsequent release of proinflammatory mediators such as eosinophilic major basic protein, eosinophilic cationic protein, leukotrienes, and platelet-activating factor. Some clinicians prefer to do intracutaneous tests only after prick or scratch tests are negative, but others do only intracutaneous testing. In any case, a positive test indicates specific binding between an allergen and its corresponding allergic antibody that had previously sensitized mast cells within the skin. Skin test reactivity, either prick or intracutaneous, may be titrated with various solutions of allergens in order to obtain a semiquantitative index of skin threshold response (4,6,7).

Certain pertinent factors must be considered in the interpretation of skin tests. In all cases, the results of the skin test should be correlated with the clinical history. A false-positive skin test may indicate the presence of specific IgE on mast cell membranes of the skin without concomitant localization in the respiratory or gastrointestinal tissues. Such a reaction may or may not predict future clinical sensitivity. False-negative reactions also occur, more commonly in the case of certain but not all food allergens. If the skin test is not confirmatory of the clinical history, organ challenge studies and other in vitro tests may be necessary.

B. Indirect Skin Tests

Indirect skin tests or passive transfer tests (sometimes referred to as the Prausnitz–Küstner or P–K reaction) should not be performed routinely in nonatopic subjects because of the hazard of transmitting serum hepatitis or human immunodeficiency virus (HIV) leading to acquired immune deficiency syndrome (AIDS) (8). Immunological specificity can sometimes be confirmed by passive transfer experiments (passive cutaneous anaphylaxis) in subhuman primates (9). It should be emphasized that this method is less sensitive and therefore a negative test does not exclude the presence of specific allergic antibody. However, at present it is the only reference method for demonstrating the presence of a heat-stable IgG-type of human allergic antibody (10). The latter antibody has short-term sensitizing properties (2 hr vs 24 hr for IgE) and is presumed but not proved to be associated with the IgG_4 subclass of human immunoglobin G.

C. Organ Challenge Tests

Organ challenge tests may be applied to the mucosae of conjunctivae, nares, or bronchi. Considerable experience with these methods is required for proper interpretation and analysis (11). The conjunctival test may have some qualitative usefulness but is subject to considerable variation and is not used frequently in modern practice. The nasal challenge test may be useful provided that the patient's nasal mucosa does not manifest nonspecific irritation responses and the results can be interpreted by objective measurements of nasal airways resistance, airflow, or allergic mediators liberated into nasal secretions after the challenge. For lower respiratory symptoms, the bronchial challenge test is most useful if performed properly. Results of this test are usually evaluated by several objective measurements of ventilatory function.

All organ challenge tests should be preceded by a control test with diluent or normal saline and, if possible, the entire testing procedure should be performed on a single-blind basis. These techniques are also helpful because they can be modified: dose-response assays and provocation concentration (PC) thresholds can be determined on the basis of the allergen concentration required to cause a 20% decrease (PC_{20}) in the forced expiratory volume in 1 sec (12). The PC_{20} dose is a measure of sensitivity and is extrapolated from the dose-response data of the challenge protocol.

D. Total IgE

Quantitative assays of total IgE may assist in determining whether a patient has an atopic susceptibility. These assays can be classified into three groups: solid-phase radioimmunoassays; radioimmunoprecipitation (double antibody) assays; and enzyme-linked solid phase (ELISA solid phase) assays (13). The common factor in all solid phase methods is the insolubilization of the monospecific anti-IgE antibody. Solid substrates that are used most commonly include Sephadex particles, methylcellulose paper, or polystyrene surfaces.

A competitive binding assay with the use of radiolabeled IgE and standards of known IgE content is commercially available and is called the radioimmunosorbent test (RIST). Monospecific anti-IgE antibodies are first covalently bound to Sephadex particles (solid phase). The concentration of IgE in the unknown sample is evaluated by its capacity to compete with a normal amount of radiolabeled IgE for binding sites on the anti-IgE molecules. This competitive capacity is then compared with that of the standard reagent of known IgE content. This method is expensive and is subject to possible errors due to nonspecific inhibition by unknown serum factors. Advantages of the method include rapidity of completion, commercial availability of reagents, and the lack of requirement for precipitating antibody.

A direct or noncompetitive radioimmunosorbent test (PRIST) is also commercially available. Unlike RIST, competition with radiolabeled IgE is not required. Instead, anti-IgE is covalently coupled to solid phase paper discs and reacted with the unknown serum sample. After being washed, the complex is incubated with radiolabeled anti-IgE and binding of the radiolabeled anti-IgE correlates with the IgE content of the unknown serum. The advantages of this assay are its greater sensitivity (as little as 1 ng of IgE can be detected) and its relative precision.

The radioimmunoprecipitation or double antibody assay for serum IgE is probably the best method with respect to both precision and reproducibility. However, after the competitive binding and incubation step is completed, a precipitating antibody is required to separate bound from unbound IgE. Because this precipitating antibody must be available in large quantities, the general applicability of the test is limited and thus the test is not commercially available. Moreover, the test requires 2 days to complete and nonspecific interference by serum factors may play a role at high serum concentrations.

An enzyme-linked immunosorbent test (ELISA) has also been designed for measuring serum IgE. This test involves only stable, nonradioactive reagents and can detect as little as 1–25 ng of IgE. Reactants are added in the following order: rabbit anti-IgE coupled to methylcellulose discs, the unknown serum, monospecific sheep anti-IgE serum, rabbit antisheep immunoglobulin conjugated to β-D-galactosidase. After several incubation and washing steps, the enzymatic activity of β-D-galactosidase in the complex is measured spectrophotometrically by hydrolysis of 0-nitrophelgalactopyranoside. The amount of hydrolysis of this substrate is directly proportional to the concentration of IgE in the serum. A dipstick modification of ELISA (Quidel) is available for total IgE and regional allergen specific screens, but the clinical validity of these screening methods has not yet been documented.

E. Radioallergosorbent Tests

Detection of specific IgE in the serum is performed most often by the RAST or radioallergosorbent test (14,15). This is a solid-phase radioimmunoassay modification of an earlier erythrocyte linked-antigen–antiglobulin reaction (RCLAAR). The original method as described by Coombs may be used to detect specific IgE antibodies to castor bean but is not practical for many other allergens because they are denatured by the conjugation procedure required for the method. The RAST technique requires structural integrity of the antigen-combining sites (Fab regions) of specific IgE molecules. Allergens coupled to solid phase paper discs are incubated with unknown serum samples. After being washed, radioactive monospecific anti-IgE is added to the substrate. The amount of specific IgE is directly proportional to the amount of radioactivity bound to the complex. Specific IgE bound to the complex may be estimated by comparing counts per minute between the unknown sample and a positive reference sample serum known to contain high concentrations of IgE specific for that particular test allergen. It should be emphasized that this assay is only semiquantitative because units of antibody are arbitrarily based on a known reference serum. Several methods of direct quantitation of RAST have been reported but these are too labor-intensive and therefore not cost–effective for routine clinical use.

The RAST technique is reliable in detecting allergic antibody to most of the pollen allergens, certain classes of foods, epidermals and insect venom allergens. It has also been used to diagnose the presence of certain drugs and chemicals. However, its sensitivity varies between categories of allergens. It is not nearly as sensitive for house dust, molds, insect venoms, drugs and chemicals as it is for pollens. There is a good correlation (65–70%) between RAST and positive prick/organ challenge tests but the RAST does not correlate well with endpoint intracutaneous skin threshold values (16). This indicates either that RAST is not as sensitive as skin tests or that absolute values of specific IgE in serum may not always reflect the amount of cell-bound specific IgE in tissue mast cells of the skin. It is also important to realize that false-positive RAST tests occur because of high concentrations of irrelevant total IgE or the presence of cross-reactive carbohydrate determinants in various allergens (17). Thus, it is crucial that this information should be known by the interpreter and that all RAST tests, including those done by commercial reference laboratories, should be performed in association with total IgE tests.

Various modifications of RAST have appeared in recent years (18). These include an enzyme-linked specific IgE test based on the same principle as described for total IgE. In addition, there is another modification as the FAST test (fluorescent allergosorbent test), which relies on a fluorogenic activator coupled to anti-IgE and a fluorescent substrate. The final test results are read in a spectrofluorometer rather than a spectrophotometer as used in the enzyme (ELISA)-coupled test. Another recent modification is the MAST test, in which a number of allergens are attached sequentially to a linear strand of methylcellulose paper substrate. This permits multiple allergen testing with a single serum specimen. At the same time, a monospecific anti-IgE antibody is coupled to the substrate so that results of the multiple allergen tests can be interpreted simultaneously with the total IgE. Finally, one modification known as the Fadal-Nalebuff technique (modified RAST) purports to increase the sensitivity of RAST by standardizing the final counting procedure for each allergen according to the time required for counting 25,000 μCi of added radioactivity (19). Indpendent groups of investigators have not confirmed that this test substantively increases the sensitivity of RAST.

F. Mediators

Quantitation of mediators released by combination of cell-bound IgE and allergens is essentially an indirect measurement of the function of IgE. Although assays of this type are good in vitro biological correlates of IgE-mediated reactions, it is important to note that they are not practical procedures because they are tedious, labor-intensive, and can only be performed with fresh specimens.

1. Histamine

Extraction and assay of histamine from leukocytes and other tissues by a fluoro-metric method is an accurate and sensitive tissue method. The technique was originally described by Shore et al. (20). The chemical basis of the fluorometric method involves extraction of histamine into N-butanol from alkalinized per-chloric acid-treated leukocytes or tissue slices, return of the histamine to an aqueous solution, and subsequent condensation with o-phthalaldehyde to yield a stable fluorescent product that can be measured in a spectrofluorometer. The assay can be performed on actively or passively sensitized leukocytes and chopped human lung fragments (21). These specimens are incubated with serial dilutions of allergens and the test results are expressed as the highest dilution of allergen capable of inducing 50% or greater histamine release. Although the specificity and accuracy of this test are good, its general use was restricted because the number of tests that could be performed in 1 day time was limited. To circumvent this technical constraint, an automated histamine-analysis system that can accommodate 30 or more samples per hour was developed (22). Samples containing as little as 0.1–15 ng of histamine can be analyzed accurately in this automated system.

In recent years, an enzyme-isotopic assay for histamine has been found to be more sensitive and specific (23). It is capable of quantitating histamine at the picogram level. This technique of histamine assay is based on the transfer of ^{14}C-labeled methyl groups from S-adenosylmethionine to unlabeled histamine by the enzyme histamine N-methyltransferase. The ^{14}C]methylhistamine formed by this reaction is separated from histamine by extraction into chloro-form. A trace amount of ^{3}H-labeled histamine is added to each sample to monitor the internal recovery, the ratio of ^{14}C to ^{3}H being proportional to the amount of unlabeled histamine in the sample. As with the fluorometric assay, the biological aspect of this technique also involves incubation of leukocytes or lung fragments with specific allergen under proper temperature and pH condi-tions. However, the significant advantage of this method is that it is sensitive enough to detect histamine in fluids such as serum, nasal, and bronchial washes.

A glass microfilter-based method of binding histamine has been reported (24). This technique is based on the fact that glass microfilters bind histamine with high affinity and selectivity. Small samples of blood are added to the microfilter incorporated into a microtiter plate. After being incubated with antigen, the released histamine is bound to the glass microfilter. Subsequently, histamine is eluted by a mixture of perchloric acid/o-phthalaldehyde and analyzed in the same manner as the chemical analysis protocol described above. This method requires only 50 μl of blood/sample and can be completed in 2½ hr.

A new radioimmunoassay assay for histamine depends on the use of a proprietary histamine antibody for the measurement of histamine (25). Further work is required to validate both the glass microfilter and radioimmunoassay histamine methods.

2. Chemotactic Factors

An assay for one of the important chemotactic factors (neutrophil chemotactic factor of anaphylaxis [NCF-A]) is performed in a Boyden chamber (26). The sample containing the NCF-A is added to the lower well of the chamber and the cells are added in the upper well. If NCF-A is present, neutrophils will migrate across the filter membrane. These are counted microscopically to determine the degree of migration through the filter. NCF-A is very stable and can be measured in serum and wash materials from various organs. Another potent neutrophil chemotactic factor (LTB$_4$), released during IgE-dependent reactions, can be measured in a similar way.

As chemical technology improves, there is a tendency to measure other mediators released by the allergic reaction. Such measurements can be made in both plasma and wash materials from various body orifices (27-29). Prostaglandin D$_2$ and sulfidopeptides (formerly known collectively as SRS-A) can be measured chemically by HPLC or radioimmunoassay. The former method is preferable. However, once one has standardized a particular measurement from a body source, the more convenient radioimmunoassay could be calibrated for routine serial measurements. These mediators can also be measured by their bioactive effects on in vitro smooth muscle preparations, but these techniques are expensive and time-consuming.

3. Platelet-Activating Factor

Platelet-activating factor is another inflammatory mediator derived from metabolism of membrane phospholipids. It is relatively unstable in various body fluids but, after proper preservation techniques, it can be measured directly by HPLC.

4. Miscellaneous In Vitro Correlates

In addition to histamine, PGD$_2$, sulfidopeptides, and PAF, enzymatic mediators such as tryptase, chymotryptase, Comrue, kinins, tosyl-L-arginine methyl esterase (Tame), and neuroendocrine peptides have been measured after controlled challenge reactions in the nose and lungs (28,30). In addition, the allergic reaction and all its release products may activate cells such as neutrophils, eosinophils, and T lymphocytes, which can be measured indirectly by erythrocyte rosetting techniques. Thus the array of diagnostic techniques, both direct and indirect, for diagnosis of IgE mediated diseases is rapidly expanding.

II. TYPE II REACTIONS

Antibody-mediated cytotoxic reactions are tested by agglutinating, hemolytic, and in situ demonstrations of antibody and complement components by fluorescein- or ferritin-conjugated antibody (31,32).

A. Hemagglutination Techniques

Classic hemagglutination techniques are used to determine ABO, Rhesus, Kell, Duffy, and MN inccompatibilities (31). These agglutination tests are performed routinely before transfusions and to prevent the occurrence of Rh sensitization in Rh-negative mothers. For example, a patient with an A phenotype in the ABO system has red cell A antigen. This would be detected by agglutination with a reference B serum containing anti-A antibodies. Likewise, Rh^+ antibodies in a Rh^- mother would be recognized by standard Rh antigen. The hemagglutination method is also the chief method of detecting other types of autoimmune hemolytic anemias, as illustrated by the direct and indirect Coombs' antiglobulin tests. These tests can determine the presence of warm-reactive antibodies reacting with the antigen at $37°C$, cold-reactive antibodies reacting with the antigen below $37°C$, or antibodies provoked by allergic reactions to drugs and chemicals. In the case of the direct Coombs' test, where antibodies have developed against specific red cell antigens (e.g., ABO or Rh), such antibodies combine with the specific red cell antigens and are detected in vitro by hemagglutination. The direct antiglobulin test can be modified as an indirect test by preincubation of patient's serum with ABO-compatible cells and subsequent addition of an antihuman IgG reagent. Similar testing procedures can be adapted to detect either warm- or cold-reactive autoantibodies. Warm-reactive autoantibody tests are performed at $37°C$ while cold-reactive reactions can be demonstrated only under cold conditions below $30°C$.

B. Complement-Dependent Cytotoxic Antibodies

Various drugs, chemicals, or their metabolites may interact with membranes of the formed components of the blood in several ways. These low-molecular-weight materials may be adsorbed onto various blood cells and the resultant membrane conjugate formed by this interaction may stimulate formation of cytotoxic antibody directed against the drug moiety on the surface of the cell. This reaction also requires fixation of complement components that ultimately lead to cell lysis. Certain chemicals (e.g., alpha methyldopa) may interact with cell membranes in such a way as to cause breakdown of self-tolerance to epitopes within the cell membrane. When this occurs, autoantibodies are produced against these modified membrane epitopes. The subsequent antigen–antibody combination and fixation of complement lead to tissue lysis.

Another method of chemically induced autotoxicity has been termed the "innocent bystander effect." In this situation, simple drugs or their metabolites form complexes with circulating specific cytotoxic antibodies. These complexes then become adsorbed to various tissue membranes via Fc receptors. This process also requires fixation of complement before tissue destruction occurs. If, in addition to adsorbed immune complexes on cell membranes, there is also an excess amount of circulating immune complexes, individual complement components such as C3 or C4 may be reduced.

C. Tissue Localization of Cytotoxic Antibodies

Cytotoxic antibodies may also localize in other tissues (32). The presence of these antibodies may be demonstrated in various tissue sites such as kidneys, skin, or lung. Frozen biopsy material from such tissue sites will determine whether there is deposition of cytotoxic antibody within vessel walls, basement membranes, or interepithelial spaces. This is accomplished by using fluoresceinated human anti-IgG, anti-IgM, or anti-C' reagents. These methods involve direct incubation of the tagged antibody with the appropriate tissue. Detection of a specific antigen localized in tissue sites may be attempted by double antibody sandwich techniques utilizing monoclonal or polyclonal antibodies specific for the antigen followed by a labeled heterologous IgG antibody.

III. TYPE III REACTIONS

A. Immune Complexes

A variety of assays have been developed to detect circulating immune complexes. The spectrum of available techniques ranges from those that estimate the degree of nonspecific physiochemical characteristics of complexes to those that selectively measure binding activity of rheumatoid factor, staphylococcal protein A, complement components, and interactions of complex-associated complement with CR1 cell receptors. Comparative investigations of these methods have revealed marked disparities that have been attributed to relative sensitivity of the method, the ability to differentiate immunoglobulin classes in the complex, and the intrinsic properties of the specific immune complex. The latter may vary depending on the stage, severity, and causes of the disease being studied (33,34). Moreover, there may be large differences between assays for immune complexes that use plasma and those that use serum, because immune complex structures are known to be modified by the processing of serum samples. Because different detection principles are used in various assays, abnormal sera may be positive in one assay but negative in another. Therefore, it may be necessary to use several assays to attain optimal diagnostic potential in a specific disease entity.

Techniques that detect specific antigens within circulating immune complexes are not generally available. However, special studies have identified antigenic constituents including DNA, viruses (*Herpes simplex*, hepatitis B, and Epstein-Barr), bacteria, carcinoembryonic antigen, a tissue glycoprotein in dermatitis herpetiformis, and food allergens (35,36). Most of the available clinical assays to detect immune complexes are not antigen-specific.

1. Cryoglobulins and Polyethylene Glycol Precipitation

The most common screening for the detection of immune complexes is a test for cryoglobulins or cold precipitable serum proteins. Immune complexes may also be detected by precipitation with polyethylene glycol (37). Both of these tests are based on changes in solubility characteristics of the IgG complexes. Precipitation in this assay occurs because of conformational changes in the complexes rather than molecular weight. It should be emphasized that neither of these tests is very sensitive and that both may trap monomeric immunoglobulins nonspecifically within the precpitate. The presence of cryoglobulinemia may be completely overlooked if the blood specimen is not collected and centrifuged under body temperature conditions prior to incubation of serum at 4°C.

2. C1q-Binding Assay

Interaction of circulating immune complexes with purified humoral substances constitutes the rationale for several important immune complex assays (Fig. 1). Two complement-dependent techniques are widely used for the clinical measurement of circulating immune complexes. The C1q-binding assay requires purification and iodination of the C1q component of complement (38). A small aliquot of [^{125}I] C1q is added to test serum. This mixture is precipitated with 3% polyethylene glycol and, after suitable incubation and centrifugation at 4°C, the supernatant is discarded and the precipitate counted in a gamma counter. The amount of [^{125}I] C1q that coprecipitates with the immune complex in the test serum is expressed as the percentage of the counts obtained in 100 μL normal human serum precipitated by 20% trichloroacetic acid. The C1q-binding assay detects activation of the classic pathway of complement by the immune complex.

3. Conglutinin-Binding Assay

Another complement-dependent assay is based on the ability of C3 (already bound to antibody in the immune complex) to bind bovine conglutinin (39). This test is known as the conglutinin-binding assay. The uptake of immune complexes is quantitated by measuring the IgG bound to bovine conglutinin by the use of radiolabeled anti-IgG. After suitable incubations and wash steps, test serum is incubated with [^{125}I] antihuman IgG. Following further incubation and wash steps, the mixture is counted in a gamma counter. The test is compared to a reference consisting of dilutions of aggregated human gamma globulin in normal human serum. Although this test might appear to have the advantage of detecting both classic and alternate complement activation by immune complexes, in practice it has not been found to detect immune complexes with the same degree of frequency as is possible with the C1q binding assay.

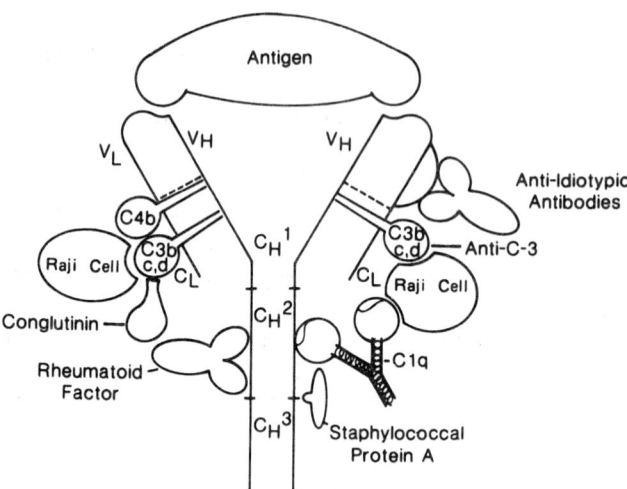

Figure 1 Binding sites of major immune complex reagents on antigen–antibody complexes. Anti-idiotypic antibodies bind to idiotopes on variable domains of antibody (V_L and V_H). C4b, C3b, and C3cd fragments bind to the first constant heavy chain domain (C_H1). Rheumatoid factor and C1q bind to the second constant heavy chain domain (C_H2). The binding site of staphylococcal protein is intermediate between C_H2 and C_H3 domains. Surface receptors of Raji cells bind either directly to C3b and/or C3c,d fragments (left), C1q alone (right) or to both C3b and C1q (right). Both conglutinin and anti-C3 antibody reagents also bind to the C3b-C_H1 complex.

Under certain conditions of active disease (e.g., serum sickness), depletion of complement components such as C3 or C4 may provide a rough estimate of complement activation and utilization during the clearance phase of the disease (40).

4. Monoclonal Rheumatoid Factor Assay

The ability of rheumatoid factor (IgM) to combine with a specific site on immune complexes (i.e., aggregated IgG) forms the basis of the monoclonal rheumatoid factor assay (41). This technique measures the ability of immune complex to inhibit the binding of labeled aggregated IgG to a monoclonal rheumatoid factor bound to a solid phase. In the past, polyclonal rheumatoid factors have been used as reactants, but such tests were found to be nonspecific. Rheumatoid factor also combines with 7S IgG, so the latter is a potential contaminant in such assays. At times preliminary dilution of test serum is required to obtain a constant IgG concentration. Another possible constraint of this technique is that the reactivity of different rheumatoid factors may vary.

5. Raji Cell Assay

The ability of certain cells and cellular components to bind immunoglobulins and complement components has been used as a basis for several important immune complex assays (42). The Raji cell assay is a cellular technique that detects immune complexes because of interaction of circulating immune complexes with CR1 complement receptors on the Raji cell surface. The Raji cell is a lymphoblastoid cell with B-cell charactistics and has very-high-affinity CR1 receptors for binding of complement. Raji cells are incubated with the test serum and then reacted with rabbit anti-human $[^{125}I]$ IgG. The amount of radioactivity is counted in a gamma counter and the amount of immune complex is compared to a standard curve constructed by the degree of anti-human IgG uptake by cells incubated with normal human serum containing various amounts of antihuman IgG. False-positive results occasionally occur if antibodies to the cellular substrate happen to be present in the test serum.

6. Staphylococcal Protein A Binding Tests

The staphylococcal protein A binding test utilizes a surface component of *Staphylococcus aureus* as a reagent for binding to the Fc portion of IgG contained in immune complexes (43). The dissociation of aggregated IgG from protein A occurs at a slower rate than that of monomeric IgG. Thus, direct binding of radioactive staphylococcal protein A to circulating immune complexes can be measured directly in a gamma counter and compared to standards similar to those used in other radioimmunoassays.

In view of the fact that the World Health Organization has not been able to recommend any single diagnostic procedure for the detection of immune complexes as having overall utility for routine clinical practice, choosing the correct procedure under specific clinical conditions can sometimes be difficult. For example, if a technique is too sensitive, it may overexaggerate the importance of transient circulating immune complexes that are physiological in almost all individuals (44). In contrast, a nonsensitive technique may obfuscate the significance of immune complexes. In addition, there is a need for further standardization of individual techniques and controls. Thus, some methods cannot differentiate true antigen–antibody complexes from endogenous aggregated IgG that may occur after heating, suboptimal storage, or freeze–thawing of serum. The significance of circulating immune complexes must always be interpreted against the background of genetic complement deficiencies that have striking associations with immune-complex disease. Furthermore, immune complexes are more likely to appear in patients who have depletion, deficiency, or reduction of access to circulating transport cells (e.g., red blood cells) that contain CR1 receptors (46). Such patients lack proper clearance mechanisms for elimination of immune complexes.

B. Interpretation of Immune Complex Tests

Because so many uncontrollable variables affect the interpretation of immune complex tests, it is argued by some that they are not particularly useful as routine clinical diagnostic tests. However, despite their limitations, they serve as useful guidelines in certain clinical situations. Positive results of immune complex tests are obtained in diseases with persistent circulating immune complexes. This may occur in persons with genetic deficiencies of various complement components and in persons whose clearance mechanisms involving CR1-bearing erythrocytes or deficient fixed macrophage clearance systems play a role (45). The presence of immune complexes may also suggest the presence of anti-idiotypic antibodies that complex with their respective idiotypic determinants within hypervariable H and L chain regions (46). This is especially likely to occur as a network aberration in patients with autoimmune diseases. Negative results of immune complex tests may be helpful at times because they exclude abnormal immunological reactions.

C. Autoantibodies

Autoantibodies are found in a variety of systemic rheumatic diseases, chronic thyroiditis, biliary cirrhosis, myocardopathies, and others. The presence of such antibodies does not necessarily indicate that they are involved in the pathogenesis of a particular disease. However, if their presence is interpreted properly, they may offer considerable assistance in the diagnosis of active disease. As previously discussed, it has also been suggested that autoantibodies could be anti-idiotypic antibodies, the internal images of which cross react with exogenous antigens such as viruses or virally induced neoantigens. Receptor autoantibodies such as have been described in newly diagnosed patients with insulin-dependent diabetes are examples of this possible linkage. These recent findings suggest that idiotypic determinants and their respective anti-idiotypic antibodies (autoantibodies) could act as toxic immune complexes under certain circumstances (46).

The most common autoantibody tests are those used to determine the presence of antinuclear antibodies in a variety of multisystem rheumatic diseases, rheumatoid factors in the diagnosis of early rheumatoid arthritis, and anti-thyroid antibodies in the diagnosis of chronic thyroiditis. The most extensively used screening test for antinuclear antibodies is the antinuclear antibody (ANA) test (47). This test is performed by incubation of test serum with commercially available mouse organ sections, which are then overlayed with fluorescent-labeled anti-IgG. It is easy to perform, relatively inexpensive, and defines antibody specificity. The different staining patterns in the ANA may be helpful in differentiating between various rheumatic diseases. The test has been further refined by the isolation and characterization of specific molecules from cytoplasm, nucleus, and cell membrane so that various staining patterns can now be identified by fluorescent antisera derived from these specific intracellular proteins.

Some of the extractable nuclear antigens include Sm antigen, ribonuclear protein (nRNP), SS–A/Ro, SS–B/La, PM-1, Scl-70, and centromere protein. Antibodies directed against double-stranded DNA are indicative of disease activity in systemic lupus erythematosus. In contrast, such antibodies are not found in drug-induced lupus erythematosus (due to hydralazine or procainamide), which is often associated with antibodies directed against histone (48,49). Rheumatoid factor tests determine circulating IgM rheumatoid factor by means of a simple latex particle test. Thyroid autoantibodies are detected by indirect immuno-fluorescence similar to that described for systemic lupus erythematosus. Interpretation of autoantibody tests requires detailed knowledge about false-negative and false-positive tests. The current available tests manifest a wide range of specificity and sensitivity; these limitations must be thoroughly understood in order to allow for proper clinical diagnosis.

IV. CELL–MEDIATED IMMUNITY TESTS

Direct patch and intracutaneous skin tests are the most convenient and cost-effective methods of evaluating delayed hypersensitivity. Patch tests are used to detect contact hypersensitivity in a wide variety of eczematous dermatitic lesions (50). Many substances including simple chemicals, proteins, and lipids may be used as test reagents. The crucial determinant in evaluating contact patch test results is the concentration of the test material. It is essential that the lowest "allergenic" threshold dose–response be obtained for each reagent in order to rule out irritant effects. Ideally, irritant threshold dose–responses for all patch test substances should be conducted in panels of both normal volunteers and patients with preexistent dermatitis.

A. Patch Tests

There are three types of epicutaneous patch tests for delayed hypersensitivity: open, closed, and prophetic. The open test is performed by applying a single drop of the suspected contactant to the skin and observing the test site 24 and 48 hr later. A modification of this test, termed the provocative or repeated open application test, has been used to minimize false-positive reactions due to non-specific irritation and the excited skin (angry back) syndrome (51). The rationale for this approach is that open testing is less likely to cause irritant reactions than closed ones. The test material is applied to forearm, antecubital fossa, or cheek twice daily for 7 days. If a strong positive test is elicited before 7 days, testing is terminated.

The closed patch test involves applying a small amount of the substance overlaid with a small adhesive patch or chamber (Finn chamber). Two closed patch systems are commonly used. In both systems aluminum is the substrate because of its low allergenicity. The "Al" test uses strips of aluminum foil with heat affixed Webril pads for allergen application. The "Finn" chamber uses 8 mm diameter aluminum chambers that are occlusive and permit more accurate quantification of the dose of allergen/unit area. Both the "Al" test and "Finn" chamber systems are applied to the skin and held in place by nonallergic adhesive tape. Many contactant allergens may be tested with either of these two methods. Less than 40 allergens produce most cases of contact dermatitis. Complex topical products may contain many potential antigens and additives. The major component of a complex mixture may not be the sensitizer. This fact has important implications for the major topic of this book, excipients. About 20–30 antigens in a usual screening panel of patch tests will probably diagnose as many as 70% of the clinically relevant cases of allergic contact dermatitis (50). A selected series has been designated by the North American Contact Dermatitis Group (Table 1). Selected panels of allergens based on the patient's history must then be used to supplement the screening panel of allergens. Petrolatum is the most widely used vehicle to disperse allergens. However, some substances do not disperse well in this medium.

Positive reactions to both open and closed patch tests range from a slight erythematous reaction to a diffuse, vesicular response with intense pruritus. The International Contact Research Group has developed a widely utilized nonlinear descriptive scale of interpretation. This scale has been almost universally accepted (50): NT, not tested; ?, doubtful reaction; 1+, weak (nonvesicular but palpable reaction); 2+, strong (edematous or vesicular reaction); 3+ extreme reaction (e.g., markedly bullous or ulcerative); IR, irritant reaction; and –, negative reaction.

The optimal reading time is 48 hr but some reactions do not peak for as long as 72 or 96 hr after application. It is estimated that 30% of relevant allergens, which are negative at a 48 hr reading, become positive at a 96 hr reading (52). Conversely, some positive reactions at 48 hr disappear by 96 hr. These are believed to represent irritant rather than allergic responses. Readings at 96 hr are conducted 48 hr after removal of the original 48 hr occlusive patch. If pruritus occurs before the closed patch test is scheduled to be read either at 24 or 48 hr, the patient is instructed to remove the patch to minimize excessive exposure to the contactant. The causes of false-positive and -negative tests are listed in Table 2.

Some substances, particularly proteins, may elicit an urticarial response known as contact urticaria (53). Such reactions could be nonspecific or associated with IgE-mediated mechanisms and should not necessarily be interpreted as evidence of contact (type IV) hypersensitivity. Several low-molecular-weight hapten substances may elicit systemic contact allergy reactions (SCAR) or flares of contact dermatitis in patients previously sensitized to such agents by the topical route (54). Among excipient substances, the two most notable examples are oral administration of hydroxyzine and butylated hydroxyanisole, which cause exacerbation in patients previously sensitized topically to ethylenediamine and butylated hydroxyanisole, respectively.

Prophetic patch tests, also known as Draize tests, are sometimes used in

Table 1 North American Contact Dermatitis Group Screening Series, 1975 (Prepared in White Petroleum Unless Specified)[a]

Ammoniated mercury, 1%	Methylparaben, ethylparaben,
Caine mixture, 8% (benzocaine, dibu-	propylparaben, butylparaben, and
caine, tetracaine, and cyclomethycaine)	benzylparaben mixture, 15% (3% of each)
Carba mixture, 3%	Naphthyl mixture, 1%
ρ-Chloro-m-xylenol, 1%	Neomycin sulfate, 20%
Disulfiram mixture, 1%	Nickel sulfate, 2.5%
Epoxy resin, 1%	Paraphenylendediamine, 1%
Ethylenediamine, 1%	Paraphenylenediamine mixture, 0.60%
Formaldehyde solution (2% aqueous)	Peruvian balsam, 25%
Lanolin, 100%	Potassium dichromate, 0.5%
Mercaptobenzothiazole, 1%	ρ-Tertiary-butyl phenol, 2%
Mercapto mixture, 1%	Thimerosal (merthiolate), 0.1%
	Turpentine, 1% (in olive oil)
	Wood alcohols, 30%

[a]May be obtained from Dermatology Services, Inc., Box 3166, Evanston, Il 60204

large groups of normal volunteers without history of prior exposure to the offending substance as a means of assessing the contact hypersensitivity potential of substances used in the formulation of topical medicinal products. Some of these test protocols also include threshold dose-response and repetitive application designs.

B. Tuberculin-Like Intradermal Tests

Systemic tuberculinlike delayed hypersensitivity is assessed by intracutaneous injection of suspected proteins or simple chemicals (55). The test is performed with the bevel of a #27 ½-inch needle directed upward and the needle held at a 15–20 degree angle to the skin of the volar aspect of the arm. The needle is inserted into the skin and channeled several millimeters through the dermis. When this is done correctly, the skin will dimple with slight pressure or movement at the tip of the needle. The injection of a 0.1 ml volume should produce a transient, mild burning discomfort and a 5–10 mm wheal in the skin.

Reactions are read at 24 and 48 hr. Positive reactions consist of indurated and erythematous areas at least 5 mm in diameter. Highly sensitive persons may exhibit bullous responses that may become necrotic. However, such extreme activity can be avoided by careful attention to the concentration of the challenge dose. Positive results of intracutaneous tests of delayed hypersensitivity may persist for as long as 96 hr. The interpretation of tuberculintype skin tests may be confused with late-onset responses mediated by IgE antibodies. In contrast to the 24–48-hour peak response of delayed reactions, IgE-mediated

Table 2 Causes of False-Positive and False-Negative Contact Dermatitis Patch Tests

Modality	False-positive	False-negative
Application technique	Irritant effect Uneven dispersion in vehicle Concentration too high Volume applied too large Volatile diluent Confounding effect of allergen in adhesive tape Reaction to vehicle	Degradation of allergen Concentration too low Volume applied too small Unsatisfactory occlusion Failure to test to ultra-violet light Age: response longer in elderly Poor dispersal in vehicle

Test Subject	Excited skin
	  concurrent derma-titis
	  multiple tests
	Pustular reaction
		Decreased reactivity
		  steroids (systemic or topical)
		  immunosuppressive drugs

Reading	Pressure effect of solid objects Koebner phenomenon of psoriatic skin Overreading of inflammation around the edge of the patch	Duration of test too short

late onset reactions begin at 4 hr and reach their maximum intensity at 8 hr, although they often persist for as long as 24–48 hr.

C. Recall Antigens Test Battery

Several in vivo techniques are available for the assessment of cell-mediated immunodeficiency or anergy (56). These tests may not be valid if patients are receiving concurrent corticosteroid therapy or if they were tested recently with homologous antigens (57). Most normal subjects will react to one or more of a battery of recall skin test antigens known to elicit delayed hypersensitivity skin responses. This battery commonly includes purified protein derivative tuberculin, histoplasmin, coccidioidin, *Candida* (*albicans*), *Trichophyton*, tetanus toxoid, and mumps skin test antigen. A "multitest" tine panel is a convenient method of assessing recall antigen sensitivity (58). At a reading time of 48 hr the "multitest" (Merieux) antigen tine panel yields an apparent reaction prevalence comparable to that obtained with tuberculintype tests but comparative biopsy data suggest that the correct "multitest" reading time may be as long as 96 hr.

D. Induction of Topical Delayed Hypersensitivity

A provocative test for competence of epicutaneous reactivity is also available but not commonly used. This consists of preliminary application of a relatively large induction dose (2,000 μg) of dinitrochlorobenzene applied to the skin of the upper arm. Two weeks later a small challenge dose (25–50 μg) is applied to the volar aspect of the arm and skin responses are read at 48 hr. Erythema and induration at the challenge site are indicative of a positive response.

E. In Vitro Correlates of Delayed Hypersensitivity

Several in vitro correlates of cell-mediated immunity may be selected to confirm the presence of specific hypersensitivity reactions. Antigen-induced lymphocyte transformation (proliferation) correlates with the delayed hypersensitivity skin test response (59). Incubation of antigen with specifically sensitized lymphocyte cultures induces lymphoblast transformation that is measured by the degree of DNA synthesis, as indexed by prior incorporation of a radiolabeled thymidine tracer in the test medium. The result of this assay is compared to a corresponding lymphocyte culture without antigen. Two other in vitro methods that detect antigen-stimulated release of lymphokines correlate better with in vivo skin tests than the antigen proliferation technique and may be available at specialized immunological centers: the macrophage inhibitory factor procedure and the leukocyte inhibitory factor test (60,61). Capillary tube and agarose methods are equally accurate (62). Determination of the macrophage inhibitory factor requires guinea pig macrophages, so its use is totally confined to university research centers. On the other hand, the leukocyte inhibitory factor tests detects a lymphokine that inhibits migration of the patient's own leukocytes (61). Therefore, it is more practical and more generally available for study. Both macrophage and leukocyte inhibitory factor tests are closely associated with in vivo cell-mediated immunity induced by the specific antigen. Both are independent of concomitant antibody production.

In vitro methods are also available to evaluate cellular immunoincompetence. An absolute lymphocyte count under 1200/mm^3 suggests an abnormal cellular immune system. The number of circulating T cells, as measured by lymphocyte binding to sheep erythrocyte (rosettes), should range between 60 and 80% of peripheral blood lymphocytes (63). Helper and suppressor T-cell populations can be differentiated by fluorescent monoclonal antibodies directed against specific membrane markers on these cells. These determinations are performed by automated flow cytometric analysis using discriminating fluorescent markers for the cell populations to be studied (64). A marked decrease in helper cell subpopulations is the hallmark of AIDS. The nonspecific functional competence of T lymphocytes may be determined by lymphocyte transformation responses to mitogens, primarily phytohemagglutinin P (PHA-P) and concanavalin A (ConA) (59). These agents stimulate T lymphocytes to change from resting small cells into metabolically active blast forms, a process that results in DNA synthesis that is quantitated by incorporation of radiolabeled thymidine in the culture system. Another method of evaluating nonspecific T-cell proliferation is the mixed lymphocyte culture that measures allogeneic stimulation of the subject's lymphocytes cocultured with lymphocytes from a histoincompatible donor.

IV. PSEUDOALLERGIC REACTIONS

A. Organ Challenge Tests

Diagnosis and confirmation of these clinical responses hinge almost exclusively on challenge tests performed with appropriate controls under single- or double-blind laboratory conditions. Since the chief manifestations of these reactions occur in the skin, eyes, respiratory tract, and gastrointestinal system, challenge tests are organ-directed. Extreme caution must be exercised in the initial determination of the concentration of substance to be tested and, wherever possible, an appropriate dose range study in normal volunteers should be conducted prior to clinical testing. Objective tests should be used to measure the adverse reaction under investigation.

1. Repeat Open Application Skin Tests

Repeat open application tests of the skin are especially useful in determining a suspected offending topical agent. These tests also identify the nonspecific urticariogenic effect of materials supplied to the skin. Repeated applications of closed patch tests may be used to determine irritant thresholds of agents used topically. These tests should always be performed in conjunction with inert and vehicle controls.

2. Double-Blind Oral Challenge Tests

Double-blind oral challenge tests are required to confirm suspected gastrointestinal or systemic symptoms occurring after ingestion of a suspected orally administered agent. The test substance is encapsulated into opaque white capsules. Control placebo capsules should be prepared with microcellulose powder or D-xylose. We prefer to avoid lactose as a placebo capsule filler because of the widespread prevalence of lactose intolerance. Dose–response testing protocols are preferred but since the administration of such tests is very time consuming it may not be possible to conduct such dose ranging in each instance. Specific test procedures have been devised for some common excipients such as tartrazine, the metabisulfites, and monosodium glutamate. The details of these specific protocols will be discussed further in the sections on these agents.

3. Conjunctival Challenge Tests

Conjunctival challenge tests, although useful for ascertaining allergenic potential of a substance, are rarely used for determining irritant properties of an offending agent. The main problem with eye tests lies in the interpretation of the reaction, because the eye has a marked irritant susceptibility that is highly dependent on concentration and pH.

4. Nasal Challenge Tests

Nasal challenge tests can be used to document both allergic and pseudoallergic reactions. However, it should be emphasized that nonspecific changes in nasal hyperreactivity may occur after application of control solutions, so it is absolutely essential that the procedure be well controlled. Relative changes in nasal airflow resistance can be documented by posterior rhinomanometry or simply by changes in airflow measured by a pneumotachograph. Nasal washes may also be examined for release of inflammatory mediators induced by certain types of nonspecific challenges (65).

5. Bronchial Challenge Tests

Bronchial challenge tests have been well systematized for the evaluation of protein materials (12). Similarly to other challenge tests, suitable controls must be done either on the same day or the day before the test. Standardization of bronchoprovocation tests with unknown chemicals is more difficult than protein challenges because there may be great variations in the irritative potential of individual chemicals. This must be ascertained on a case-by-case basis.

6. Systemic Testing

Although anaphylactic reactions are known to occur on a pseudoallergic basis, intravenous challenge tests are not recommended because of the inherent danger of such tests. Rarely, such nonimmunological reactions may activate complement and complement-derived anaphylatoxins by way of the alternate pathway so that depletion of C3 and/or decrease of total complement may provide adjunctive evidence that a systemic reaction is occurring. However, one rarely has the opportunity to apply these tests on a prospective basis.

VI. IMMUNOTOXICOLOGICAL SURVEYS

Although the concept of immunoxicological evaluation of xenobiotics has been supported by the United States National Toxicology Program and the Environmental Protection Agency, such protocols have not yet been extended to excipient xenobiotics with one notable exception, saccharin. Extensive studies were conducted in rats to determine the carcinogenic effect of this compound. In the course of these studies, immunotoxicologic parameters such as macrophage or NK-cell-dependent cytotoxicity, primary immunization with sheep cell erythrocytes, and effects of T- and B-cell mitogens were assessed to detect possible immunotoxicological effects of saccharin, both in vitro and in vivo (66). While in vitro exposure of rat lymphoid cells to pure saccharin at concentration ranges between 0.1 and 2 mg/ml did not modify macrophage or NK-cell-dependent cytotoxicity, a marked inhibition in responsiveness of rat lymphoid cells to phytohemagglutinin (PHA), a T-cell mitogen, and lipopolysaccharide (LPS), a B-cell mitogen, was observed. Chronic feeding of animals with 1–5% saccharin diets did not cause detectable changes in macrophage and NK-cell host resistance parameters or antigen-induced delayed typed hypersensitivity but was associated with decreased primary antibody response to sheep erythrocytes. These results suggested that repeated exposure to relatively high doses of saccharin in experimental animals may be associated with immunotoxicological risk. However, extrapolation of these data to humans is not possible for several reasons: the dose effects were selective and observed only at high saccharin concentrations that are not achieved in humans under normal dietary consumption conditions; the effect of PHA and LPS on human lymphocytes was not affected when these cells were exposed in vitro to the identical concentrations used in rat experiments; and comparative saccharin feeding experiments in rats and humans suggest that saccharin distribution to tissues is at least several orders of magnitude higher in rats than humans. Similar intraspecies differences apply to other xenobiotics. It is therefore apparent that animal screening cannot predict the occurrence of human immunotoxicological effects; it can only provide insight into the potential immunotoxicological effects of a substance.

Two strategies have been developed to demonstrate the immunotoxicological potential of xenobiotic substances. Immunotoxicologists have developed and validated a two-tiered panel of methods that is reproducible between laboratories. This panel is designed to characterize inappropriate humoral and cell mediated immune responses following in vivo exposure to test substances. The second initiative was to demonstrate that the immune system was a more sensitive indicator of toxicity than classic toxicological methods for studying injury at cellular and functional levels.

A. Two-Tiered System of Immune Function Testing

The two-tiered system of immune function testing was developed by the United States National Toxicology Program as an outgrowth of its earlier carcinogenic studies (67). Thus far, the method has been standardized and validated in the mouse. Experimental mice receive subcutaneous injections of xenobiotics dissolved in corn oil over a 14-day period. Immunological assays are performed 2–5 days after administration of the final dose. The overall objectives of immune tests are to assess immunopathology, immune function, and host resistance, Tier I assays consist of gross and microscopic pathological examination of lymphoid organs, humoral antibody responses (i.e., plaque-forming assays of sensitized spleen cells and ELISA tests), macrophage function, and cell-mediated immunity (i.e., mixed lymphocyte cultures). If no abnormalities appear in this panel of tests, further testing is not necessary. If positive responses occur, tier II assays are performed to determine the mechanisms responsible for these immunological effects. Immunopathological aberrations are investigated further by histochemical determination of lymphocyte cell populations, T- and B-cell quantitation by means of monoclonal antibodies to lymphocyte CD antigens, and architectural studies of lymphoid organs and cells. Humoral abnormalities are investigated further by tests of secondary antibody responses to sheep erythrocytes. Functional abnormalities of cell-mediated immunity are determined by mitogenic responses of lymphocytes in vitro and cytotoxic T-cell assays including antibody-dependent cell cytotoxicity tests. Finally, host resistance models include challenge with viruses, bacteria, and tumor cell lines. In the bacterial resistance model, xenobiotic-treated and control animals are treated with *Listeria monocytogenes* and susceptibility differences between treated and control groups of animals are compared. Tumor resistance is assessed by comparing the percentage of successful tumor transplants between xenobiotic-treated and control mice. Finally, a panel of immunologic tests (NK-dependent cytotoxicity, lymphocyte cytotoxicity, mixed lymphocyte culture, PHA- and LPS-stimulated in vitro lymphocyte proliferation) are compared between *Listeria*-, influenza, virus- and tumor transplant-treated mice and untreated controls.

B. Experimental Contact Hypersensitivity

Experimental contact sensitivity in guinea pigs and humans has been utilized to estimate the contact allergenic properties of low-molecular-weight xenobiotics (68). The guinea pig patch test procedure is designed to serve as a prescreen prior to human repeated insult patch tests and other types of human topical exposures. Single occlusive patches with the solubilized test material are applied to gunea pigs at weekly intervals for 3 weeks. The elicitation challenge with the highest nonirritating concentration of the same test material is conducted during the 5th week. Patch test sites are graded 24 and 48 hr after application of the challenge patch. The degree of erythema observed is graded on a scale of 0-3. The incidence of sensitization is expressed as the fraction of tested animals responding with greater severity than the controls. If the test substance exhibits a high degree of guinea pig contact sensitization, further testing in humans is probably not advisable. However, further tests in humans are usually performed with substances showing minimal delayed hypersensitivity reactions in guinea pigs. In human tests it is important to test not only with the specific xenobiotic but also the vehicle with which it will be used in clinical practice. One hundred to 200 subjects are used for human repeated insult patch tests (69,70). Occlusive patches are placed three times a week for 3 weeks. Two elicitation challenges are conducted, one in the original site of application and the other on the opposite arm. Interpretation of these tests may vary among individuals because of prior exposures, genetic susceptibilities, or differences in vehicle formulation. In some cases, sensitized test subjects may be used for further provocative tests with "low potential" sensitizers. The lack of response in such individuals is good confirmation of the low allergenic potential of a test material. Both guinea pig and human models are useful for risk assessment of the potential allergenicity of a chemical. However, neither method can predict the occurrence, incidence, or severity of contact dermatitis when the substance is subsequently introduced into wider consumer use. Under these circumstances of protracted use, uncontrolled variables such as exposure conditions, concentration of a particular formulation, number of individuals using the preparation, and genetic susceptibility singly, or in combination, determine the occurrence of contact sensitivity.

C. Experimental Respiratory Sensitization

Although it is possible to sensitize several animal species by inhalation and tracheal instillation of low-molecular-weight chemicals, neither the incidence of human sensitization nor the immunological sequelae of these procedures after humans are exposed by the same route can be predicted. Moreover, the skin-sensitizing potential of a particular substance does not predict the occurrence of pulmonary sensitization to that chemical. Thus, there are no accepted experimental models of respiratory sensitization nor can one predict the allergenic potential or incidence of sensitization in humans by current animal models of respiratory sensitization. One recent exception to this principle may be the induction of pulmonary hemorrhagic lesions in rats after inhalation of trimellitic anhydride (71). This animal model strongly resembles the hemorrhagic pulmonary lesions occurring in some workers after heavy occupational exposure to trimellitic anhydride. However, it is noteworthy that this model was developed only after this unusual respiratory syndrome had been observed in several sensitized workers. In this instance, the predictive potential was reversed; human respiratory disease predicted that a similar pathologic process could be induced in animals.

REFERENCES

1. Vanselow, N.A. Skin testing and other diagnostic procedures. *In* A Manual of Clinical Allergy (J.M. Sheldon and K.P. Mathews, eds.), W.B. Saunders, Philadelphia, p. 62. (1967).
2. Lockey, R.F., Benedict, L.M., Turkeltaub, P.C. and Bukantz, S.C. Fatalities from immunotherapy (IT) and skin testing (ST). J. Allergy Clin. Immunol. 79:660–677 (1987).
3. Squire, J.R. The relationship between horse dandruff and horse serum antigens in asthma. Clin. Sci. 9:127–150 (1950).
4. Bernstein, I.L. Proceedings of the Task Force on Guidelines for Standardizing Old and New Technologies Used for Diagnosis and Treatment of Allergic Diseases. J. Allergy Clin. Immunol. 82(3)Part 2, 487–526 (1988).
5. Dolovich, J., Hargreave, F.E., Chalmers, R., Shier, K.S., Gauldie, J. and Bienenstock, J. Late cutaneous allergic response in isolated IgE-dependent reactions. J. Clin. Immunol. 52:38–46 (1973).
6. Hordle, D.A., Mehta, V., Tomenen, B. and Wainscott, G. Development of the prick test for allergen assay. J. Immunol. Methods 75:369–382 (1984).
7. Turkeltaub, P.C., Rastogi, S.C., Baer, H. et al. A standardized quantitative skin test assay of allergen potency and stability: studies on the allergen dose-response curve and effect of wheal, erythema and patient selection on assay results. J. Allergy Clin. Immunol. 70:343–352 (1982).

8. Prausnitz, C. and Küstner, H. Studien uber ueberempfindlichkeit. Zentralbl. Bakteriol. 86:160 (1921).

9. Patterson, R. and Kelley, J.F. Animal models of the asthmatic state. Annu. Rev. Med. 25:53 (1974).

10. Parish, W.E. Short term anaphylactic IgG antibodies in human sera. Lancet 2:591–592 (1970).

11. Bernstein, I.L. Allergy of the respiratory tract. In Textbook of Pulmonary Diseases (G. Baum, ed.), Little, Brown, Boston, pp. 279–338 (1965).

12. Chai, H., Farr, R.S., Forehlich, L.A., Mathison, D.A., McLean, J.A., Rosenthal, R.R., Sheffer, A.L., Spector, S.L. and Townley, R.G. Standardization of bronchial inhalation challenge procedures. J. Allergy Clin. Immunol. 56: 323–327 (1975).

13. Adkinson, N.F.,Jr. Measurement of total serum immunoglobulin E and allergen-specific immunoglobulin antibody. In Manual of Clinical Laboratory Immunology (N.R. Rose, H. Friedman and J.L. Fahey, eds.), American Society for Microbiology, Washington, D.C., pp. 664–669 (1986).

14. Ibid, pp 670–674.

15. Wide, L., Bennich, H. and Johansson, S.G.O. Diagnosis of allergy by an *in vitro* test for allergen antibodies. Lancet 2:1105–1107 (1967).

16. Perera, M.G., Bernstein, I.L., Michael, J.G. and Johansson, S.G.O. Predictability of the radioallergosorbent test (RAST) in ragweed pollenosis. Am. Rev. Respir. Dis. 111:605–610 (1975).

17. Schellenberg, R.R. and Adkinson, N.F.Jr. Assessment of the influence of irrelevant IgE on allergic sensitivity to two independent allergens. J. Allergy Clin. Immunol. 63:15–22 (1978).

18. Hamilton, R.G. and Adkinson, N.F.Jr. Serological methods for the assessment and management of IgE-mediated diseases. Clin. Immunol. Newsletter 7:1 (1987).

19. Nalebuff, D.J., Fadal, R.G. and Ali, M. IgE investigation and management of atopic disorders: Recent advances. J. Cont. Ed. ORL Allergy 40:47 (1978).

20. Shore, P.A., Burkhalter, A. and Cohn, V.H.Jr. A method for the fluorometric assay of histamine in tissues. J. Pharmacol. Exp. Ther. 127:182–186 (1959).

21. Lichtenstein, L.M. and Osler, A.G. Studies on the mechanisms of hypersensitivity phenomena IX. Histamine release from human leukocytes by ragweed pollen antigen. J. Exp. Med. 120:507–530 (1964).

22. Siraganian, R.P. An automated continuous-flow system for the extraction and fluorometric analysis of histamine. Anal. Biochem 57.:383–394 (1974).

23. Beaven, M.A. and Horakova, Z. The enzymatic isotopic assay of histamine. In Handbook of Experimental Pharmacology New Series, Vol. 18/2, Histamine II and Antihistamines (m. Rocha de Silva, ed.), Springer-Verlag, Berlin, pp. 151–173 (1978).

24. Skov, P.S., Mosbech, H., Norn, S. et al. Sensitive glass microfibre-based histamine analysis for allergy testing in washed blood cells. Allergy 40:213–218 (1985).

25. Immunotech patent No. 84.05783.
26. Maderazo, E.G. and Woronick, C.L. Micropore assay of human granulocyte locomotion: Problems and solutions. Clin. Immunol. Immunpathol. 11: 196-211 (1978).
27. Bernstein, I.L. Bronchoalveolar lavage and asthma: Sampling the humors speeds up. J. Allergy Clin. Immunol. 69:320-323 (1987).
28. Naclerio, R.M., Meier, H.L., Kagey-Sobotka, A., Adkinson, N.F., Meyers, D.A., Norman, F.S. and Lichtenstein, L.M. Mediator release after nasal challenge with allergen. Am. Rev. Respir. Dis. 128:597-602 (1983).
29. Murray, J.J., Tonnel, A.B., Brash, A.R. et al. Release of prostaglandin D_2 into human airways during acute antigen challenge. N. Engl. J. Med. 315: 800-804 (1986).
30. Walker, K.B., Serwonska, M.H., Valone, F.H. et al. Distinctive patterns of release of neuroendocrine peptides after nasal challenge of allergic subjects with ryegrass antigen. J. Clin. Immunol. 8:108-113 (1988).
31. Wells, J.V., Isbister, J.P. and Ries, C.A. Hematologic diseases In Basic and Clinical Immunology, 6th ed. (D.P. Stites, J.D. Stobo and J.V. Wells, eds.), Appleton & Lange. Norwalk, Connecticut pp. 386-419 (1987).
32. Valenzuela, R. and Deodhar, S.D. Tissue immunofluorescence. In Manual of Clinical Laboratory Immunology, 3rd ed. American Society for Microbiology, Washington, D.C., pp. 923-925 (1986).
33. Theofilopoulos, A.N. and Dixon, F.J. Detection of immune complexes: Techniques and implications. Hosp. Pract. 107-121, 1980.
34. Lambert, P.H., Dixon, F.J., Zubler, R.H. et al. A WHO collaborative study for the evaluation of eighteen methods for detecting immune complexes in serum. J. Clin. Lab. Immunol. 1:1-15 (1978).
35. Theofilopoulos, A.N., Eisenberg, R.A. and Dixon, F.J. Isolation of circulating immune complexes using Raji cells: Separation of antigens from immune complexes and production of antiserum. J. Clin. Invest. 61(1): 1570-1581 (1978).
36. Leary, H.L. and Jalsey, J.F. An assay to measure antigen-specific immune complexes in food-allergy patients. J. Allergy Clin. Immunol. 74:190 (1984).
37. Inman, R.D. and Day, N.K. Immunologic and clinical aspects of immune complex disease. Am. J. Med. 70:1097-1106 (1981).
38. Casah, P., Bossus, A., Carpentier, N.A. and Lambert, P.H. Solid-phase enzyme immunoassay of radioimmunoassay for the detection of immune complexes based on their recognition by conglutinin: conglutinin-binding test. A comparative study with ^{125}I-labelled Clq binding and Raji cell RIA tests. Clin. Exp. Immunol. 29:342-354 (1977).
39. Eisenberg, R.A., Theofilopoulos, A.N. and Dixon, F.J. Use of bovine conglutinin for the assay of immune complexes. J. Immunol. 118:1428-1434 (1977).
40. Frank, M.M. Complement in the pathophysiology of human disease. N. Engl. J. Med. 316:1525-1530 (1987).
41. Luthra, H.S., McDuffie, F.C., Hunder, G.G. and Samayoa, E.A. Immune complexes in sera and synovial fluids of patients with rheumatoid arthritis. J. Clin. Invest. 56:458-466 (1975).

42. Theofilopoulos, A.N., Wilson, C.B. and Dixon, F.J. The Raji cell radio-immunoassay for immune complexes in human sera. J. Clin. Invest. 57: 169–182 (1976).

43. McDougal, J.S., Redecha, P.B., Inman, R.D. and Christian, C.L. Binding of immunoglobulin G aggregates and immune complexes in human sera to Staphylocci containing protein A. J. Clin. Invest. 63:627–636 (1979).

44. Husby, S., Oxelius, V.A., Teisner, B., Jensenius, J.C. and Svehag, S.E. Humoral immunity to dietary antigens in healthy adults. Occurrence, iso-type and IgG subclass distribution of serum antibodies to protein antigens. Int. Arch. Allergy Appl. Immunol. 77:416–422 (1985).

45. Schifferli, J.A., Ng, Y.C. and Peters, D.K. The role of complement and its receptor in the elimination of immune complexes. N. Engl. J. Med. 315: 488–495 (1986).

46. Cooke, A., Lydyard, P.M. and Roitt, I.M. Autoimmunity and idiotypes. Lancet 2:723–724 (1984).

47. Fritzler, M.J. Antinuclear antibodies in the investigation of rheumatic diseases. Bull. Rheum. Dis. 35:1–10 (1985).

48. Budinsky, R.A., Roberts, S.M., Coats, E.A. et al. The formation of procain-amide hydroxylamine by rat and liver microsomes. Drug Metab. Dispos. 15:37–43 (1987).

49. Portanova, J.P., Arndt, R.E., Tan, E.M. et al. Anti-histone antibodies in idiopathic and drug-induced lupus recognize distinct intrahistone regions. J. Immunol. 138:446–451 (1987).

50. Fisher, A.A. Contact Dermatitis, 3rd ed. Lea & Febiger, Philadelphia (1986).

51. Bruynzeel, D.P. and Maibach, H.I. Excited skin syndrome (angry back). Arch. Dermatol. 122:323–328 (1986).

52. Mathias, C.G.T. and Maibach, H.I. When to read the patch test? Int. J. Dermatol. 18:127–128 (1979).

53. von Krogh, G. and Maibach, H.I. The contact urticaria syndrome—an up-dated review. J. Am. Acad. Dermatol. 5(3):328–342 (1981).

54. Menne, T. and Maibach, H.I. Reactions to systemic exposure to contact allergens: Systemic contact allergy reactions (SCAR). Immun. Allergy Pract. IX:373/17–385/29 (1987).

55. Sokal, J.E. Measurement of delayed skin-test responses. N. Engl. J. Med. 293:501–502 (1975).

56. Ahmed, A.R. and Blose, D.A. Delayed-type hypersensitivity skin testing. Arch. Dermatol. 119:934–942 (1983).

57. Threstrup-Peterson, K. Suppression of tuberculin skin reactivity by prior tuberculin skin testing. Immunology 28:343–348 (1975).

58. Dunn, J.A. and Johnson, A.J. Comparison of the tine and Mantoux tuber-culin skin tests. Br. Med. J. 1:1451–1453 (1978).

59. Oppenheim, J.J., Dougherty, S., Chan, S.P. and Baker, J. Use of lympho-cyte transformation to assess clinical disorders. In Laboratory Diagnosis of Immunologic Disorders (G.N. Vyas, D. Stites and G. Brecher, eds.), Grune & Stratton, New York p. 87 (1975).

60. Rocklin, R.E., Reardon, G., Sheffer, A. et al. Dissociation between two *in*

vitro correlates of delayed hypersensitivity: absence of MIF in the presence of antigen-induced incorporation of ^{3}H-thymidine. In Proceedings of the Fifth Leukocyte Culture Conference. Academic Press, New York, p. 639 (1970).

61. Mirza, A.M., Perera, M.G., Maccia, C.A. et al. Leukocyte migration inhibition in nickel dermatitis. Int. Arch. Allergy. Appl. Immunol. 49:782–788, 1975.

62. Borish, L., Liu, D., Remold, H. et al. Production and assay of macrophage migration inhibitory factor, leukocyte inhibitory factor and leukocyte adherence inhbitory factor. In Manual of Clinical Laboratory Immunology (N. Rose, H. Friedman, J. Fahey, eds.), American Society Microbiology, Washington, D.C., 3rd ed., p. 282 (1986).

63. Winchester, R.J. and Ross, G.D. Methods for enumerating cell populations by surface markers with conventional microscopy. In Manual of Clinical Immunology (N. Rose, H. Friedman, J. Fahey, eds.), American Society Microbiology, Washington, D.C., 3rd ed. (1986).

64. Jackson, A.L. and Warner, N.L. Preparation, staining and analysis by flow cytometry of peripheral blood leukocytes. In Manual of Clinical Laboratory Immunology (N. Rose, H. Friedman and J. Fahey eds.), American Society Microbiology, Washington, D.C., 3rd ed. (1986).

65. Togias, A.G., Naclerio, R.M., Proud, D. et al. Nasal challenge with cold, dry air results in release of inflammatory mediators. J. Clin. Invest. 76:1375–1381 (1985).

66. Spreafico, F., Vecchi, A., Sironi, M. et al. Problems in immunotoxicological assessment: Examples with different classes of xenobiotics. In Immunotoxicology (G.G. Gibson, R. Hubbard and D.V. Parke, eds.), Academic Press, London, pp. 2343–357 (1983).

67. Dean, J.H., Luster, M.I., Murray, M.J. et al. Approaches and methodology for examining the immunological effects of xenobiotics. In Immunotoxicology (G.G. Gibson, R. Hubbard and D.V. Parke, eds.), Academic Press, London, pp. 205–218, (1983).

68. Buehler, E.V. Experimental contact sensitivity. In Immunotoxicology (G.G. Gibson, R. Hubbard and D.V. Parke, eds.), Academic Press, London, pp. 131–147 (1983).

69. Magnusson, B. and Kligman, A.M. The identification of contact allergens by animal assay. The guinea pig maximization test. J. Invest. Dermatol. 52: 268–276 (1969).

70. Buehler, E.V. and Griffith, J.F. Relevance to human dermatopharmacology and dermatotoxicity. In Animal Models in Dermatology (H.I. Maibach, ed.), Churchill Livingstone, New York, pp. 56–66 (1975).

71. Zeiss, C.R., Levitz, D. and Leach, C.L. et al. A model of immunologic lung injury induced by trimellitic anhydride inhalation: Antibody response. J. Allergy Clin. Immunol. 79:59–63 (1987).

Part II
Adverse Effects of Excipients by Class of Excipient

Chapter 6   Adverse Effects: Bulk Materials   89

Chapter 7   Adverse Effects: Coatings   121

Chapter 8   Adverse Effects: Flavoring Agents   133

Chapter 9   Adverse Effects: Coloring Agents   159

Chapter 10   Adverse Effects: Other Products   167

6

Adverse Effects: Bulk Materials

I. Oral   90
   A. Solid formulations   91
   B. Liquid formulations (solvents)   97
II. Topical   102
   A. Solids (gels, ointments, creams)   103
   B. Liquids (lotions, emulsions, suspensions)   106
III. Parenterals   109
IV. Suppositories   113
   References   113

Bulk materials in medication are the most obvious of excipients and, to the extent that they are the "carriers" of active medication, some definitions would consider the term excipients to be best exemplified by the bulk materials discussed in this section.

Many modern medications involve doses of active ingredient that are too small to handle as such. They therefore require some type of carrier. Pharmaceutical scientists are of necessity concerned about the mixing of large amounts of solid bulk excipient with small amounts of active ingredients. Homogeneity in the final mix is critical to dependable dosage. A bulk filler that cannot be properly mixed or does not "run" well on machinery can be a poor and potentially dangerous excipient, even if it is in itself intrinsically nontoxic.

Not all the bulk materials used in modern pharmaceuticals are simple "carriers" or "fillers." Some are binding agents selected and handled to achieve a form of controlled release. The selection of bulk fillers often involves a wide variety of considerations, such as the need for and compatibility with other additives to obtain flow characteristics, stability, or compressibility essential to the manufacture and suitability of the final formulation. Whatever the purpose, the potential for adverse reaction needs to be considered.

An obvious factor critical to the selection of bulk fillers is the route of administration. By any route, including intravenously, carriers can influence the effect of the medication. Whether the surface the medication reaches is gastrointestinal mucosa (oral medication), some integumental structure (topical preparations), or even an intramuscular or subcutaneous site, the filler can make a difference in the fate of the active ingredient.

Since there are marked differences in the potential for reaction to any particular bulk filler as a consequence of the site and manner of administration, the following review of fillers will be made under the headings "Oral", "Topical," and "Parenteral," with appropriate subdivisions.

Fillers, particularly for oral and topical use are themselves often formulations of several ingredients designed to have properties useful to the manufacture and stability of the final dosage form. Manufacturers like to have more than one supplier, and often the suppliers themselves use different sources for their materials. The nature and degree of product refinement are generally determined by the costs involved and the significance of the refinement to the quality of the final product.

It may seem disturbing that the final dosage forms of many currently marketed products contain hundreds of substances, many of which arrive by way of the bulk filler (1). On the other hand, every time a leaf of lettuce or a slice of bread is consumed, hundreds of chemical moieties are ingested. The fact that most of them are "natural" is no guarantee that they are harmless (see discussion in the Introduction). Bulk fillers may, but need not be, pure single chemical entities in order to be safe and useful components of medications.

I. ORAL

For most systemic medications, the oral route is by far the preferred method of administration, and solid dosage forms are by far the easier to handle, transport, and store. Tablets or capsules usually present less taste and stability problems than liquids. On the other hand, liquids are sometimes easier to administer and have no disintegration/dissolution problems that may compromise bioavailability. They also permit, at least theoretically, any degree of fine adjustment of dosage. The user of tablets or capsules is confined to multiples of the available unit formulations. Powders in bulk or packaged in unit dose papers or envelopes, once a popular form of oral medication, are only occasionally used today. Usually they are intended for suspension or dissolution of each dose in water or other appropriate liquid just before consumption. Occasionally, effervescent tablets are similarly used, and special formulations may be designed to make tablets chewable to avoid problems of swallowing and disintegration (2).

By and large, the potential for side effects from oral solid bulk fillers is the same whether the final product is a capsule, tablet, or powder. Individual excipients used for oral preparations will be reviewed under a general classification of solid and liquid excipients.

A. Solid Formulations

Modern pharmaceutical production methods demand that solid formulations be capable of "running" dependably and reproducibly on high-speed machinery. Thus, while clinical safety of a bulk excipient is a fundamental requirement, it is only one of several. The general public and medical practitioner are concerned only with the properties of the final product. The pharmaceutical specialist must spend much effort on determining how an acceptable final product can be achieved. Selection of the proper solid bulk excipient is critical to a successful formula. At times, an excipient that seems ideal from the point of view of safety simply cannot be used for technical reasons.

The following is a review of specific materials commonly used to achieve the desired bulk of a solid oral formulation.

1. Starch

Starch used as an excipient is derived primarily from corn (maize) and occasionally from rice, potato, and wheat. It consists of several polysaccharides of alpha-glucose such as amylose and amylopectin, and takes up water as a function of humidity.

Starch is one of the most commonly used excipients for solid oral medicinals. It is contained in over 2000 prescription drugs marketed in the United States and has a well-deserved reputation for safety.

Oral starch causes no ill effect unless massive doses are given, to the point of bowel obstruction by "starch calculi" (3). It can cause granulomatous reactions when applied to the peritoneum (4-6) or the meninges (7) via powdered surgical gloves or if insufflated onto injured tissue in the ear when used, for example, as a carrier for an antibiotic preparation (7). These observations are of little relevance to its potential for harm as an excipient in oral preparations.

There is some concern about the ability of starch to serve as a medium for growth of microorganisms, particularly if it is moist. Experimental studies have shown that the notorious carcinogenic aflatoxins can form in starch inoculated with the appropriate organisms, leading to the recommendation that starch should be stored dry (humidity below 12%) (8). However, there have not been reports of detectable trace amounts of aflatoxin in starch used for medication as there have been for many common foods, including legumes and milk (9).

Earlier reports of allergic reactions to cornstarch (10) are not well supported by subsequent experience. The possibility of trace residues of corn protein acting as a significant allergen in medicinal starch is remote. Nevertheless, there are instances in which subjects presumably intolerant to corn starch have no difficulty with potato starch. An orally less allergenic material would probably be hard to find.

A wide variety of treated starches have been prepared and some of these have been evaluated for digestibility and toxicity by the World Health Organization (11,12). Among the derivatives found suitable for use without limit are starches that have been treated with acid or alkali, blanched, and oxidized; mono- and distarch phosphate; acetylated distarch phosphate; distarch glycerol; hydroxypropyl distarch glycerol; hydroxypropyl starch; phosphated distarch phosphate; and starch acetate.

2. Lactose

For many years, lactose was considered as safe an excipient as mother's milk, which contains about 6.5 g of this sugar per 100 ml. It is a simple disaccharide of glucose and galactose that is absorbable only after hydrolysis of the disaccharide in the intestinal tract to those two hexoses by the enzyme lactase (13).

The discovery of a syndrome of abdominal pain, flatulence, distention, and diarrhea associated with a deficiency in intestinal lactase has precipitated concern among nutritionists about intolerance to milk and among medicinal specialists about the use of lactose as an excipient. There is an extensive literature on the consequences of this problem in child nutrition for which milk is so critical (14) and in the elderly (15), since milk products are a prime source of calcium for these populations. The elderly, who have a particular need for calcium to avoid the consequences of osteoporosis, also have a high incidence of lactase deficiency (16).

Lactose is said to be present in over 20% of all prescription drugs (17). Consequently, the problem of reactions to lactose used as an excipient is of considerable importance. Anecdotal reports (18,19) are not adequate to determine whether symptoms are induced by ingestion of small amounts of lactose used as bulk fillers.

The pathophysiological mechanism responsible for instances of intolerance to lactose does not involve an allergic immunologic phenomenon. When a disaccharide such as lactose fails to be hydrolysed and absorbed, it passes on to the large intestine where it is attacked by colonic bacteria that convert it to acidic trioses and related derivatives including lactic acid, carbon dioxide, and hydrogen gas. These derivatives are irritating to the colon and acidify its contents. In fact, the disaccharide, lactulose, for which there is no intestinal hydrolyzing enzyme equivalent to lactase, is clinically useful as a laxative in doses of 10–20 g, and also serves as an ammonia trap to help control the symptoms of portal systemic encephalopathy (20). In subjects with complete lactase deficiency, administration of lactose can be expected to yield consequences similar to the effects of lactulose in normal subjects.

Numerous studies of the degree and incidence of lactase deficiency among different populations and different age groups confirm that it is a common condition that varies widely with race (16) and becomes more common with increasing age. Based on a breath hydrogen test that differentiates sugars that undergo complete absorption and metabolism from those that are unabsorbed and possibly broken down in the colon, a 1 g/kg, lactose dose showed complete absorption in children under 2 years of age, with an increasing incidence of malabsorption reaching essentially adult levels (some degree of deficiency in 85-89%) by age 6 (21).

Lactase deficiency may be primary (i.e., unrelated to active gastrointestinal disease) or secondary (i.e., presumably related to some acquired gastrointestinal disturbance) (22). A rare but severe deficiency occurs as a congenital phenomenon (13). Estimates of the degree of lactase deficiency can be made by direct assay of intestinal villa biopsy material or indirectly by identifying the absorbed products of hydrolysis in the blood, (i.e., galactose or glucose) (23-25). Another useful measure is hydrogen gas in the expired breath, since H_2 gas is generated by bacterial action in the colon when lactose reaches the colon intact (26-28). In general, controlled studies trying to match clinical symptoms with lactose deficiency show poor correlations.

Lactose can result in galactosemia in subjects who may have normal lactase activity but are unable to handle galactose normally. Like other sugars, it may not be well tolerated in rare glucose–galactose malabsorption syndromes.

Some studies suggest that a dose equal to the contents of a glass of milk (over 10 g lactose) is generally required to create significant clinical symptoms in most lactase-deficient subjects. This is consistent with what is known to be the laxative dose of lactulose (10-20 g). Since most drug formulations using lactose as an excipient use a fraction of a gram per dose, it is indeed the rare individual among lactase-deficient subjects who will suffer significantly from a medication because of its lactose content. However, there are wide individual differences in the dose necessary to cause symptoms (16,18,29). Reports of reactions to as little as 100-200 mg lactose (19) are difficult to evaluate.

3. Calcium Salts

Calcium salts are used both as excipients and for a variety of medicinal purposes. Since their medicinal use is commonly over prolonged periods and in relatively large doses, the smaller amounts generally used as excipients are considered to be essentially without toxic protential. However, calcium salts used as excipients can have significant physiological effects and their potential influence on the bioavailability of active ingredients must be considered.

A variety of calcium salts are used as excipients for different purposes. The acetate is added to food as a preservative. The sulfate is used in tablets prepared by direct compression. The hemihydrate of calcium sulfate is plaster of Paris. Various calcium phosphate salts are used in baking, as an abrasive in toothpaste, as a nonhygroscopic diluent for powders, and also as an excipient for tablets to be compressed in preparation for coating.

The presence of calcium in formulations of active agents with which it can form complexes may seriously alter the bioavailability of the agent, since the calcium complex often has different solubility and absorption characteristics from the agent itself. Tetracycline is a notorious example of a drug that becomes poorly absorbable when formulated with calcium salts. The reaction is of such importance that patients are frequently cautioned not to consume calcium-containing foods such as dairy products within 1 hr of taking oral tetracycline.

Another well-publicized example of calcium altering absorption is the experience in Australia, when lactose replaced calcium sulfate as a filler in the formulation of hydantoin used to control epilepsy. The reformulated product caused a flood of adverse effects (30) as a consequence of the more complete absorption achieved when the calcium salt was eliminated from the formulation. There have also been instances, such as with the drug sulfinpyrazone, in which a formulation containing a calcium salt successfully passed standard dissolution tests but had to be rejected when in vivo bioavailability studies showed poor absorption. The problem was easily corrected by eliminating the calcium salt.

Most information about toxicity of calcium salts comes from its purposeful use as an active ingredient, rather than as an excipient. Frequently calcium and magnesium salts are balanced in antacid preparations to offset the presumed bowel-stimulating effect of magnesium and the constipating effect of calcium.

Absorption of calcium salts is rarely complete, and the levels observed in plasma are more the result of mechanisms that influence calcium metabolism such as thyroid, parathyroid, and vitamin D status than of calcium intake. The insolubility of calcium as the oxalate or phosphate, or complexed with polyphosphates commonly in the diet, such as phytic acid (31), make it difficult to quantify what constitutes a toxic oral intake of calcium. While "excess calcium" has been held responsible for many ill effects, including myocardial infarction (32), hypertension (33), congenital defects (34) and the spectrum of observations labeled "calciphylaxis" by Selye (35), problems attributable to calcium toxicity from the use of calcium salts as excipients in oral preparations are rare. There are special cases in which calcium intake needs to be controlled (33,36). However, clinical calcium-related problems arise more from the use of massive amounts of antacids (37,38) or in their use in renal dialysis solutions (39) than from their use as excipients.

4. Citric Acid

Citric acid and its effervescent salts are used as excipients to adjust pH and to prepare effervescent tablets. Its use as an anticoagulant in the collection of blood reflects its capacity to bind calcium, a phenomenon that anticipates concern that its excessive use might lead to tooth erosion (40) and local irritation by complexation, with the possible induction of trace metal deficiency (41). Sodium or potassium salts of citric acid are alkalinizing and could cause hypernatremia or hyperkalemia if administered in sufficiently large amounts (42).

Citric acid induces cough in 90% of human subjects (42A). The response is rapid but transient. Both high osmolarity and acidity of citric acid aerosol solutions probably account for the irritation of cough receptors.

Effervescent formulations using citric acid or its salts need to be evaluated for the amounts involved to avoid problems, particularly in patients with pH and electrolyte sensitivity or balance problems. A more detailed discussion of excessive sodium and potassium intake is included in the following section on bicarbonate salts.

5. Bicarbonate Salts

Bicarbonate salts of sodium and potassium are generally used to create effervescent tablets and to develop or maintain a more alkaline pH. They are generally preferred to the corresponding carbonates, which, if not adequately diluted or neutralized by other components of the formulation, can be caustic.

The key problem in the use of these agents as excipients is their potential effect on electrolyte balance, which in turn is a function of two important variables: the amount used and the clinical condition of the patient.

The clinical problems associated with the excessive ingestion of sodium bicarbonate are well known and documented in standard medical texts. Patients with congestive heart failure, hypertension, renal or hepatic decompensation, and a variety of other edematous or hypernatremic conditions frequently need to limit sharply their sodium intake. Consequently, formulation of medications intended for such patients should avoid significant amounts of sodium salts if possible. In general, preparations with even modest amounts of sodium bicarbonate should be labeled to indicate the amount of sodium that will be ingested with each unit dose.

When sodium bicarbonate is ingested, the absorbed bicarbonate becomes a part of the body pool, controlled by respiratory CO_2 excretion, while the absorbed sodium is eliminated by renal excretion. The urine becomes more alkaline, the rate of renal excretion of some coadministered drugs may be altered, and the solubility of solutes in the urine may change. Systemic alkalosis is also a potentially significant complication.

To avoid enhancing the sodium burden, acidic compounds are often prepared as potassium rather than sodium salts, and potassium rather than sodium bicarbonate is used in some formulations. However, excessive potassium intake is also potentially dangerous, especially in subjects with renal insufficiency and various forms of dehydration. As with sodium, control of potassium intake is frequently medically important so that its use as an excipient in formulations needs to be quantitatively limited.

The ill effects of excessive potassium are described in standard texts and numerous reports. Symptoms generally become apparent when plasma potassium levels exceed 6.5 mEq/L (43), with weakness, lassitude, and neuromuscular deficits. More immediately life threatening are the cardiovascular effects, particularly if there is an underlying cardiovascular disturbance. Electrocardiographic changes (peaking T wave) may become apparent when plasma potassium levels reach 5.5 mEq/L, and arrhythmias may develop at these levels. Patients treated with digitalis may be particularly sensitive to abnormal blood and tissue potassium levels.

To avoid the possible local irritating and ulcerogenic effects of potassium chloride when used as a medication, it may be formulated with enteric coating or extended-release formulations to be taken with food or a full glass of water. When used as an excipient in oral formulations, the amount involved is not likely to be significantly irritating to the gastrointestinal mucosa.

6. Dextrose

Dextrose is generally produced by the hydrolysis of starch. It is commonly used as a filler, particularly for chewable tablets when sweetness is desired. Dextrose excipient, a USP product, is a monohydrate of dextrose. Like other USP products, its definition of acceptability limits the allowable content of identified significant impurities such as heavy metals and sulfites.

Dextrim (starch gum) is a "halfway" dextrose produced by the partial acid hydrolysis of starch. It is a handy binding and thickening agent and is also used as an adhesive and to stiffen surgical dressings. The fact that it is a component of infant feeding formulations reflects its safety as an excipient in oral formulations.

Other USP hydrolysis products of starch (dextrates) are enzymatically produced purified mixtures of saccharides that are standardized in terms of dextrose equivalence. They are essentially nontoxic, nonparenteral excipients.

The potential of dextrose to enhance the development of dental caries and to complicate the control of diabetes is well recognized and discussed elsewhere.

There are some reports of dubious significance suggesting that the ingestion of dextrose can influence several aspects of the electrocardiographic pattern (44) in some women, and may induce a "dumping syndrome" in gastrectomized subjects (45). Large doses of glucose, especially when administered parenterally, can produce hyperkalemia in diabetics (46,47) although in normal subjects a glucose drink can result in lower serum potassium levels (46). Marked glucose intake in pregnant women may stimulate insulin release, resulting in hypoglycemia in the fetus (48,49).

In spite of these phenomena occurring with administration of large doses, glucose remains a fundamental nutrient and an excipient of unquestioned safety.

Other sugars, such as sucrose, mannitol, and sorbitol, also used in solid formulations, are discussed elsewhere.

7. Cellulose

Microcrystalline cellulose is a partially depolymerized acid hydrolysis product of purified wood cellulose, which is prepared in water-dispersible and nondispersible forms. Besides functioning as a filler, nondispersible cellulose is used as a lubricant for tablets and to adsorb water-soluble ingredients before compression. Colloidal cellulose, with or without other cellulose derivatives such as carboxymethyl cellulose or hypromellose, commonly serves as a suspending agent.

Since the celluloses are not absorbed, they are essentially devoid of systemic toxic potential when orally administered. They may have a bulk laxative effect in adequate dosage and might conceivably be broken down by bacteria in the large bowel (see discussion of lactose in subjects with lactase deficiency, above). However, they can generally be ruled out as a source of side effects in oral medications.

B. Liquid Formulations (Solvents)

Liquid medicines for oral use are still used in spite of the general inconvenience of shipping and storing, and the greater likelihood of problems with stability and contamination. When liquid dosage is relatively small, there is the possibility of significant loss or delay in the oropharynx and esophagus with a corresponding effect on the amount of drug reaching the absorbing gastrointestinal mucosa. The problem is rarely seen if the liquid dose is several milliliters and is followed by the patient drinking several ounces of an aqueous drink. However, small volumes of viscous or oily formulations can have bioavailability problems and may cause local irritation of tissues to which they may adhere.

Liquids are particularly useful for patients who have difficulty in swallowing a solid dosage form. They also permit fine gradation of dosage. Most liquid formulations are perceived as being more readily bioavailable because dissolution is not a problem. Even liquid suspensions have the advantage over solid dose forms of not having to undergo disintegration. However, the fact that an agent is formulated in true solution is no guarantee that it will be absorbed.

There are liquid formulations in which active drug is entrapped or coupled with an excipient to form an unabsorbable complex. At times this is deliberately designed so that "controlled release" takes place, to allow a slower, more prolonged period of absorption. When it is an inadvertent consequence of the excipients in the liquid formulation, it can seriously compromise bioavailability and efficacy.

Aqueous and other liquid formulations may include as solutes salts and other materials discussed in the prior section.

Side effects may result not only from the bulk liquid excipient itself, but also from the products of its possible interactions with specific drugs. Some agents are liable to hydrolysis in aqueous solutions over a period of time, especially at elevated temperatures.

A particular concern is the "leaching" of potentially toxic agents from container walls. These will be reviewed below under the heading of specific materials used as containers, some of which are also involved in the coating of solid medication and for microencapsulation of both liquid and solid dosage forms.

1. Water

Water, the universal solvent of living matter, is also the prime solvent for medicinals. In considering water as an excipient, it is essential to pay attention to a series of characteristics that influence the nature of water and its properties. Water invariably contains solutes from its containers and its atmosphere in spite of undergoing purification procedures such as distillation and filtration. The hydrogen (pH) and other ion concentrations, tonicity, oxidation potential, trace metal content, and other factors can vary and influence dissolved medicinals.

With oral aqueous solutions there is seldom a problem related to water per se. A key concern is that the aqueous medication not serve as a culture medium for microorganisms and that the water used contains no pathogens. Relatively large deviations in the pH of plain water to be used as an excipient may be of little consequence, since the medicinal solutes dissolved in the water generally are the predominent determinants of pH. Similarly, total ionic strength of plain water is so low as to generally be overwhelmed by the components added. In any event, the minor amounts of solutes responsible for the pH and ionic strength of "pure" water used for oral medication, if not overcome by the solutes added, is readily overwhelmed by the contents of the gastrointestinal tract after the medication is ingested. Consequently, minor differences in ionic strength and the pH of the water used as an excipient for oral medicinals has essentially no potential for harm. Only if very large volumes of hypotonic aqueous solutions are administered might there be problems associated with diuresis or volemia.

2. Alcohol

By far the most common alcohol used as an excipient in oral liquid medications is ethanol (ethyl alcohol). Methyl alcohol is notoriously toxic, leading to blindness and death when consumed in sufficient amounts. In most instances such consumption is inadvertent. Isopropyl alcohol, commonly used externally as "rubbing alcohol," is considerably more toxic than ethanol taken orally, and has no features that warrant its oral use over ethanol.

Alcohol itself, or diluted to highly variable degrees with water, is used to enhance solubility. Historically many natural products were extracted with alcohol to obtain the desired active ingredient, and the resulting alcoholic product was often the basis of the final formulation. Alcoholic beverages such as wine are used as palatable and convenient excipients. Alcoholic solutions of medications referred to as tinctures were the elegant formulations of pharmacy. Some of them, like tincture of camphorated opium (i.e., paregoric), are clear alcoholic solutions, but form a precipitate on contacting water. They were nevertheless therapeutically convenient and effective formulations.

A spectrum of elixirs (sweetened alcoholic solutions) are used as vehicles and range from about 75% ethanol with glycerol and no water to as little as 8% ethanol, some glycerol, and mostly water with dissolved sucrose. Agents such as codeine phosphate dissolve readily in a small volume of water and can then be added to an elixir such as terpin hydrate to make a clear, precipitate-free formulation. In contrast, solid codeine phosphate added directly to elixir terpin hydrate remains undissolved, resulting in a cloudy suspension. Such particular characteristics of altered solubility of alkaloids in various types of vehicles can cause concern that the preparation may be flawed and perhaps dangerous. While this is rarely the case, formulations with varying patterns of solubility state can be disconcerting.

The toxic effects of ethanol are well known and will not be reviewed here in detail. The amounts used as excipient can be significant in some instances, and particularly in patients who are "supersensitive" to alcohol, such as those being medicated with disulfiram, an agent that blocks the normal breakdown of acetaldehyde. Accumulation of this intermediate in the metabolism of alcohol can cause severe symptoms (50).

3. Syrups

Syrups are aqueous solutions of sugar, usually sucrose, that are commonly used as vehicles because of taste (see below). They also serve as demulcents and their viscosity can be a desired property compared to more freely running solutions. Sucrose, a disaccharide, is readily hydrolyzed in the gut to its absorbable monosaccharides, glucose and fructose. It is sometimes subjected to acid hydrolysis in vitro to form invert sugar.

Caloric (i.e., absorbable) sugars in medicinals are generally considered undesirable for diabetics. The relationship of sucrose to dental caries (51) is another argument against its use as an excipient, particularly with formulations such as lozenges that require prolonged mouth contact.

Some individuals suffer sugar intolerance because of specific enzyme deficiencies. Children with hereditary intolerance to fructose lack the hepatic enzyme fructose-1-P-aldolase (52) and are sensitive to modest doses of that sugar (52). They may show increased lactic acid and uric acid production (53). Hypoglycemia (i.e., low glucose blood levels) may accompany increases of fructose blood levels in such individuals. In general, the dangers of fructose are far more apparent as a consequence of intravenous fructose infusion (54) than from oral fructose or the disaccharide sucrose, which is hydrolyzed by intestinal sucrase to glucose and fructose. Toxic potential exists when the rate of fructose presentation to the liver exceeds its metabolizing capacity, i.e., either fructose levels accumulate, leading to a mild osmotic diuresis, or the intermediate fructose-1-phosphate accumulates, with a toxic potential to liver and kidney (55). Neither of these phenomena are likely from oral fructose. However, fructose is to be avoided in patients recognized to be intolerant.

Glucose (dextrose) the cheaper, less sweet hydrolysis product of starch that is also used for syrups, is discussed above.

4. Glycerin (Glycerol)

Glycerin is used in oral liquid preparations primarily to enhance the solubility of active ingredients. It can also serve as a sweetening agent. It is readily miscible with other solvents such as water, alcohol, and propylene glycol, but is not compatible with oxidizing agents.

Glycerin is a basic component of normal carbohydrate and fat metabolism. It is the backbone to which fatty acids are esterified to form natural fats and oils. It can therefore be expected to undergo the same fate as metabolically derived glycerol.

Dogs and rats fed 35-40% glycerol diets for 40-50 weeks showed normal growth and reproduction (56). Its use is permitted as a solvent for foods with the precaution that impurities such as the butanetriols should not be present in an amount exceeding 0.2%.

When administered orally in relatively high concentration (40%) and large doses, glycerin can be irritating to the gastric mucosa of animals (57). Its irritating effect on the lower bowel contributes to the use of glycerin rectally to promote evacuation.

Large oral doses in humans may result in gastrointestinal symptoms (nausea, vomiting, and diarrhea) and signs suggesting metabolic/electrolyte disturbances. Central nervous system (CNS) disturbances such as confusion, euphoria, drowsiness (58), and metabolic disturbances, particularly in diabetic subjects and subjects with glaucoma (59,60) have been reported. However, these clinical events were observed in situations in which glycerol was used in very large dose doses as a therapeutic agent, generally to dehydrate acute edematous lesions (61). Glycerol has also been recommended therapeutically in place of sugar, with the claim that it reduces ketosis and glycosuria in diabetics, presumably because it is a caloric carbohydrate that may not be insulin dependent (62).

The amounts of glycerol used as excipients in oral formulations rarely approach the quantities needed for the development of clinical side effects.

5. Glycols

Polyethylene glycols (PEG) (macrogol; Carbowax) are polymeric alcohols with the structure $H(O-CH_2-CH_2)_nOH$, where n is four or more. They could be classified as surfactants rather than bulk excipients. However, they are so frequently the material that gives the preparation its bulk characteristic that they are perhaps better discussed in this category. Varieties of PEG are generally classified in accordance with their average chain length or molecular weight. With increased chain length, the preparation takes on the characteristics of a gel rather than a liquid. The polymers are not orally absorbed.

The monomer, ethylene glycol, is notoriously toxic, being the solvent used to make an "elixir" of sulfanilamide that killed over 100 people in 1937 and precipitated new food and drug laws (63,64). Propylene glycol is less toxic (65), but its oral use is also associated with ill effects (66,67), particularly in persons with renal disease (68). However, the unabsorbed polymers are considered sufficiently safe for the Food and Drug Administration (FDA) to have recently approved the oral administration of high-volume doses of products containing many grams of PEG per dose to help retain water and flush out the the bowel in preparation for gastrointestinal radiologic and endoscopic studies (69).

Although there have been some rare reports of reactions to large doses of PEG (95), there are no reports of the oral absorpiton of PEG by patients with ulcerative gastrointestinal disease leading to renal toxicity characteristic of ethylene glycol. Such reports have appeared in burn patients who were treated with large amounts of PEG-based creams topically applied to denuded areas (70). Parenteral effects of PEG are reviewed elsewhere.

6. Unabsorbed Monosaccharides

Unabsorbed monosaccharides such as sorbitol, mannitol, and xylitol are used in place of the absorbable sugars in some formulations, largely to overcome the problem of sugar in diabetics. It remains to be established whether these sugars are significantly less capable of serving as substrates for organisms held responsible for the production of dental caries.

Reports of side effects after infusion of large doses of these sugars are not likely to be relevant to their oral toxicity. Nevertheless, it may be of interest to note that patients receiving such intensive infusions (of the order of 100 g/day) may suffer encephalitic reactions that have been associated with the unusual phenomenon of cerebral deposition of calcium oxalate crystals (71). Unabsorbed sugars such as lactulose are useful orally as laxatives and to control portal systemic encephalopathy, presumably because they are broken down to small acidic metabolites by colonic bacteria, resulting in the neutralization of ammonia and possibly other basic derivatives that contribute to the encephalopathic syndrome (72). Some unabsorbed monosaccharides might have a similar fate and effect if administered orally in sufficiently large quantities.

7. Oils

Many oils used as foods would appear to be intrinsically safe excipients for oral medications provided that spoilage (oxidation, rancidity) is prevented and there is no significant interaction between the medication and the oil vehicle.

Fractionated coconut oil is sometimes preferred for oral formulation of drugs that are unstable in water. It is prepared from coconut oil by hydrolysis, separation of the free fatty acids and reesterification to yield largely triglycerides of medium chain length that are more easily hydrolyzed and less dependent upon normal intestinal enzyme function. Increased absorption of calcium and magnesium, particularly the former, has been reported to result from a high dietary content of fractionated coconut oil (73).

Some subjects react to coconut oil derivatives with diarrhea and abdominal cramps. However, it generally seems to be well tolerated even in cirrhotic subjects with portal-systemic encephalopathy (74).

II. TOPICAL

Topical application probably is the route of treatment by which it is most difficult to separate components into "active" and "excipient." Of course the steroid in a hydrocortisone cream or the antibiotic in neomycin ointment are active ingredients. But their activity is critically dependent on the nature of the vehicle. How deeply into the skin does the material penetrate? Does it wash off easily? Is the preparation occlusive? Studies have shown that the "placebo" base of such preparations with only "excipients" applied topically can indeed by therapeutic (75). It is noteworthy that as of 1986 the FDA did not require the listing of excipients on labels for oral prescription preparations, but did require that excipients of topical prescription preparations be listed on the labeling.

The materials used as topical excipients would ideally exclude any component that may be a primary irritant or sensitizer. Topical excipients are selected to achieve a desired pattern of characteristics. Some can make almost invisible "vanishing" formulations, while others are designed to act as thick occlusive dressings. If these agents are improperly designed, prepared, or used, the intended purpose can be compromised and undesired reactions can result.

A frequently discussed aspect of topical formulation excipients is their contribution to the "penetration" of the active ingredient. Too often the critical question "penetration to where?" is not asked. Some formulations may allow their active ingredient to penetrate so thoroughly that measurable blood levels and systemic effects result. In fact, very special topical drug delivery systems for nitroglycerin, estrogens, and scopolamine have been designed and are marketed for controlled release and systemic action achieved through the intact skin. These agents are of sufficiently high potency to require low milligram dosage and readily penetrate the skin. A key characteristic of these percutaneous drug delivery systems is that the rate-limiting factor of drug delivery is the mechanics of the system by which the drug is delivered to the skin, rather than the time necessary to penetrate through the skin and into the circulating blood.

The most common intent of a topical formulation is to achieve a response within the topical structure to which it is applied, that is, the skin itself. In this respect, the goal of a "penetrating" topical formulation is to transport the medication into underlying local structures such as pesumably inflamed muscles, tendons, or joints rather than into the systemic circulation. However, it is often not clear if and to what extent the penetrated active ingredient enters and remains at underlying structures rather than being absorbed into the circulation. There are few examples in which it has been objectively shown that a topical formulation delivers its contents directly to organs underlying the skin.

When an adverse reaction to a topical preparation is observed, excipients are as suspect as active ingredients. This has lead to the development of a "vehicle tray" for patch testing subjects who show an adverse response to a topical preparation (76).

Topical preparations for ophthalmologic use are essentially similar to other topical formulations, and may be aqueous or oily solutions, emulsions, suspensions, or ointments. However, they require particular attention to tonicity, pH, sterility, and particularly delivery and packaging techniques that exclude the possibility of cross-contamination. Primary irritation is also likely to be of greater concern in ophthalmic than in other topical formulations.

A. Solids (Gels, Ointments, Creams)

The distinction between solids and liquids for topical formulations is often unclear. With the exception of materials formulated as dusting powders, most "solid" topical preparations are ointments, creams, gels, or other materials that take the shape of the vessel into which they are pressed. For the sake of this discussion topical materials that do not "run" when they are poured will be considered to be solids.

1. Petrolatum Hydrocarbons

The so-called mineral hydrocarbons include a wide variety of materials extracted from crude petroleum and classified in accordance with an equally wide variety of physical and chemical characteristics, including liquid, semiliquid, or solid, and white or yellow. The fractions prepared from mineral hydrocarbons that are used as excipients include:

1. Mineral oil, composed of the more liquid hydrocarbons, and also known as liquid petrolatum and liquid paraffin. It is classified as heavy or light, white or yellow.
2. Petrolatum or Vaseline, a purified mixture of semisolid hydrocarbons that has served for years as a cheap, nonaqueous topical ointment base.
3. Hard paraffin or paraffin wax, the solid fractions, composed mostly of n-alkyl compounds. They are used to stiffen ointment bases and for wax baths.

Other classifications of petrolatum are reviewed in Part III.

While adequately purified and standardized liquid petrolatum (mineral oil) is used orally or by suppository as a lubricant or laxative, its inclusion in foods or cooking is generally forbidden. Its repeated oral use is discouraged because it may interfere with the absorption of fat-soluble vitamins. However, it is allowed in concentrations of a fraction of a percent in some food products and as a component of preserving covers for whole pressed cheese and chewing compounds. The processing of petroleum into the products used for medicinals and even for machinery lubrication (77) is believed to remove components of the crude oil that might have carcinogenic potential.

Mineral oil is no longer used as a solvent for the active ingredients of nose drops or to lubricate nasopharyngeal structures because of the danger of lipoid pneumonia and lipoid granulomata when even small amounts of such materials are deposited into small airways and alveoli (78).

While absorption of mineral oil is minimal, it can be irritating and, if emulsified, may cause local granulomatous reactions (79).

Granulomatous reactions (paraffinomas) to the more solid petroleum fractions, particularly hard paraffin, is recognized as a consequence of its injection into tissue for cosmetic purposes or for pain relief (80-83).

2. Glycols

Major characteristics of the glycols have been discussed above. In topical preparations, propylene glycol has been described as both irritating and sensitizing (84-90). The nature and incidence of contact sensitivity to propylene glycol are reported to be low (91,92) but higher than that of glycerol; this subject is reviewed in detail in section III. Glycol is classified as "a minimal irritant" compared to other dermatologic excipients (93). The use of glycol as a solvent in ear drops under circumstances that permit the material to reach the middle ear has led to deafness (94). There is little information concerning the effects of butylene glycol.

The consequences of polyethylene glycol (PEG) absorption from burn-denuded skin is a serious concern when large amounts of topical preparations are applied (70). A recent FDA report cautions practitioners about the use of burn preparations and antimicrobial creams containing glycols (96). In the usual situation of topical formulations applied to essentially intact skin, these pharmaceutically helpful excipients are apparently reasonably safe. However, even the polymeric forms such as PEG can be absorbed from denuded skin and undergo enzymatic depolymerization to the systemically dangerous monomer.

3. Lanolin

This USP standardized material (97) is commonly used because of its emollient action on the skin and ability to form emulsions. It is essentially immiscible with water. Preparations of so-called hydrous wool fat (USP) are made by mixing 65-70% wool fat with paraffin and water or olive oil and water. The resulting ointment, while still essentially insoluble in water, is preferred for some formulations. Anhydrous wool fat contains no more than 0.25% water.

Allergic reactions to lanolin are reviewed in detail in Part III. They are apparently largely due to its aliphatic alcohols (98-100) and are affected by the presence of detergents that are used to recover the "wool grease" from wool (101-103). About 5-10% of eczematous patients have positive patch test reactions to lanolin (104,105).

Lanolin alcohol (wool alcohol) is a high-cholesterol (over 30%) material obtained by the saponification of lanolin. It has some capacity to absorb water, which can be useful in its role as ointment base, and can be used to prepare water-in-oil emulsions. Patch tests of 30% wool alcohol in soft paraffin did not yield particularly high incidences of positive skin sensitivity tests (106,107). The relatively high concentrations of antioxidants (up to 0.1%) added to these materials are a theoretical basis for concern.

4. Silicates

Inorganic agents such as aluminum magnesium silicate and bentonite (soap clay), which is a colloidal hydrated aluminum silicate, are used in medicated jellies and ointments and as suspending agents. Pharmaceutical grade materials are usually heat-treated to destroy spores. If cationic antibacterial preservatives are used in formulations with bentonite, they may be adsorbed and lose their efficacy.

The capacity of bentonite to absorb water and form solids or gels makes it particularly useful for aqueous external preparations such as calamine lotion. It is also useful for oil-in-water emulsions and for suspending powders.

While silicates in the lungs and in tissues are prone to cause reactions, they are generally innocent agents in topical preparations nor are they likely to be troublesome in the amounts used in oral formulations.

5. Beeswax

Beeswax, obtained from the honeycomb of bees, is prepared in yellow and white (bleached) forms and is used in ointments and in cosmetics. Reports of adverse reactions are rare. Work-up of a dermatitis reaction in a beeswax handler indicated the sensitivity to be due to the poplar resin in the crude wax, with no reaction to the purified beeswax (108).

B. Liquids (Lotions, Emulsions, Suspensions)

1. Water

Water is probably the most common excipient in topical liquid preparations and water per se is rarely a cause of reactions when reasonable precautions are taken to ensure adequate purity. The trace materials responsible for its pH rarely influence the final pH of the preparation, which is generally controlled deliberately or incidentally by other ingredients. When other ingredients are present only in very low concentration, the pH, minerals, and other trace components in water might influence these other ingredients and become significant.

With topical preparations, and especially eye preparations, sterility is particularly important. Pathogens growing in aqueous eye solutions have led to disastrous consequences. There is some concern that topical aqueous formulations such as ophthalmic solutions that are improperly sealed or are stored open may be subject to evaporation and can result in critical changes in the effective concentration of ingredients. Thus eye preparations formulated as aqueous solutions must be sterile and properly sealed.

With other topical aqueous preparations the need for sterility varies with the nature of the product. In general, water used in topical aqueous medicinal solutions should be selected and handled with essentially the same precautions as water for parenteral preparations (see below).

2. Alcohol

The toxicity of several alcohols was briefly discussed above. The use of methyl alcohol (wood alcohol, methanol) is generally discouraged even in strictly topical formulations because of the serious consequences of inadvertent oral ingestion. Isopropyl alcohol is perhaps the most common topically applied alcohol. However, it is used mostly for topical sterilization or as a cooling or soothing "rubbing alcohol" rather than as an excipient. Higher alcohols are used as excipients largely to achieve a desired consistency and "feel," as well as to help solubilize active ingredients. It is sometimes difficult to determine whether altered reactions to an alcoholic formulation are due to the excipient per se or to the change in the topical fate of the dissolved ingredient.

3. Oils

Because of problems concerning active ingredient solubility, stability, the need for prolonged surface contact and pharmaceutical elegance, many topical preparations are lotions, emulsions, or suspensions rather than simple aqueous solutions. Many of the oils used as excipients for these purposes are of natural origin and varying degrees of purity. Their potential for causing adverse reactions therefore is variable.

Oils are frequently recovered or purified by organic solvent extractions. Such extraction generally excludes aquaphilic proteins, peptides, and related potential allergens but may extract lipophilic irritants or leave harmful solvent residues. In each instance, experience with a particular material rather than hypothesis is a prime basis for evaluating potential for adverse reactions.

Liquid mineral oils (i.e., hydrocarbons extracted from petroleum) are used in topical preparations, most commonly in solid or semi solid forms. Adverse reactions have been reviewed previously.

The following are some of the more commonly used nonmineral oils and their characteristics relevant to side reactions.

a. Cottonseed oil

Cottonseed oil as a component of topical formulations has rarely been associated with side effects when properly sterilized, sealed, and stored at temperatures between 10 and 40°C (see discussion of intravenous toxicity below).

b. Coconut oil

Coconut oil and fractionated coconut oil (hydrolyzed and reesterfied) are medium-chain triglycerides, generally C_8-C_{10}. While some gastrointestinal symptoms may occur when these oils are consumed in large quantities, this class of triglycerides has found therapeutic usefulness and good tolerance in several clinical conditions involving disturbed fat metabolism, including severe liver dysfunction (74). There are essentially no safety problems in its use as a topical excipient. It is commonly used as an oral excipient.

c. Corn oil (maize oil)

Corn oil (maize oil) is widely used in foods and special diets as a fat rich in unsaturated fatty acids. Topically it is also essentially without side effects.

d. Olive oil

Olive oil is used topically as an emollient, a lubricant, and to soften skin, crusts, and ear wax. It is essentially devoid of side effects.

e. Sesame oil (gingilli oil)

Sesame oil is used particularly in liniments and as a solvent for steroids. While the oil itself seems to be devoid of toxicity, an impurity identified with it, tricresyl phosphate, is a dangerous neurotoxin. It has been responsible for polyneuropathy when consumed orally in gingilli oil (109) and is the prime cause of the widespread "ginger jake paralysis" seen particularly in alcoholics

(110). There is no significant problem in the use of sesame oil as an excipient according to U.S. National Formulary specifications. However, there are allergens in sesame oil capable of causing contact dermatitis (111).

f. Hydrogenated castor oil

Hydrogenated castor oil is used externally in ointments and tablet coatings and also as a solvent for intramuscular injectables (112). Its laxative effect in adequate oral doses is well recognized. The castor bean (*Ricinus communis*) from which it is derived can be a potent and even fatal substance (113) and is highly allergenic (114) to the point of anaphylaxis (115). However, as used for tablet coatings, the properly prepared oil is not likely to create problems, nor is its use in topical preparations likely to be troublesome.

While other vegetable oils such as persic oil from peaches and poppyseed oil are also harmlessly used as excipients, some others are generally avoided. Rapeseed oil, sometimes substituted for olive oil, is known to have toxic–allergic potential (139). Safflower oil which is mostly linoleic acid, can change its consistency and become rancid on exposure to air.

Several more or less specific fatty acid preparations are used to replace vegetable oils in formulations, particularly to resist oxidation and avoid rancidity. The high-molecular-weight materials, isopropyl myristate and isopropyl palmitate, are examples. While they are generally considered nonirritating and nonsensitizing, there has been a report of contact dermititis in patients using an antibiotic spray with isopropyl myristate. This is discussed further below (140).

4. Glycerin (Glycerol)

Glycerin is used topically not only as an excipient to carry active agents but also for its own humectant (water-retaining) and emollient (softening or soothing) properties. However, at high concentrations it can act as a drying agent since it is hygroscopic. It also has preservative properties when used in concentrations over 20%.

Glycerin is commonly used in facial creams, jellies, and soaps as well as dermatologic preparations and ear drops, where it helps soften wax and is weakly antimicrobial, besides acting as a vehicle solvent for antimicrobial and other active agents.

Experience with glycerin orally and parenterally attest to its systemic safety. Reactions to its use intravenously are essentially irrelevant to its topical application. It is unremarkable in standard hypersensitivity/irritation skin tests (84). Glycerin in water (50%) in 420 patients with eczema was also nonirritating and nonsensitizing topically, although one "allergic reaction" has been reported (116).

5. Dimethylsulfoxide

Dimethylsulfoxide (DMSO) is a relatively small uncharged molecule with a checkered medical history. Its strong characteristic odor is a limiting factor in its use as a solubilizing agent. It can dissolve highly lipophilic materials and is completely miscible with water. It readily penetrates cell membranes (117) and exerts an osmotic influence. This property may contribute to the alleged beneficial effect of topically applied DMSO in musculoskeletal inflammatory disease.

The safety of systemic DMSO is reflected in numerous animal studies as well as in its use for the preservation of blood and bone marrow components (118). Relatively large amounts are infused intravenously with these components, apparently without ill effect.

DMSO is an excellent solvent for many substances and it is assumed that its penetrating ability may carry some solutes with it (119). Consequently, the toxic potential of an agent dissolved in DMSO and applied to the skin might be different from that of the same agent dissolved in a solvent with less penetrating capacity.

Although DMSO has little systemic toxicity (120,121), when used topically it is classed as a primary irritant (119,122). There are a variety of special concerns about skin effects of DMSO on intracellular viruses and viral genomes, which are not well understood (123).

III. PARENTERALS

A key requirement of any parenteral formulation is that it must be capable of being prepared and kept in a sterile state. Special requirements apply for materials to be injected intravenously, and tolerance of tissue at the local site of injection is critical. These factors will be considered for each of the solvents to be discussed.

While water is the predominant solvent for parenterals, nonaqueous solvents have a place despite their potential dangers. Besides their inherent toxicity, they can significantly alter the pharmacological response to the active agents for which they serve as vehicles (124).

1. Water

The sterility and purity of water for injection must be ensured, and it should be pyrogen-free. With solutions for injection, and especially with highly active medicaments present in low milligram or microgram amounts, or with enzymatically or hormonally active agents, trace metal impurities in water can critically influence the state of the active ingredient, even though they are not likely to cause side effects per se.

The tonicity of the aqueous solution can be a critical factor. There are several important differences in the characteristics of aqueous solutions for intravenous (IV) vs intramuscular (IM) or subcutaneous (SC) administration.

a. Intramuscular and subcutaneous

Aqueous solutions given SC or IM that are not close to physiological tonicity can be significantly more painful than isotonic solutions. Intramuscular injection of lyophylized material that is intended to be dissolved in saline but is instead dissolved in sterile water can create considerable discomfort. Some nursing schools used to arrange for students to experience the painful consequences of an IM injection of 1 ml of sterile distilled water so that they would appreciate the importance of distinguishing between water and saline when it is necessary to dissolve an injectable medication stored in solid form.

b. Intravenous

Hypertonic solutions infused slowly IV are generally well tolerated, although even modest volumes of hypotonic solution or water given intravenously can result in significant hemolysis, especially if injected rapidly. The need to emphasize this point is illustrated by the anecdote about a medical student whose supervising resident physician asked him to write an order of intravenous fluids for a newly admitted diabetic patient in congestive heart failure who could not tolerate fluids by mouth. The student reasoned that he did not want to infuse glucose to a hyperglycemic diabetic, or salt to a patient in congestive heart failure, so instead of the usual 5% glucose or 0.9% saline for IV infusion, he ordered sterile water. The resident physician had to point out that in spite of the apparent logic of his thinking, water alone infused intravenously will result in hemolysis. If the volume and speed of infusion are sufficiently rapid, it could be fatal. The formulation of potent medications intended for intravenous use must be carefully prepared to ensure that the final solution is not dangerously hypotonic. In contrast, hypertonic solutions are not absolutely contraindicated for intravenous use. If administered slowly, they do not, as a rule, present a problem of hemolysis.

Solutions for IV use must avoid antioxidants and preservatives often used safely in preparations for SC and IM injection. Since intravenous medications are commonly given in 5% glucose solutions, it is noteworthy that such solutions are more likely to cause thrombophlebitis if they are sterilized by autoclaving rather than filtration (125), possibly because of the lower pH of autoclaved glucose solutions. Autoclaving results in the production of several acids, including formic acid, levulinic acid, furfural, and particularly 5-hydroxymethyl furfural (126, 127). Raising the pH with sodium bicarbonate (128) or neutralizing with phosphate buffer (pH 6.8) essentially eliminates the occurrence of thrombophlebitic reactions (125).

Intravenous glucose solutions have been reported to suppress gastric secretion, influence gastric function tests, and affect the absorption of some drugs (129). Isotonic salt solution used intravenously did not have these actions.

1. Glycols

Toxic effects with some glycol formulations were at first ascribed to the active ingredient dissolved in the glycol (130) but were later shown to be due to the glycol itself (131). It is now apparent that large doses of parenterally administered polyethylene glycol (PEG) can be expected to be toxic as a consequence of enzymatic hydrolysis of the polymer in vivo to mono, di, and triethylene glycol (see above). By analogy with ethylene glycol, PEG is believed to be oxidized in the body to acid alcohols and diacids, which are potent calcium chelators and are toxic to renal epithelial cells (63). The consequences of systemic absorption or injection of excessive quantities of PEG include elevated osmolarity, acidosis, elevated total plasma calcium, and renal dysfunction due to the toxic depolymerized species that are chemically identifiable in the plasma and urine. These consequences require many grams of absorbed or injected PEG, so that the modest quantities used to solubilize medication for small-volume injections have not been associated with detectable toxicity. However special caution is required for injectables intended for patients with renal impairment (132) and for infants since, on a per kilo basis, dangerously large amounts of solvent may be administered with serious consequences (133,134). There may also be local irritations at the site of injection if the amounts are excessive (135).

Propylene glycol is less toxic than ethylene glycol, but has been reported to be responsible for acute cardiovascular collapse when used as a solvent for some parenteral preparations (136) and is of particular concern in patients with renal impairment (89).

While there has been some discussion about the carcinogenic potential of macrogels (56,137), this is not significant. Discussions of these agents used orally were presented previously.

2. Glycerin (Glycerol)

Because of its efficacy as a solvent, glycerin is used in parenteral preparations, but with several precautions, since it is capable of causing intravascular hemolysis, hematuria, renal damage, and hyperglycemia (61).

The hyperosmolality resulting from large doses of glycerol administered intravenously represents the prime mechanism for its adverse effects as well as its systemic use as a therapeutic agent. When large intravenous doses are given in an effort to reduce intracranial pressure, hemolysis may occur (138). However, limiting the infusion rate to under 10 g/hr (diluted in isotonic saline) seems to avoid this problem (139). A tabular summary of adverse effects reported following IV glycerin presented by Frank et al. (61) supports the importance of infusion rate/dose. Adverse systemic effects of excessive glycerol have been discussed above.

While a suspension of red blood cells in isoosmotic glycerol (2.6%) is reported to result in hemolysis (140), glycerol–saline solutions are used routinely by blood banks to prepare red blood cells for freezing. The high glycerol content of these cells makes freeze preservation possible, and the thawed cells are deglycerinated stepwise with hypertonic saline to prepare them for infusion as viable isotonic cells. Thus there is no fundamental incompatibility between glycerin as such and red blood cells. In fact, cryoprotection can be added to the long list of uses for glycerol (141).

Glycerol has essentially no toxic potential when used in the small amounts involved in the usual type of intravenous preparation with glycerol as a solvent.

3. Other Nonaqueous Solvents

A wide variety of nonaqueous solvents are used as excipients for parenteral products. These include fats of the type generally considered nutrients, so called fixed oils, and nonglyceryl esters of fatty acids such as ethyl oleate, isopropyl myristate, benzyl benzoate, dicrolenes, and others (56).

Some formulations of fat-soluble (and water-insoluble) vitamins and other medications are well tolerated intravenously. It is difficult to determine whether reports of unusual reactions to some of these preparations, such as rectal itching after Mephyton, a clear, water-miscible K_1 oxide preparation, are due to the active ingredient itself or the nature of the formulation. In any event, the fact that a solvent or other useful excipient is not miscible with water does not automatically rule out its potential to be formulated for parenteral use.

Several oils, including cottonseed oil and Pitkin menstruum have a long and dubious history of use as solvents intended to result in delayed absorption from the site of intramuscular injection. Local reactions, often painful and prolonged, have been the rule rather than the exception. Absorption rates are likely to be erratic. A commonly overlooked phenomenon is the tissue binding and subsequent slow release of some materials injected intramuscularly in simple aqueous solution, so that formulation into nonaqueous solvents is not necessary or rational. An intramuscular preparation should not be formulated with oils unless and until it is demonstrated that the absorption pattern following the use of appropriate aqueous solvents is unacceptable.

Polyethoxylated castor oil (Cremophor EL) has been used as a solvent for an intravenous steroid anesthetic and for miconazole. Apparently in large doses it can cause a hepatitislike reaction (142). Castor oil has been discussed previously.

With the development of lipid preparations for parenteral nutrition, the possibility of using such formulations as vehicles becomes a distinct possibility. While the early fat emulsion preparations for intravenous feeding caused significant side effects, current formulations are considered safe, even though there are concerns about their effect on platelets (143).

Preparations made of cottonseed oil for intravenous nutrition can cause an "overload syndrome", presumably as a result of fat embolism, and attributed to failure of the emulifying/stabilizing agent rather than the oil itself (144).

The National Formulary (NF XVI, 1985) describes products of glycerin esterified with acetic acid and fatty acids from edible fat called diacetylated monoglycerides. There is little information about their safety. Similarly, little is known about the potential side effects of gels of aluminum monstearate used suspended in oil to adsorb active components (112).

IV. SUPPOSITORIES

Suppositories are generally fatty preparations with melting points below body temperature and solidification points above room temperature. These characteristics are dictated by the need to have a reasonably solid dose form on insertion and a liquid form for absorption, since achieving dissolution or enzymatic degradation of an excipient in the rectum is difficult.

The lipidic bases used are almost all triglycerides, usually from vegetable fats, but also specific mixtures of mono-, di-, and triglycerides and their hydrogenated or ethoxylated derivatives (145). Beeswax is also occasionally used (see above). Emulsifying bases with PEG and water-soluble bases are prepared from various polyethylenes, glycerin, and gelatin. Glycerin suppositories as such are used to induce bowel movement, probably reflecting both a mildly irritating and lubricating action.

There is little literature to indicate side effects specific to suppository excipients. Some suppository formulations include detergents, some of which can apparently influence drug absorption via the rectum without the type of intestinal mucosal damage sometimes otherwise seen as a response to detergents (146).

REFERENCES

1. Lockey, S.D., Sr. Reactions to hidden agents in foods, beverages and drugs. Ann. Allergy 29:461 (1971).
2. Darkwala, J.B. Chewable tablets. *In* Pharmaceutical Dosage Forms: Tablets (Lieberman, H.A. and Lachman, L, eds.). Marcel Dekker, New York pp. 289–337 (1980).
3. Warshaw, A.L. Diagnosis of starch peritonitis by paracentesis. Lancet 2: 1054–56 (1972).
4. Sternlieb, J.J. Starch peritonitis and its prevention. Arch. Surg. 112:458–461 (1977).
5. Michaels, L. and Shah, N.S. Dangers of corn starch powder. Br. Med. J. 2: 714 (1973).

6. Neely, J. and Davis, J. Starch granulomatosis of the peritoneum. Br. Med. J. 3:625–29 (1971).

7. Dunkley, B. and Lewis, T.T. Meningeal reaction to starch powder in the cerebrospinal fluid. Br. Med. J. 2:1391–1392 (1977).

8. Fernadez, G.S. and Genis, M.Y.C. Formation of aflatoxin in different type of starches for pharmaceutical use. Pharm. Acta Helv. 54:78–81 (1979).

9. Detroy, R.W., Lillehoj, E.B. and Ciegler, A. Aflatoxin and related compounds. In Microbial Toxins (Ciegler, A., Kadis, S. and Ajl, S.J., eds.). Academic Press, New York, pp. 3–178 (1971).

10. Randolph, T.G. Allergy to so-called "inert ingredients" (excipients) of pharmaceutical preparations. Ann. Allergy 7:519–529 (1950).

11. Toxicological evaluation of hdyroxypropyl distarch phosphate. WHO Fd. Ad. Ser. No. 5, 355–357 (1974).

12. Toxicological evaluation of oxidized starch. WHO Fd. Ad. Ser. No. 5, 365–367 (1974).

13. Dahlquist, A. The baric aspects of the chemical background of lactase deficiency. Postgrad. Med. J. 53:57–62 (1977).

14. American Academy of Pediatrics. Committee on Nutrition. The practical significance of lactose intolerance in children. Pediatrics 62:240–245 (1978).

15. Bridge, S.J., Keutmann, H.T., Cuatrecasas, P. and Whedon, G.D. Osteoporosis, intestinal lactose deficiency and low dietary calcium intake. N. Engl. J. Med. 276:445–448 (1967).

16. When does lactose malabsorption matter in adults? Br. Med. J. 2:351–352 (1975).

17. Brown, J.L. Health hazard of unlabeled ingredients in pharmaceuticals. Pediatrics 73:402–404 1984.

18. Lieb, J. and Kazinko, D.J. Lactose filler as a cause of drug induced diarrhea. N. Engl. J. Med. 299:314 (1978).

19. Gundmand-Hower, E., Dahlquist, A. and Jarnum, S. The clinical significance of lactose malabsorption. Am. J. Gastroenterol. 53:460–471 (1970).

20. Conn, H.D. and Lieberthal, M.M. The Hepatic Coma Syndromes and Lactulose. Williams & Williams, Baltimore (1979).

21. Nose, O., Iida, Y., Kai, H., Harada, T., Ogawa, M. and Yabauchi, H. Breath hydrogen test for detecting lactose malabsorption in infants and children. Arch. Dis. Child. 54:436–440 (1979).

22. Newcomer, A.D. disaccharidase deficiencies. May Clin. Proc. 48:648–652 (1973).

23. Isokoski, M., Jussila, J. and Sarna, S. A simple screening test for lactose malabsorption. Gastroenterology 62:28–32 (1972).

24. Saki, T., Isokoski, M., Jussila, J., Launiala, K. and Pyorala, K. Recessive inheritance of adult-type lactose malabsorption. Lancet 2:823–826 (1973).

25. Saki, T. Lactose absorption in populations in Finland. Scand. J. Gastroenterol. 9:303–308 (1974).

26. Calloway, D.H., Murphy, E.L. and Bauer, D. Determination of lactose intolerance by breath analysis. Am. J. Dig. Dis. 14:811–815 (1969).

27. Newcomb, A.D., McGill, D.B., Thomas, P.J. and Hoffman, A.F. Prospective comparison of indirect methods for detecting lactose deficiency. N. Engl. J. Med. 293:1232–1235 (1975).
28. Metz, G., Jenkins, D.J.A., Peters, T.J., Newman, A. and Blendis, L.M. Breath hydrogenes or hapnotic method for hypolactasia. Lancet 1:1155–1157 (1975).
29. Lactose malabsorption and lactose intolerance. Lancet 2:831–832 (1979).
30. Tyrer, J.H., et al. Outbreak of anticonvulsant intoxication in an Australian city. Br. Med. J. 4:271 (1970).
31. Wise, A. Influence of calcium on trace metal-phytate interactions. In Phytic Acid: Chemistry and Applications (Graf, E., ed.). Pilatus Press, Minneapolis, pp. 151–160 (1986).
32. Elwood, P.C., Sweetman, P.M., Beasley, W.H., Jones, D. and France, R. Magnesium and calcium in the myocardium: Cause of death and area differences. Lancet 2:720–722 (1980).
33. Blum, M., Kirsten, M. and Worth, M.H., Jr. Reversible hypertension caused by the hypercalcemia of hyperthyroidism, vitamin D toxicity and calcium infusion. JAMA 237:262–263 (1977).
34. Heinonen, O.P., Slone, D. and Shapiro, S. Inorganic compounds and certain vitamins. In Birth Defects and Drugs in Pregnancy (Kaufman, D.W., ed.). Publishing Sciences Group, Littleton, Massachusetts pp. 401–408 (1977).
35. Selye, H. Calciphylaxia. University of Chicago Press, Chicago (1982)
36. McGuigan, J.E. Consequences of excess hormonal secretion in digestive disease. May Clin. Proc. 48:634–636 (1973).
37. Stiel, J.N., Mitchell, C.A., Radcliff, F.J. and Piper, D.W. Hypercalcemia in patients with peptic ulceration receiving large doses of calcium carbonate. Gastroenterology 53:900–904 (1967).
38. Robson, R.H. and Heading, R.C. Obsolete but dangerous antacid preparation. Postgrad. Med. J. 54:36–37 (1978).
39. Ginsburg, D.S., Kaplan, E.L. and Katz, A.I. Hypercalcemia after oral calcium carbonate therapy in patients on chronic hemodialysis. Lancet 1:1271–1274 (1973).
40. Douglas, N.A. Enamel erosion with lemon juice. Br. Dent. J. 122:300–302 (1967).
41. Nishi, Y., Kittaka, E., Fukuda, K., Hatamo, S. and Usmi, T. Copper deficiency associated with alkali therapy in a patient with renal tubular acidosis. J. Pediatr. 98:81–83 (1981).
42. Wilson, R.G. and Farndon, J.R. Hyperkalemic cardiac arrhythmia caused by potassium citrate mixture. Br. Med. J. 284:197–198 (1982).
42a. Pounsford, J.C., Birch, M.J. and Saunders, K.B. Effect of bronchodilators on the cough response to inhaled citric acid in normal and asthmatic subjects. Thorax 40:662–7 (1985).
43. Newmark, S.R. and Dluhy, R.G. Hyperkalemia and hypokalemia. J.A.M.A. 231:631–633 (1975).
44. Ostrander, L.D. The effect of glucose ingestion upon electrocardiograms in an epidemiological study. Am. J. Med. Sci. 251:399–404 (1966).

45. Naumann, H.N. Glucose tolerance and "dumping" syndrome. J.A.M.A. 195:700–701 (1966).
46. Viberti, G.C. Glucose-induced hyperkalaemia: A hazard for diabetics? Lancet 1:690 (1978).
47. Goldfarb, S., Cox, M., Singer, I. and Goldberg, M. Acute hyperkalemia induced by hyperglycemia hormonal mechanisms.? Ann. Intern. Med. 84: 426–432 (1976).
48. Light, I.J., Keenan, W.J. and Sutherland, J.M. Maternal intravenous glucose administration as a cause of hypoglycemia in the infant of a diabetic mother. Am. J. Obstet. Gynecol. 113:345–350 (1972).
49. Kenepp, N.B., Shelley, W.C., Grabbe, S.G., Kumar, S., Stanley, C.A. and Gutsche, B.B. Fetal and neonatal hazards of maternal hydration with 5% dextrose before cesarean-section. Lancet 1:1150–1152 (1982).
50. Fuller, R.K., Branchey, L., Brightwell, D.R., et al: Disulfiram treatment of alcoholism. J.A.M.A. 256:1449–1455 (1986).
51. Yudkin, J. Sugar and disease. Nature 239:197–199 (1972).
52. Black, J.A. and Simpson, K. Fructose intolerance. Br. Med.J. 4:138–141 (1967).
53. Mehnert, H. and Forster, H. Fructose-induced hyperuricaemia. Lancet 2: 1205 (1967).
54. Editorial. Fructose infusion hazards. Can Med. Assoc. J. 108:1208 (1973).
55. Hazards of fructose infusion. Comments section. Med. J. Aust. 2:1220–1221 (1972).
56. Spiegel, A.J. and Noseworthy, M.M. Use of non-aqueous solvents in parenteral products. J. Pharm. Sci. 52:917–927 (1963).
57. Staples, R., Misher, A. and Wardell, J., Jr. Gastrointestinal irritant effect of glycerin as compared with sorbitol and proylene glysol in rats and dogs. J. Pharm. Sci. 56:398–400 (1967).
58. MacLaren, N.K., Cowles, C., Ozand, P.T., Shuttee, R. and Cornblath, M. Glycerol intolerance in a child with intermittent hypoglycemia. J. Pediatr. 86:43–49 (1975).
59. Oakley, D.E. and Ellis, P.P. Glycerol and hyperosmolar nonketotic coma. Am. J. Ophthalmol. 81:469 (1976).
60. D'Alena, P.T. and Ferguson, W. Arch. Ophthalmol. 75:201 (1966).
61. Frank, M.S.B., Nahata, M.C. and Hilty, M.D. Glycerol: Review of its pharmacology, pharmacokinetics, adverse reactions and clinical use. Pharmacotherapy 1:147–160 (1981).
62. Freund, G. The metabolic effects of glycerol administered to diabetic patients. Arch. Intern. Med. 121:123 (1968).
63. Beasley, V.R. and Buck, W.B. Acute ethylene-glycol toxicicosis: A review. Vet. Hum. Toxicol. 22:255–263 (1980).
64. Drug bioequivalence—A report of the office of Technology Assessment Drug Bioequivalence Study Panel. Office of Technology Assessment, Washington, D.C., July 15, 1974.
65. Weil, C.S., Woodside, M.D. Smyth, H.F., Jr. and Carpenter, C.P. Results of feeding PG in the diet to dogs for 2 years. Fd. Cosmet. Toxicol. 9:479–490 (1971).

66. Axulanatham, K. and Genel, M. Central nervous system toxicity associated with ingestion of propylene glycol. J. Pediatr. 93:515–516 (1978).
67. Hannuksela, M. and Forstrom, L. Reactions to peroral propylene glycol. Contact Derm. 4:41–45 (1980).
68. Cate, J.C. and Hedrick, R. Propylene glycol intoxication and lactic acidosis. N. Engl. J. Med. 303:1237 (1980).
69. Meadows, J.O. and Conyers, C.T. Golytely: Preparation of choice for colonoscopy. Gastrointest. Endosc. 29:256 (1983).
70. Herold, D.A., Rodeheaves, G.T., Bellamy, W.T., Fitton, L.A., Bruns, D.E. and Edlich, R.F. Toxicity of topical PEG. Toxicol. Appl. Pharmacol. 65: 329–335 (1982).
71. Peiffer, J., Danner, E. and Schmidt, P.F. Oxalate induced encephalitic reactions to polyol-containing infusions during intensive care. Clin. Neuropathol. 3:76 (1984).
72. Conn, H.O. and Lieberthal, M.M. The Hepatic Coma Syndrome and Lactalose. Williams & Wilkins, Baltimore (1979).
73. Tantibhedhyangkul, P. and Hashim, S.A. Medium-chain triglyericde feeding in premature infants: Effects on calcium and magnesium absorption. Pediatrics 61:537–545 (1978).
74. Halary, M.M., Bolton, C.H., Morris, J.S. and Read, A.E. Medium chain triglycerides and hepatic encephalopathy. Gut 15:180–184 (1974).
75. Eaglestein, W.H. and Mertz, P.M. Effect of topical medicaments on the role of repair of superficial wounds. In The Surgical Wound (Dineen, P. and Dildrick-Smith, G., eds.). Lea & Febiger, Philadelphia, pp. 150–170 (1981).
76. Fisher, A.A., Pascher, F. and Kanof, N.B. Allergic contact dermatitis due to ingredients of vehicles. A "vehicle tray" for patch testing. Arch. Dermatol. 104:286–290 (1971).
77. Risk of contact with mineral oils used in engineering. Br. Med. J. 3:44 (1973).
78. Varkey, B. and Kutty, A.V.P. Lipoid pneumonia with lipoid granulomata in scalene node. Ann. Intern. Med. 84:176–177 (1976).
79. Mazier, W.P., Sun, K.M. and Robertson, W.G. Oil-induced granuloma (eleoma) of the rectum. Dis. Colon Rectum 21:292–294 (1978).
80. Lame, E.L., Sohn, S.S. and Levin, D.W. Calcified paraffinomas of the subcutaneous tissues: Case report. Milit. Med. 139:818–819 (1974).
81. Bolem, J.J. and van der Waal, I. Paraffinoma of the face. Oral Surg. 38: 675–682 (1974).
82. Crosbie, R.B. and Kaufman, H.D. Self-inflicted oleogranuloma of breast. Br. Med. J. 3:840–841 (1967).
83. Arouete, M.H. and Grupper, C. Vaslinome de la paupière. Bull. Soc. Fr. Dermatol. Syphiligr. 77:808–810 (1970).
84. Fisher, A.A. Reactions to popular cosmetic humectants. Part III: Glycerin, propylene glycol and butylene glycol. Cutis 26:243 (1980).
85. Fisher, A.A. The management of propylene glycol-sensitive patients. Cutis 25:24 (1980).
86. Fisher, A.A. Propylene glycol dermatitis. Cutis 21:166 (1978).

87. Hannuskela, M. Allergic and toxic reaction caused by cream bases in dermatological patients. Int. J. Cosmet. Sci. 1:257–263 (1979).

88. Hannuksela, M., Pirilla, V., and Salo, O.P. Skin reactions to propylene glycol. Contact Derm. 1:112–116 (1978).

89. Demey, H., Daelemans, R., DeBroe, M.E. and Bossaert, L. Propylene glycol intoxication due to intravenous nitroglycerin. Lancet 1:1360 (1984).

90. Fisher, A.A. and Brancaccio, R.R. Allergic contact sensitivity to propylene glycol in a lubricant jelly. Arch. Dermatol. 115:1451 (1979).

91. Angelini, G. and Meneghini, C.L. Contact allergy from propylene glycol. Contact Derm. 7:197–198 (1981).

92. Hannuksela, M. Allergic and toxic reactions caused by cream bases in dermatological patients. Int. J. Cosm. Sci. 1:257–263 (1979).

93. Trancik, R.J. and Maibach, H.I. Propylene glycol: Imitation or sensitization? Contact Derm. 8:185–189 (1982).

94. Monzono, T. and Johnstone, B.M. Ototoxicity of chloramphenical ear drops with propylene glycol as solvent. Med. J. Aust. 2:634–638 (1975).

95. Marsh, W.H., Bronner, M.H., Yantis, Y.L. et al.: Ventricular ectopy associated with peroral colonic lavage Gastrointest. Endosc. 32:259–263 (1986).

96. Topical PEG in burn ointments. FDA Drug Bull. 12:25 (1982).

97. USP specifications for lanolin USP XXI, p. 582–583 (1985) or lanolin, lanolin anhydran. Anhydrous lanolin. USP XXI: 583 (1985).

98. Briet, R. and Bandmann, H.-J. Contact dermatitis XXII Dermatitis from lanolin. Br. J. Dermatol. 88:414–415 (1973).

99. Lanolin Allergy. Br. Med. J. 2:379–380 (1973).

100. Schlossman, M.L. and McCarthy, J.P. Lanolin and derivatives chemistry. Relationship to allergic contact dermatitis. Contact Derm. 5:65–72 (1979).

101. Clark, E.W., Cronin, E. and Wilkinson, D.S. Lanolin with reduced sensitizing potential. Contact Derm. 3:69–74 (1977).

102. Bourrinet, P. and Berkovic, A. Cutaneous hypersensitivity test in guinea pig of lanolin and derivatives. Ann. Pharm. Fr. 38:483–492 (1980).

103. Takano, S., Yamanaka, M., Okamoto, K. and Saito, F. Allergens of lanolin. Part I. Isolation and identification of the allergens of hydrogenated lanolin. Part 2. Allergenicity of synthetic alkane -B-diole and alkane -W-diole. J. Soc. Cosmet. Chem. 34:99–125 (1983).

104. Wereide, K. Contact allergy to wool-fat ("lanolin"). Acta. Derm. Venerol. 45:15–18 (1965).

105. Clark, E.W. Estimation of the general incidence of specific lanolin allergy. J. Soc. Cosmet. Chem. 26:323–335 (1975).

106. Bandmann, H.J., Calnan, C.D., Cronin, E., Hjorth, N., Magnusson, B., Maibach, H., Malten, K.E., Meneghini, C.L., Pirilla, V. and Wilkinson, D.S. Dermatitis from applied medicaments. Arch. Dermatol. 106:335–337 (1972).

107. Hannuksela, M., et al. Sensitivity due to wool alcohol. Contact Derm. 2:105 (1976).

108. Rothenborg, H.W. Occupational dermatitis in beekeepers due to popular resins in beeswax. Arch. Dermatol. 95:381–384 (1967).
109. Senayake, N. and Jeyaratnam, J. Toxic polyneuropathy due to gingilli-oil contaminated with tri-cresylphosphate affecting adolescent girls in Sri Lanka. Lancet 1:88 (1981).
110. Ramirez, M. and Eller, J.J. "Patch" test in "contractile dermatitis" (dermatitis venenata). Allergy 1:489 (1930).
111. Neering, H., Vitanyi, B.E.J., Malten, K.E., Van Ketel, W.G. and van Dijk, E. Allergens in sesame oil contact dermatitis. Acta. Derm. Venerol. 55: 31–34 (1975).
112. Deasy, P.B. Coating properties. In Microencapsulation and Related Drug Processes (Deasy, P.B. ed.). Marcel Dekker, New York, pp. 22–25 (1984).
113. Knight, B. Ricin—potent homicidal poison. Br. Med. J. 1:350–351 (1979).
114. Wolfromm, R., Gubert, L., Rivolier, J. and Tournier, J. Epidemic of ricinus allergy in Dieppe. Presse Med. 75:2157–2160 (1967).
115. Lockey, S.D. and Dunkelberger, L. Anaphylaxis from an Indian necklace. J. A. M. A. 206:2900–2901 (1968).
116. Hannuksela, M. and Forstrom, L. Contact hypersensitivity to glycerol. Contact Derm. 2:291 (1976).
117. Franco, R.S., Wagner, K., Weiner, M. and Martelo, O.J. Preparations of low affinity red cells with DMSO-mediated IHP incorporation. Am. J. Hematol. 17:393–400 (1984).
118. Appelbaum, F.R., Herzig, G.P., Ziegler, J.L., Graw, R.G., Levine, A.S. and Deisseroth, A.B. Successful engraftment of cryopreserved autologous bone marrow in patients with malignant lymphoma. Blood 52:85 (1978).
119. Danober, R. Idoxuridine in herpes zoster: Further evaluation of intermittent topical therapy. Br. Med. J. 2:526–527 (1974).
120. Brobyn, R.D. The human toxicology of dimethyl sulfoxide. Ann. N.Y. Acad. Sci. 243:497–506 (1975).
121. Kligman, A.M. Topical pharmacology and toxicology of dimethyl sulfoxide—1 & 2. J.A.M.A. 193:796–807 (1965).
122. Malten, K.E. and Arend, J.D. Topical toxicity of various concentrations of DMSO recorded with impedence measurements and water vapor loss measurements. Contact Derm. 4:80–92 (1978).
123. Handschumacher, R.E. Aspects of pharmacology pertinent to the skin. Clin. Pharmacol. Ther. 16:865–868 (1974).
124. Spiegel, A.J. and Noseworthy, M.M. Use of nonaqueous solvents in parenteral products. J. Pharm. Sci. 52:917–929 (1963).
125. Vere, D.W., Skykes, C.H. and Armitage, P. Venous thrombosis during dextrose infusion. Lancet 2:627–630 (1960).
126. Taylor, R.B. and Sood, V.C. An HPLC study on the initial stages of dextrose decomposition in neutral solution. J. Pharm. Pharmacol. 30:510–511 (1978).
127. Ogata, M., Shikazaki, T., Matsuura, T. and Shimada, F. Furqural as a new decomposition product of glucose solution under oxygen atmosphere. J. Pharm. Pharmacol. 30:668 (1978).
128. Fonkalsrud, E.W. Neutralization of IV fluids. N. Engl. J. Med. 280:1480 (1969).

129. Moore, J.G. Gastric acid suppression by intravenous glucose solution. Gastroenterology 64:1106–1110 (1973).
130. McCabe, W.R., Jackson, G.G. and Grieble, H.G. Treatment of chronic pyelonephritis. 2. Short-term intravenous administration of single and multiple antibacterial agents—Acidosis and toxic nephropathy from a preparation of intravenous nitrofurantoin. Arch. Intern. Med. 104:710 (1959).
131. Spiegel, A.J. and Noseworthy, M.M. Use of non-aqueous solvents in parenteral products. J. Pharm. Sci. 52:917 (1963).
132. McCabe, W.R., Jackson, G.G. and Grieble, H.G. Treatment of chronic pyelonephritis. Arch. Intern. Med. 104:710–719 (1959).
133. McKean, D.L. and Pesce, A.S. Determination of polysorbate in ascites fluid from a premature infant. J. Anal. Toxciol. 9:174–176 (1985).
134. Martin, G. and Finberg, L. Propylene glycol: A potentially toxic vehicle in liquid dosage form. J. Pediatr. 77:877–878 (1970).
135. Carpenter, C.P. and Shaffer, C.B. A study of polyethylene glycols as vehicles for IM and SC injectins. J. Am. Pharm. Assoc. Sci. Ed. 41:27–29 (1952).
136. Gross, D.V.M., et al. Cardiovascular effects of I.V. propylene glycol and of oxytetracyclene in proprylene glycol in calves. Am. J. Vet. Res. 40:783 (1979).
137. Greene, M.H., Young, T.I. and Eisenbarth, G.S. Polyethylene glycol in suppositories: Carcinogenic? Ann. Intern. Med. 93:781 (1980).
138. K. Hagnevik, et al. Lancet 1:75 (1974).
139a. Tabuenca, J.M. Toxic-allergic syndrome caused by ingestion of rapeseed oil denatured with aniline. Lancet 2:567–568 (1981).
139b. Mateo, I.M., Izquierdo, M. et al. Toxic epidemic syndrome: musculoskeletal manifestations. J. Rheumatol. 11:333–338 (1984).
139c. Solis-Herrugo, J.A., Vidal, J.V. et al. Nodular regenerative hyperplasia of the liver associated with toxic oil syndrome: Report of 5 cases. Hepatology 6:687–693 (1986).
140. Hammarlund, E.R. and Pedersen-Bjergaard, K. Hemolysis of erythrocytes in various iso-osmotic solutions. J. Pharm. Sci. 50:24 (1961).
141. Pegg, D.E. Advances in cryobiology. Practitioner 221:543 (1978).
142. Lawler, P.G.P., McHutchon, A. and Bamber, P.A. Potential hazards of prolonged steroid anesthesia. Lancet 1:1270–1271 (1983).
143. Burnham, W.R., Cockbill, S.R., Heptinstall, S. and Harrison, S. Blood platelet behavior during infusion of an intralipid based intravenous feeding mixture. Postgrad. Med. J. 58:152–155 (1982).
144. Goulon, M., Barois, A., Grosbuis, S. and Schortgen, G. Fat embolism after repeated perfusion of lipid emulsion. Nouv. Presse Med. 3:13–18 (1974).
145. Ritschel, W.A. Advanced Biopharmaceutics. University of Cincinnati Press, Cincinnati (1974).
146. Tsuchiya, S., Aramaki, Y., Ozawa, S. and Matsumaru, H. Effects of polyoxytethylene cetylether on the absorption of $3'$–$4'$ dideoxykanamycin B from rat rectum. Int. J. Pharm. 14:279–290 (1983).

7
Adverse Effects: Coatings

I. Capsules   121
II. Tablet coatings   123
III. Containers for liquids   126
    A. Plastics   126
    B. Glass   127
IV. Microencapsulation   127
    References   128

The coatings to be reviewed in this section include not only the materials used to cover dosage units, such as capsules and tablets, but also the containers for liquids (glass and plastic) as well as materials used to "microencapsulate" active ingredients to make them suitable to the objectives of the formulation, including solubility, flow characteristics, and availability for absorption (controlled release).

The reason for interest in the toxic potential of coatings that are ingested with the medication is obvious. For containers that are presumed to be merely inert vessels, there would seem to be little basis for concern. However, experience teaches that very few materials are really "inert." It took centuries to discover that water running through lead pipes can be dangerously contaminated, and that toxic amounts of other metals such as cadmium can be leached from metal alloy containers by acidic solutions.

This discussion will review the potential for adverse effects from materials used in capsules, tablet coatings, containers for liquids and creams, and microencapsulations. A recent review (1) includes a tabulation of some 60 commonly used "film-formers" used for microencapsulation and related applications.

I. CAPSULES

Capsules are small, unit-dose containers that are premanufactured and then filled with medication. They obviate the need to compress material with adequate firmness to maintain a solid shape, as with tablets. Consequently, capsules are

121

less likely to have dispersion problems once dissolution of the capsule itself takes place, and dissolution is a function of the capsule itself independent of its contents. Local irritation may occur at a site where a tablet of aspirin or potassium chloride may lodge (2), but such local irritation is less likely to occur with capsules.

In recent times, the potential for criminal tampering with gelatin capsules has led to a preference for tablets, even though gelatin capsules are a more rational pharmaceutical form when rapid disintegration and dispersion are desired.

Most capsules are made primarily of gelatin, a protein derived by the partial hydrolysis of collagen obtained from connective tissue in the skin and bones of animals. Commercial gelatin may be prepared by acidic or basic treatment (Pharmagel A and B) and may contain several additional products, such as surfactants, coloring agents, and antimicrobial agents. Gelatin preparations with excessive amounts of sulfur dioxide (more than 0.15% according to USP XXI) are not considered suitable (see Chapter 5 for a discussion of sulfites).

Gelatin capsules may be hard or soft, depending on whether they are treated with hardening agents such as sucrose, or plasticized into thicker, softer capsules by the addition of polyols such as glycerin or sorbitol (3).

Gelatin is used in the form of an absorbable sponge or film to place over wounds for surgical hemostasis. There are apparently no direct undesired side effects as a consequence of this application. However, gelatin or collagen dressings that are not changed at frequent intervals can be a nutrient source for microorganisms that may contribute to local infection. Side effects from the intravenous infusion of gelatin as a plasma expander (4) (discussed elsewhere), is not relevant to its use as a coating for oral medications.

The major use for gelatin as an excipient is in oral preparations, particularly as both hard and flexible gelatin shells or capsules. Gelatin characteristically takes on several times its weight in water, becoming soft and swollen, and releasing its contents even though its solubility in the absence of proteolytic enzymes in cold water is poor. Gelatin desserts are made by dissolving powdered gelatin in hot water. On cooling, the solution solidifies into a characteristic semisolid commonly referred to as "gelatinous." From the pharmaceutical point of view, the easy disturbance and breakdown of hydrated gelatin make it an ideal ingestible, single-dose container.

There are rare episodes of gelatin capsules adhering to the esophageal lining in people with anatomical and motility disturbances of the gastrointestinal tract. The contents of the lodged capsule could then become locally irritating. However, compressed tablets represent a greater danger, so capsules are preferred when there is concern about local irritation before a formulation is disintegrated and dispersed.

The risks of systemic side effects from gelatin as an oral excipient are essentially nil. Tolerance problems related to its parenteral use are not relevant to its use in oral preparations.

II. TABLET COATINGS

A wide variety of polymers are used as coating materials for tablets. These include newer synthetic materials that may be basic such as poly-l-lysine or acidic such as carboxyvinyl polymers (carbomer). Materials more commonly used for tablet coatings in the past are shellac, acacia, gluten, paraffin, and a variety of resins and silicones. By and large these agents are stable on storage, are not absorbed, and have shown little toxic potential. However, many of them have not been subjected to full toxicological evaluation of the type currently required of new agents.

1. Shellac

Shellac is largely a fatty-acid material obtained from the resinous secretions of an insect. It has long been popular as a coating for tablets. As a component of tablet-coating mixtures with oils, stearic acid, or isopropyl myristate, it improves the stability of the tablet. The concentration of shellac in the coating mixture is a controlling factor in the rate of disintegration (5). However, with aging of the tablet, this characteristic may change significantly.

A variety of grades of shellacs are used for microencapsulation preparations (6). Pathologic pulmonary reactions to some hair sprays have been attributed to shellac (7,8). However, such effects are probably of no relevance to the toxic potential of shellac in orally ingested formulations.

2. Silicones

The silicones include a spectrum of agents used not only as film formers for tablets and microencapsulations (10) but also in topical preparations (i.e., dimethicone [9]) intended as barrier formers; as lubricants and coatings for glass syringes, vials, and rubber stoppers; and as antifoaming agents. They are polymeric chains prepared from chlor and dichlor methylsilane ($[CH_3]_2SiCl$ or Cl_2), which on hydrolysis form active SiOH (simalol) groups that polyermize by condensation.

The use of one form of silicone—simethacone—in oral doses of 2 g/day to control flatulence attests to its general safety. However, various reactions have been reported with nonpharmaceutical uses of silicone. Repeated injections of a fluid form of silicone to reshape breasts have caused granulomatous mastitis (11) as well as hepatic and pulmonary lesions (12). Following the perfusion of dimethyl polysiloxane fluid with silica as an antifoaming agent during open heart surgery, plugs of the material were found in the retinal vessels (13). Dialysis patients have been reported to have refractile particles in marrow cells and macrophages as well as granulomatous lesions, possibly from silicones used in the dialysis equipment (14). Reports of granulomatous reactions to silicones used in a variety of applications continue to appear (15-17).

Rare reports of allergic reactions to silicone (18) are reviewed in Part III.

3. Mucilages and Gums

These agents are common components of coating preparations. Their potential toxicity is reviewed below, which discusses their use as suspending, emulsifying, and stiffening agents.

4. Gluten

The term gluten describes a mixture of wheat proteins and is also applied to proteins from other grains such as rye, oats, and barley. It is commonly used to form films for microencapsulation and related drug processes.

Gluten sensitivity is well recognized and is particularly important and persistent in celiac disease. Patients on a gluten-free diet are warned to avoid medications formulated with gluten (19). In the clinical management of gluten intolerance it may be helpful to differentiate transient gluten intolerance from celiac disease (20,21).

The role of gluten in celiac disease and its management is complex (22,23). The high incidence of malignant degeneration in patients with celiac disease does not seem to be influenced by following a gluten-free diet (24). However, the occurrence of dermatitis herpetiformis does seem to be related to gluten intake (25,26). Claims that gluten may influence schizophrenia (27) and the behavior of autistic children (28) are not well founded.

In general, gluten in medicinal formulations poses a minor problem compared to that of dietary gluten for the sensitive individual.

5. Acidic Polymers

The weakly acidic polymer, poly-(vinyl methyl ether/maleic acid) mono ester resin, also used as a coating material (6) shows no acute toxic responses in oral, eye, and skin tests in animals. The most commonly used acidic polymers are the carbomers (carbopol), described below.

6. Basic Polymers

The basic polymer, poly-l-lysine, is also used as a coating material (6). Renal perfusion technique studies showed that it caused anatomical ultrastructural changes and decreased stainability of anionic sites that were largely reversible by subsequent perfusion with a polyanion (heparin) (30). Guinea pig studies show that poly-l-lysine causes changes resembling those induced by neomycin (31), an agent with well-recognized ototoxicity attributed to effects on phosphinositide monolayers and cochlear microphonic potentials. Poly-l-lysine has also been described as an excellent carrier for electrophilic haptens capable of eliciting allergic skin sensitivity reactions (32).

7. Carboxyvinyl Polymers (Carbomer)

Carbomer is a high-molecular-weight cross-linked acrylic acid material with acidic properties due to its numerous carboxyl groups. It is a readily soluble agent commonly used in oral and topical formulations. It is the basis of the numbered carbopol preparations that differ in physical characteristics to serve a variety of purposes including control of viscosity, as a suspending agent at concentrations up to 0.4%, and to form a gel or aqueous ointment at higher concentrations. Being acidic, it may react with basic drugs to form prolonged action preparations.

Carbopols are frequently formulated with antimicrobial preservatives and antioxidants to control the consequences of exposure to light. When the agent is used as a suspending agent, the concentrations required are low (a fraction of 1%). Concentrations of 0.5–5% are used to make an aqueous ointment base.

The safety of these agents administered orally is reflected in their use in 1–3 g doses as a bulk laxative. Such doses are rarely achieved in medications that include the carbomers for formulation purposes. Thus the carbopols are described as essentially nontoxic (29).

8. Cellacephate

Cellacephate is a particularly useful excipient for enteric coating since it will not dissolve in acid media but will soften and swell in neutral or alkaline solution. It is essentially cellulose that is partly acetylated and esterified with phthalic acid. There are several formulations of cellaphate, particularly with plasticizers to form tablet-coating solutions or enteric varnish.

Reactions to enteric-coated formulations relate primarily to deviations from the desired release pattern of the active ingredient. Cellacephate per se is essentially free of any history of causing side effects.

9. Paraffins

These solid hydrocarbon products from petrolatum are used in tablet formulations. The potential of paraffins to cause adverse reactions is reviewed above. The quantity and the nature of paraffin use in tablets are not likely to cause any significant adverse effects unless abused parenterally by "kick" seekers, who crush tablets of stimulant drugs prepared for oral use and inject the contents intravenously.

10. Waxes

Beeswax, discussed previously, and vegetable waxes such as carnaubawax NF (33), used in tablet coating, have essentially no history of creating adverse responses when used for this purpose.

III. CONTAINERS FOR LIQUIDS

A. Plastics

Plastics are a heterogeneous group of materials defined chemically as products of condensation or polymerization and structurally as materials that can be molded. They may contain additives such as plasticizers (particularly phthalate derivatives) lubricants, antioxidants, and ultraviolet absorbers. Among the plastics of medicinal interest are polyvinyl chloride (PVC), polystyrene, polyethylene, and polypropylene.

In general, plastics appear to be biologically inert unabsorbed agents that pose no problems of systemic or even local toxicity, although there are reports alleging the induction of malignant change around some chronically implanted plastics (34). Besides additives, these polymeric materials may contain varying amounts and kinds of monomeric or other impurities, some of which, even in concentrations of a few parts per million, can be of clinical concern. In evaluating these findings, it is helpful to know the identity of the impurity, its concentration in the plastic material as used, and the fraction of that concentration that may become available for absorption or interaction.

Plastics are involved as excipients in two ways: as containers for liquid and other formulations into which potentially toxic materials may be leached, and as components of fluid formulations that make possible delayed absorption by controlled release of active ingredients (see Chapter 12). The Food and Drug Administration (FDA) has ruled that plastic contact lenses are to be considered drugs capable of causing chemically induced reactions (35). However, lenses and other plastic devices will not be reviewed here.

In an attempt to determine an index of the toxic potential of various plastics, a series of procedures have been developed that involve extraction of plastics in various solvents (isotonic saline, alcohol, polyethylene glycol, vegetable oil) or the injection or implantation of strips of plastics into animals (36). The conclusions to be drawn from such testing are, of necessity, guarded.

When plastic containers are used for preparations going through the FDA approval process, the nature of the container is a component of the safety evaluation and information is required to ensure that the contents are not adversely altered by its container. A recent USP publication (37) on the use of plastic prescription bottles for oral liquids states:

> In view of the fact that there are many formulations of pharmaceuticals on the market with different solvents and concentrations that might theoretically extract plasticizers, etc., from the plastic or, conversely, show a loss of potency, color, flavor, etc., through sorption by some types of plastic, USP cannot recommend use of these containers by dispensers.

Experience with a variety of materials used for dialysis membranes is also of interest. The older cellulose acetate membranes seem to be less likely to be associated with problems reported to occur with cuprammonium cellulose materials used in hollow-fiber dialyzers (38,39), particularly if these are not adequately rinsed. Infrequent but serious anaphylactic and other reactions, including neutropenia, alleged to be associated more frequently with cuprammonium cellulose, are discussed in Part III.

B. Glass

It is almost axiomatic that glass containers, properly washed, are safe for housing medicinals because of their insolubility and impermeability. The dangers of glass ingestion are essentially from its physical form and the physical damage it can do. The likelihood of the wall of a glass container interacting with its medicinal contents is very remote. Nevertheless, in dealing with low concentrations of highly potent materials, it may be wise to check for adherence to the surface that could influence potency. The grades and types of glass used as vessels for medicinals have essentially no other toxic potential.

Standard stability study techniques often require that the containers used be made of the same material as that to be used commercially. This requirement is probably more important for containers other than glass, and glass is usually the standard against which other packaging materials are tested.

IV. MICROENCAPSULATION

While the formulation techniques used for microencapsulation are often ingenious and complex, the materials currently used for microencapsulation (6) are essentially those already discussed, particularly involving plastics and proteins of animal (albumin, gelatin) and vegetable origin, sometimes combined with acacia.

Pharmaceutical grades of albumin are prepared from bovine and human sources. A foreign protein such as bovine albumin cannot be safely used parenterally in humans. Human albumin preparations are commonly used intravenously as plasma expanders, and occasionally cause reactions (40-43). Many drugs bind to albumin, which may markedly influence the disposition and response to the drug. However, human albumin is not often added as a drug carrier for parenteral drugs, since drugs that bind to albumin will do so in vivo when the concentration of albumin in plasma is about 5 g/dl.

The reactions to parenteral albumin are irrelevant to the use of albumin or other proteins in oral formulations, which are not more likely to cause ill effects than eating beef or other foods of animal origin.

Newer microencapsulation techniques currently under development involve a variety of other materials (44) including both natural and synthetic phospholipids and cholesterol to create lipid vesicles or liposomes that are formulated to imitate natural cell membranes and are targeted by one or another method to specific structures (45). Many aspects of the safety of such microencapsulations remain to be worked out, even though their foodlike nature and origin suggest that they should be well tolerated.

Some experimental techniques use microorganisms to house medication. Even human red cells and red cell "ghosts" have been used to "encapsulate" one or another medication (46). The targeting of medication to specific structures for specific purposes is an active field of research.

Microencapsulation is also accomplished with nonbiodegradable materials (47) such as methyl methacrylate, a copolymer of methacrylate esters such as polymethyl methacrylate (PMMA). While there is little evidence of ill effects from such oral formulations, the use of these materials in contact lenses and as a base cement has lead to several reports of hazards, ranging from cystitis, granuloma, and urinary bladder carcinoma in people who work with the material repeatedly (48) to acute symptoms (dizziness, dyspnea, nausea, and vomiting) in operating room personnel handling the material (49). Recipients may experience hypotension (50) and other manifestations of cardiovascular toxicity (51). Fat embolism with cerebral infarction (52), bladder cancer (53), and contact dermatitis (54) have all been reported after use of PMMA cement. A major factor could be the 3–5% of free monomers in PMMA, since the monomer is corrosive to mucosa and skin (48). While as little as 12.5 ppm of methyl methacrylate in the air is enough to cause significant symptoms if inhaled for 20–30 min, it is difficult to translate these observations into an estimation of risk from the use of PMMA in microencapsulation for oral sustained-release or film coating.

REFERENCES

1. Deasy, P.B. Coating Properties. *In* Microencapsulation and Related Drug Processes (Deasy, P.B., ed.). Marcel Dekker, New York, pp. 22–25 (1984).
2. Delany, T. and Hoxworth, P.I. Enteric coated potassium chloride enteropathy. Surg. Gynecol. Obstet. 127:76 (1968).
3. USP XXI/NFXVI. Pharmaceutical dosage forms. Supplement 3, p. 2074, Rockville, Maryland (1986).
4. Ring, J. and Messmer, K. Incidence and severity of anaphylactoid reactions to colloid volume substitutes. Lancet 1:466–469 (1977).
5. Shellac specifications. NF XVI, p. 1601 (1985).
6. Deasy, P.B. Coating properties. *In* Microencapsulation and Related Drug Processes (Deasy, P.B., ed.). Marcel Dekker, New York, pp. 24–25 (1984).
7. Hirsch, E.F. and Russell, H.B. Chronic exudative and indurative pneumonia due to inhalation of shellac. Arch. Pathol. 39:281–286 (1945).

8. McLaughlin, A.I.G., Bidstrup, P.L. and Konstam, M. The effects of hair lacquer sprays on the lungs. Food Cosmet. Toxciol. 1:171–188 (1963)
9. NF XVI Official Monographs, p. 1558, Rockville, Maryland (1986).
10. Polystyrene use in microencapsulation. NCR, U.S. Patent 3, 336, 155. The process of coating particles with a polymer. Egbert Rowe (inventor). National Cash Register Corporation, Dayton, Ohio (1967).
11. Symmers, W. St. C. Granulomatous mastitis by injection of silicone in breast. Br. Med. J. 3:19 (1968).
12. Ellenbogen, R., Ellenbogen, R. and Rubin, L. Injectible fluid silicone therapy: human morbidity and mortality. J.A.M.A. 234:308–309 (1975).
13. Williams, I.M. Retinal vascular occlusion in open heart surgery. Br. J. Ophthalmol. 59:81–91 (1975).
14. Boomer, J., Ritz, E., Waldherr, R. Silicone-induced splenomegaly. Treatment of pancytopenia by splenectomy in patients on hemodialysis. N. Engl.J. Med. 305:1077-1079 (1981).
15. Travis, W.D., Balogh, K., et al. Silicone granulomas. Hum. Pathol. 16:19 (1985).
16. Kozeny, G.A., Barbato, A.L., et al. Hypercalcemia associated with silicone-induced granulomas. N. Engl. J. Med. 311:1103 (1984).
17. Sollitto, R.J. and Shonkweiler, W. Silicone shard formation: A product of implant arthroplasty. J. Foot. Surg. 23:362 (1984).
18. Fellner, M.J. and Rudikoff, D.A. Adverse reaction following silicone infections. Int. J. Dermatol. 18:375–376 (1979).
19. Gluten in medicines. Br. Med. J. 2:185 (1976).
20. Walker-Smith, J.A. Gastrointestinal allergy. Practitioner 220:562 (1978).
21. Jonas, A. Wheat-sensitive—but not coeliac. Lancet 2:1047 (1978).
22. Management of coeliac disease. Br. Med. J. 2:130–131 (1973).
23. McNeish, A.S. Coeliac disease: Duration of gluten-free diet. Archs. Dis. Child. 55:110–111 (1980).
24. Holmes, G.K.T., Stokes, P.L., Soraham, T.M., Prior, P., Waterhous, J.A.H. and Cook, W.T. Celiac disease gluten-free diet, and malignancy. Gut 17: 612–619 (1976).
25. Dermatitis herpetiformis—the thin veneer? Lancet 2:458–459 (1978).
26. Ljunghall, K. and Tjernlund, U.M. Diagnosis of dermatitis herpetiformis. Lancet 2:1003–1004 (1978).
27. Gluten and schizophrenia. Lancet 1:844 (1976).
28. McCarthy, D.M. and Coleman, M. Response of intestinal mucosa to gluten challenge in autistic subjects. Lancet 2:877–878 (1979).
29. Gosselin, R.E., Smith, R.P. and Hodge, H.C. Clinical Toxicology of Commercial Products. 5th Edition. Williams & Wilkins, Baltimore, 1984.
30. Seiler, M.W., Venkatachalem, M.A. and Cotran, R.S. Glomerular epithelium: Structure alterations induced by polycations. Science 189:390–393 (1975).
31. Takada, A., Lodhi, S., Weiner, N.D. and Schecht, J. Lysine and polylysine: Correlation of their effects on polyphosphoinositides in vitro with ototoxic action in vivo. J. Pharm. Sci. 71:1410–1411 (1982).

32. Petit, L., Gervais, P. and Denuc, A.M. Chemical allergy to electrophilic haptens bound to poly-L-lysine. Bull. Med. Leg. Toxciol. 21:759–763 (1978).

33. National Formulary XVI specifications regarding carnauba wax, p. 1617 (1985).

34. Rigdon, R.H. Plastics and carcinogenesis. South. Med. J. 57:1459–1465 (1974).

35. Soft contact lenses. Br. Med. J. 1:608–609 (1976).

36. USPXXI/NFXVI Containers. Biologic tests—plastics. Supplement 3, 2047 (1985).

37. USP D1/Update No. 4. Use of plastic prescription bottles for oral liquids. 4:49 (1985).

38. Daugiras, J.T., Ing, T.S., et al. Severe anaphylactoid reactions to cuprammonium cellulose hemodialysis. Arch Intern. Med. 145:489 (1985).

39. Iranovich, P., Cemoweth, D.E., et al. Utersuchungen zur ventraglichkeit von zellulose-azetort und cuprophan-dialysemembranen. Dtsch. Gesundh. 39: 420 (1984).

40. Paul, K., Schlesinger, R.G., Schanfield, M.S. and Harbich, J. Reaction to albumin. J.A.M.A. 245:234–235 (1981).

41. Weaver, D.W., Ledgerwood, A.M., Lucas, C.E., Higgins, R., Bouwman, D.L. and Stemple, D.J. Pulmonary effects of albumin resucitation for severe hypovolemic shock. Arch. Surg. 113:387–391 (1978).

42. Dahn, M.S., Lucas, C.E., Ladgerwood, A.M. and Higgins, R.F. Negative inotropic effect of albumin resucitation for shock. Surgery 86:235–241.

43. Paton, C.J. and Kerry, P.J. Prekallikrein activation in human albumin. Lancet 2:747 (1981).

44. Johnson, J.C. (Ed.). Sustained release medications. Noyes Data Corp., Park Ridge, New Jersey (1980).

45. Tom, B.H. and Six, H.R. (Eds.). Liposomes and Immunobiology. Elsevier/ North Holland, Amsterdam (1980).

46. Green, R., Lamon, J. and Curran, D. Clinical trial of desferrioxamine entrapped in red cell of hosts. Lancet 2:327 (1980).

47. Deasy, P.B. Polymerization procedures for nonbiodegradable micro- and nanocapsules and particles. In: Microencapsulation and Related Drug Processes (Deasy, P.B., ed.), Marcel Dekker, New York, pp. 203–218 (1984).

48. Routledge, R. Possible hazard of contact lens manufacturer. Br. Med. J. 1:487–488 (1973).

49. Burchman, S. and Wheater, R.H. Hazard of methyl methacrylate to operating room personnel. J.A.M.A. 235:2652 (1976).

50. Brittain, G.J.C. and Ryan, D.J. Hypotension and methylmethacrylate cement. Br. Med. J. 4:667–668 (1972).

51. Wong, K.C., Martin, W.E., Kennedy, W.F., Akamatsu, T.J., Convery, R.F. and Shaw, C.L. Cardiovascular effects of total hip placement in man with

observation on the effect of methylmethacrylate on the isolated rabbit heart. Clin. Pharmacol. Ther. 21:709 (1977).

52. Adams, J.H., Graham, D.I., Mille, E. and Sprunt, T.G. Fat embolism and cerebral infraction after use of methylmethacrylic cement. Br. Med. J. 3: 740–741 (1972).

53. Wines, R.D. Possible hazard of polymethyl methacrylate. Br. Med. J. 3:409 (1973).

54. Fries, I.B., Fisher, A.A. and Saluvati, E.A. Contact dermatitis in surgeons from methylmethacrylate bare cement. J. Bone Joint Surg. 57:547–549 (1975).

8

Adverse Effects: Flavoring Agents

   I. Sweetening Agents   135
  II. Inorganic salts   140
 III. Fruit flavors   141
 IV. Aromatic (essential) oils   146
  V. Synthetic (imitation) flavors   152
      References   154

Of all the excipients used for medicinals, natural flavoring agents are probably the least well defined. By and large they are produced by establishments that cater primarily to the food industry with pharmaceutical flavoring a relatively minor and commercially unimportant market.

In recent years the use of synthetic, chemically well-defined flavoring agents has increased considerably. It is paradoxical that these are looked upon with more suspicion and concern for toxicity than the ill-defined concoctions prepared from botanical materials by methods that are more historic art than modern science. These latter are "natural" products and therefore considered historically "safe", in spite of a relative paucity of information about the four cardinal criteria by which medicinal materials are defined: identity, strength, quality, and purity.

A variety of sophisticated modern techniques ranging from accurate pH measurements to recognition of a characteristic high-performance liquid chromatography (HPLC) pattern are used in the quality control of some of these natural products. However, the inadequacy of these high-technology tests are demonstrated by the fact that some suppliers insist on using a panel of sophisticated "tasters" or "smellers" to confirm that a new batch is up to the standards of previous materials that had proved satisfactory in the marketplace. Regardless of pH, HPLC, or other findings, if the panel of tasters and smellers does not approve, the material is not acceptable. Perhaps this is not really unique among pharmaceuticals, since the standards by which essentially all pure active ingredients as well as excipients are characterized include subjective descriptions of appearance (color, etc.) and odor.

Many flavor producers are reluctant to reveal anything about their products other than the most basic and obvious characteristics. They consider their know-how concerning the selection of raw materials, production, handling, and measures for quality control of their products to be critically important trade secrets, and would rather forfeit pharmaceutical use if such use required public disclosure of these details. As a rule, the amount of flavoring consumed with medication is a minor fraction of that used for foods, and it would seem irrational to forbid the use of a flavor in medicine that is freely permitted in foods. On the other hand, interactions of any excipient with an active ingredient leading to altered absorption are far more important for drugs than for foods.

Historically, medications were mostly liquids and often nasty tasting. For a long time the public had generally been more willing to accept a nasty-tasting medicine than bad-tasting food. In fact, the bad taste or odor was sometimes the hallmark of "strong medicine," probably contributing to the placebo effect. Nevertheless, skillful flavoring was and continues to be an important component of the art of formulation.

Today a more sophisticated public expects pharmaceutical experts to overcome palatability problems. For some products, manufacturers go to great lengths to identify the particular flavor and intensity that is preferred. In general, children will prefer sweet, fruity flavors while adults like more acidic, tangy tastes and the elderly may prefer winelike flavors.

The nature of the unpleasant taste to be masked can be an important guide to the flavor selected. Thus bitter drugs tend to be best masked by mint and citrus flavors, and acidic taste by other fruit flavors. Salty drug tastes are often hidden by butterscotch and caramel flavors. It is rare for one flavor to be chosen over another because of concern for possible side effects due to the flavoring.

Most modern oral medications for adults are solid formulations, usually in capsules or coated tablets that protect the patient from exposure to bad-tasting materials. In some instances the drug is formulated as a relatively insoluble and therefore tasteless salt, thus avoiding the need for flavoring agents in liquid formulations. The same procedure is also used to permit oral liquid formulations of drugs that are unpleasantly topically anesthetic to the mouth. For example, imipramine formulated as the less-soluble palmitate salt will not produce the oral anesthesia seen with liquid formulations of the readily soluble hydrochloride.

There still remain a significant number of liquid or chewable tablet formulations, for both pediatric and adult use, for which flavoring is important. Sublingual and other mouth-absorbed medications may need flavoring. Oral lozenges and other semimedicinal preparations such as mouth washes and medicated (fluorinated, etc.) toothpastes constitute a major group of materials for which flavoring is of prime importance. It therefore behooves us to review the nature of currently used flavoring agents and our knowledge about their toxic potential, limited as it may be.

Flavoring agents are generally classified on the basis of their source and the nature of their use rather than their chemistry or the sensory systems by which they are perceived. Taste in the sense of stimulation of taste buds of the tongue is largely confined to sweet, sour, bitter, and salty (80). Texture contributes to acceptability or palatability, as do sensations generated over the whole oral mucosa by some substances such as the more potent spices. Materials that are topically anesthetizing obviously influence taste. However, the important subtleties of flavoring are generally the result of olfactory perceptions coupled with oral and lingual sensations.

Flavoring may include ingredients to achieve a tart or sour quality for some adult tastes. That sensation is largely a consequence of pH of the final preparation. The pH of a formulation can adversely effect the intent of the medication. These effects are reviewed below.

Bitterness, a sensation perceived by buds at the back of the tongue, is usually a quality of medication that one wishes to mask rather than impart with an excipient. There are occasions when bitterness may be added to discourage misuse or create matching flavors for controlled clinical drug studies. Minute amounts of very bitter substances such as aloe may be used. There is essentially no evidence to suggest any significant adverse effects from the tiny quantities involved in such formulation additions.

The classification of flavors in this section follows common practice and lends itself to discussion of adverse reactions in an organized fashion. Materials involved in the tongue sensations of sweet and salty are reviewed. Agents that create sour or bitter tastes are seldom added as excipients, since these sensations are rarely among the desired goals of flavoring. Most flavoring materials are syrups or oils from plants, synthetic agents, or synthetically modified natural substances.

I. SWEETENING AGENTS

1. Sugars

Of the many natural sugars, the most commonly used are the disaccharide, sucrose, generally derived from sugar cane or beets, and the monosaccharide, glucose (dextrose, invert sugar) generally derived by hydrolysis of various starches.

Gram for gram, sucrose is sweeter than glucose, but it is also more expensive so that glucose is sweeter dollar for dollar. Glycerin may be looked upon as a sugar, specifically a triose, which also imparts sweetness in addition to its usefulness as a solvent. The potential adverse reactions from these agents, are reviewed in detail in the previous section on bulk fillers.

Other sugars that add sweetness may be used simply because they are components of natural product materials used as excipients. For example, fructose is found in honey and in many flavor preparations made from fruits. Sweetness is a major contributing factor in the use of these preparations as excipients. Fructose also appears as one of the two monosaccharides to which the disaccharide, sucrose, is hydrolyzed before it is absorbed.

The relative sweetness of the commonly used sugars, with sucrose scored as 100, is: fructose 173, glucose 74, maltose 32, galactose 32, and lactose 16 (1,2).

It is sometimes assumed that sugars other than glucose do not share in the problems involved in diabetes mellitus, the hallmark of which is elevated blood sugar (i.e., glucose) levels. However, it is known that other monosaccharides are caloric, entering cells and becoming involved in carbohydrate metabolism, presumably without the aid of insulin (3). Nevertheless, the administration of fructose does cause an elevation in blood glucose levels. Consequently, the substitution of this sugar for glucose or sucrose as a sweetening agent does not obviate the concerns about sugar in formulations to be consumed by diabetics or others with disturbed carbohydrate metabolism. The monosaccharides, sorbitol (4) and xylitol (5), are used as sweeteners in lozenges and chewing gum with the notion that they will not disturb the carbohydrate control of diabetics. When taken in large doses, they may cause an osmotic diarrhea.

An unabsorbed sweet sugar has long been sought, particularly among disaccharides and higher sugar polymers, as a food ingredient for baking and as an excipient with the physical properties of sugar, but without adding calories. Many long-chain polysaccharides are not hyrolyzable by gastrointestinal enzymes are are therefore not absorbed (e.g., cellulose, dextran). But they are also not very sweet. There are unabsorbed disaccharides that are sweet, such as lactulose, but these are generally attacked by colonic bacteria in a manner that yields colonic irritants with a significant laxative effect. Consequently, they cannot be used in quantity as a nonabsorbed and therefore noncaloric sweetening agent. The fate of the disaccharide lactose (milk sugar) in lactase deficiency, common among the elderly, is very similar to that of lactulose in normal persons (see above). Fermentable sugars that reach the colon unabsorbed can be the cause of cramping, diarrhea, and flatulence from the products of decomposition by colonic organisms, particularly *E. coli*. However, this is far more likely to result from consuming several ounces of such carbohydrates than from the small amounts of these sugars generally used for sweetening tablets, lozenges, or liquids prescribed in teaspoon doses.

Some forms of sugar are truly flavoring agents rather than just sweeteners. These include caramel, made by heating sucrose or glucose, sometimes with the addition of an inorganic acid or alkaline agent during the heating process. Other syrups used for flavoring, such as maple syrup, owe their characteristic flavor to components other than their sugar content.

2. Artificial Sweeteners

The use of artificial sweeteners rather than sugar has become popular largely because of an interest in avoiding the contribution of sugars to caloric intake and disturbances in the control for subjects with carbohydrate dysfunction, such as diabetics. Other factors favoring artifical sweeteners are adverse dental effects of sugar, particularly with lozenges, mouthwashes, etc.; bulk- and viscosity-related formulation problems, and the propensity of sugar to support microbiological growth. The potent artificial sweeteners are essentially noncaloric and do not significantly influence factors such as the viscosity and flow characteristics of the formulations to which they are added. In food preparation, sugars often serve to supply both sweetness and desired bulk-texture qualities. In pharmaceutical preparations, however, when sweetness per se is the objective, the lack of bulk is more likely to be an advantage than a handicap.

Major research efforts are underway to understand the conformational characteristics of the sweetness receptors (6). The ultimate goal is the development of more potent, safe, and economical sweetening agents.

The three major nonnutritive sweeteners to be considered are saccharin, cyclamate, and aspartame. Both cyclamate and saccharin are noncaloric and do not undergo metabolic conversion in the body. They are found unchanged in the urine. In contrast, aspartame is a methyl ester of a dipeptide of aspartic acid and phenylalanine (Fig. 1), which does not survive the intestinal tract intact. The methyl group is hydrolyzed off to methanol by esterases in the lumen, and the remaining dipeptide is hydrolyzed to its component amino acids by mucosal

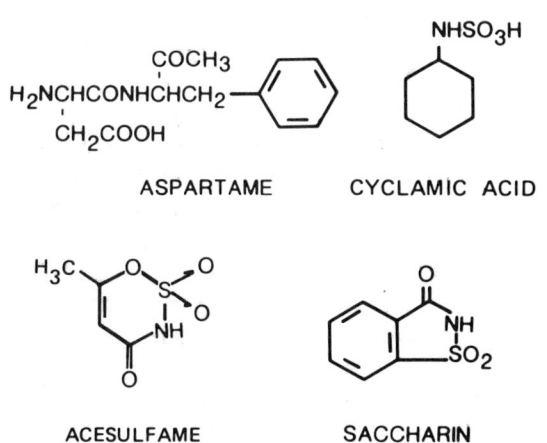

Figure 1   Chemical structures of sweetening agents.

dipeptidases (7). While these products are technically caloric, the calories involved are quantitatively insignificant, since the amount of aspartame consumed is measured in milligrams. Aspartame is almost 200 times sweeter than sucrose.

The safety of agents currently used as artificial sweeteners has been the subject of considerable controversy and there are still major differences of opinion concerning their potential influence on consumers. The problem arises because their use tends to be widespread, continuous, and in relatively large amounts by people of all ages and with a wide variety of health problems. The results of animal studies involving very large doses over prolonged periods have been interpreted by some as indicating a carcinogenic, or at least a tumorigenic, potential. However, these agents have been used for decades by millions of people with only the flimsiest evidence of adverse effects.

Cyclamate and saccharin The depth of the controversy about cyclamate and saccharin is well illustrated by the fact that the FDA currently (1987) bans cyclamate and, in keeping with measures taken by United States Congress, continues to allow the widespread use of saccharin. In contrast, the Canadian Health Protection Branch forbids the use of saccharin but permits the general use of cyclamate. Both of these scientifically advanced nations have spent a great deal of time and effort reviewing years of accumulated data, and seem to have settled on contradictory regulatory actions in pursuit of their mission to protect the public.

Whenever a public health decision to ban use of an agent is considered, it is critical to take into account what will be used in its place. The seriousness of obesity as a health hazard is well established (8) and the appropriate dietary measures to control obesity are well known. While there is no doubt about the medical wisdom of quenching thirst with plain calorie free water, the public demand for sweet drinks and its concern about caloric sugar is such that no government has found it expedient to ban all artificial sweeteners. In the absence of any clear data to indicate that one of the sweeteners in question is more dangerous than the others, perhaps the best action in the interest of the public health would be to allow the availability of a spectrum of such sweeteners in order to reduce the amount of any one of them that is likely to be consumed.

It would serve no useful purpose to review again here the controversial data on the carcinogenic potential of saccharin and cyclamate that are covered in detail elsewhere (9-15). Certainly the clinical data cited are far from convincing. The human data on bladder malignancy show peculiar sex and regional differences that make doubtful the presumed relationship to the artifical sweetener. The bladder malignancies reported in rats seem to be associated with urinary levels of cyclamate much higher than any achievable with doses in human use. It may be important that at these high urine levels in rats, cyclamate is present as a complex that apparently does not form in human urine. Studies of the effects of the urinary complex found in bladder epithelium of rats might help to resolve whether the rat data have any relevance to species such as humans, in whom the complex is not found in the urine.

When used as excipients in medicinals, the amount of the sweeteners involved and the dosage consumed is so small compared to their use in foods that it can hardly be considered a potential health hazard. Unfortunately, regulatory language often makes yes–no statements and the propensity for lawsuits can override the scientific logic of giving formulation experts a freer hand in using both of these agents in medicinal formulations.

Aspartame A major limiting factor in the use of aspartame as a sweetener, particularly in medicinals, is its instability in solution. With elevated temperatures, and particularly at pH values below 3.9 or above 4.3, it converts to a presumably harmless but no longer sweet diketopiperazine derivative (16). It is therefore not surprising that there has not been a dramatic medicinal switch to aspartame, an agent with no demonstrated tumor-causing potential (17) and with a presumed additional property of enhancing certain fruit flavors (18). However, aspartame is not without potential side effects, particularly when overused and in persons with certain medical conditions. Granulomatous panniculitis has been reported to be associated with aspartame (19,20). Its aspartic acid metabolite, especially in concert with another dicarboxylic acid, glutamic acid, is reported to be epileptogenic (21) and potentially neurotoxic in young children. The phenylalanine component has been considered as possibly harmful in phenylketonurics and in pregnant women carrying a phenylketonuric fetus (22,23). These risks are of doubtful practical importance (24,25) even when huge doses are used, and are insignificant when dealing with amounts likely to be used to sweeten medicines. Recent observations suggest that aspartame may be linked with headaches (26,27). However, a double-blind crossover trial in which 40 subjects who reported having headaches repeatedly after consuming products with aspartame failed to show a difference in the incidence of headache or any other symptom after 30 mg/kg aspartame compared with placebo (28).

While all three potent artificial sweeteners are soluble and can generally be added to liquid formulations without significant side effects or alteration of the fundamental characteristics of the formulation, there is reason for concern that they, like any other component of a formulation, might interact with an active ingredient. It has been found, for example, that the use of cyclamate in a sugarless liquid formulation of the antibiotic, lincomycin, apparently resulted in an unabsorbable complex that seriously compromised the bioavailability of the antibiotic (29,30). This example illustrates that liquid formulations, including true solutions, are not necessarily free of bioavailability problems. In fact, it is conceivable that the use of a soft drink sweetened with cyclamate to "chase down" an ordinary solid dosage form of lincomycin might interfere with the absorption of the drug. Overall, such events appear to be rare but deserve consideration. While a generalized concept of excipient–active drug interaction has been developed in some areas, such as impaired absorption by calcium complexing, no such generalization is currently available for sweetener-drug interactions. There is, however, a warning of "limited compatibility" of calcium cyclamate with potassium salts, carbonates, citrates, phosphates, sulfates, and tartrates (1). (See Chapter 7.)

Recently a new sweetening agent, the potassium salt of acesulfame, has been released for bulk sale to food processors. Chemically, acesulfame resembles cyclamate and saccharin in that it is an aminosulfate derivative. It is estimated to be about 200 times sweeter than sucrose and to be synergistic with sugars in its sweetening action. It apparently does not undergo metabolic conversion in the body and is excreted unchanged. It is stable to heat so that it can be used in food processing that involves cooking and baking. While available data have been judged to prove the safety of this agent for general use, some consumer groups are questioning the adequacy of the testing to date. There is as yet very little experience with its use as a pharmaceutical excipient.

II. INORGANIC SALTS

1. Sodium Chloride

Salt (sodium chloride) is occasionally used to improve the palatability of medicinals. It is also added to achieve a desired tonicity for solubility or other formulation purposes. Modest amounts are present in some flavoring preparations derived from natural sources. Other standard flavoring preparations are deliberately formulated with salt as an added ingredient. For example, the NF XVl (1985) formulation for cocoa syrup includes 2% sodium chloride.

The adverse reactions to ordinary sodium chloride are well recognized to be a function of dose and are highly dependent on the clinical status of the patient, particularly in relation to hypertensive, cardiovascular, hepatic, and renal diseases. When flavoring products include significant amounts of sodium, this fact should be noted, particularly for patients on a sodium-restricted diet.

2. Potassium Chloride

Potassium is a common component of fruit flavors, but the amount is rarely enough to be of clinical significance. A variety of potassium salts are used therapeutically, but they are seldom added to formulations for flavoring purposes. Occasionally a potassium-containing flavor preparation is selected because its potassium content is perceived to contribute favorably to therapeutic goals. The significance of potassium intake in relation to digitalis administration and mineralocorticoid disturbances is well recognized. Both hyper- and hypopotassemia are potentially dangerous. However, the flavorings used for medicines rarely contribute significantly to potassium imbalance.

Other salts used primarily for purposes other than flavoring are bulk materials such as calcium and magnesium salts, and buffers such as phosphate salts. These are discussed in other sections.

III. FRUIT FLAVORS

Several dozen fruit flavors prepared from natural sources have been used for centuries. They frequently are prepared as syrups and are assumed to be as nontoxic as the fruits from which they are derived. However, botanical preparations can have considerable pharmacological activity, and food allergies to fruits are well known. It is no surprise that people allergic to a particular fruit may also be allergic to the flavoring products prepared from it if sufficient amounts of protein/carbohydrate are carried over into the final product.

In recent years considerable information has been gathered concerning the chemical composition of natural flavors. A key source is Fenaroli's *Handbook of Flavor Ingredients* (22), which tabulates and quantifies the ingredients analyzed in natural flavor preparations.

Naturally occurring components of strawberry aroma, for example, include 19 different alcohols, 15 carbonyl compounds, 27 esters, 13 organic acids, plus 12 other identified moieties that do not fall into any of the above classes, including 3 sulfides. A formula used to imitate strawberry flavor is made with 30 ingredients, including 8 different ethyl esters, 4 methyl esters, and 2 essential oils. Such formulae are based on ingredients making up the relative contribution of components found in the natural product.

The FDA lists flavors that may be used, some of which are identified by a numbering system. For example cherry flavors include F232, FMC#8513, N2753, imitation cherry, mint imitation, raspberry imitation, wild cherry, artificial wild cherry, and anise PFC9758. A tabulation of the components of sour cherry flavor (22) lists 22 identified chemical entities.

Sweet cherry flavor is prepared with a similar number of ingredients, 16 of which are the same and 6 different from those of sour cherry flavor.

Other FDA-approved multi-ingredient formulations include "fantasy" formulations such as tutti frutti and bubble gum. Some of these are used as bases to which some natural flavors are added, leading to a naming of the product according to the natural flavor, even though the amount of the natural flavor would be inadequate in the absence of added artificial fantasy flavoring.

The components identified in natural cocoa aroma require almost four pages of two columns each merely to name the compounds found and give reference numbers to the publications reporting their presence (22, pp. 654–657). An attempt to study the toxic potential of each component of such natural products is obviously beyond the bounds of practicality. Yet many of the agents identified have structures that would arouse the suspicion of toxicologists if they were presented as new synthetic entities intended for human consumption. Once again, the quantities involved are generally low enough not to be harmful, but there can be no guarantee of absolute safety under all circumstances. Identification of components responsible for sensitization reactions is exceedingly difficult.

To assist in the evaluation and diagnosis of allergic reactions to foods, the American Academy of Allergy and Immunology in collaboration with the National Institute of Allergy and Infectious Diseases has prepared a volume (31) that includes a classification of plant products in related groups. It may be useful to review flavoring agents prepared from fruit and other plant products in such botanical groups.

Table 1 shows a list of fruit flavors used in medicinals approved by the regulatory authorities. In many instances, a particular chemical of known structure or a particular chemical class has been identified as the prime contributor to the characteristic flavor. In others, the components responsible for the flavor are

Table 1 Sources of Natural Flavors

Family	Source of flavor preparation
Apple	Apple, pear, quince
Beech	Beechnut, chestnut
Birch	Hazel nut, wintergreen (betula)
Citrus	Orange, lemon
Cola nut	Chocolate (cocoa), cola
Ginger	Cardamon, arrowroot, ginger
Grape	Grape, wine, raisin
Heath	Blueberry, cranberry, wintergreen (pyrola)
Laurel	Sassafras, cinnamon
Lily	Aloe, sarsaparilla
Mint	Basil, lavender, mint, peppermint, spearmint, sage, thyme
Myrtle	Clove, myrtle
Olive	Jasmine, olive
Orchid	Vanilla
Parsley	Anise, caraway, dill
Pea	Acacia, licorice, peanut, tragacanth
Plum	Almond, cherry, plum, peach
Rose	Rose, raspberry, strawberry, blackberry
Sunflower	Absinthe (wormwood), camomile, chicory

multiple and complex. Some well-identified chemical entities of known structure are recognized as playing an important role in imparting a variety of flavors (see Fig. 2). For example, piperonal, a methylene dioxy derivative of benzaldehyde, is an important component of the characteristic flavor of both vanilla and cherry (32).

The intensity of a flavor is often critical to its perception as pleasant or unpleasant. It is not unusual for a concentrate to be pungent and even revolting, while the adequately diluted agent tastes very pleasant. This creates an element of built-in protection against excessive and possibly toxic doses, since the purpose of the flavoring agent is defeated if too much is used.

The components of fruits vary with the seasons, weather, geography, and time of harvesting as well as species and variety. With time and under various conditions of storage, a multitude of complex chemical reactions may take place in natural flavor extracts. Wine and various fruit liquors serve as well-studied examples of these phenomena and are often used as flavored vehicles for medicinals. Besides ethyl alcohol, a spectrum of higher alcohols, aldehydes, esters, and ethers may be present in these products. Some, like absinthe made from wormwood, have been sufficiently toxic to be banned. The generation or addition of methanol (methyl alcohol) in substantial amounts is a real and recurring source of danger (see above). From time to time instances of the accidental or clandestine addition of methanol to products are reported. Some such adulterated products may be destined to be used as vehicles for drugs. Acute poisoning with methanol can be fatal or lead to irreversible blindness (33). Fortunately, the dosage likely to be consumed in the use of adulterated wines and liquors used for medicinals is generally low. Nevertheless, methanol in more than trace amounts is not an acceptable component of an excipient. As little as 30 ml has been reported to be fatal.

As with the sweetening agents, the amounts of natural fruit flavors consumed in medicinals are generally far less than the amounts in foods, so that their use as excipients is not likely to be responsible for significant adverse toxic effects. In rare instances in which even minor amounts of sugar or ethanol consumption may be a problem, the use of flavoring products that contain sugar or alcohol may have to be tempered.

Fruit-flavored preparations may require precautions against deterioration and microbiological contamination. Concentrated syrups that have a "preservative" quality may lose that quality when diluted in a formulation. Consequently, modern stability studies are essential to characterize such preparations. Once opened, bottles of fruit syrup containing liquid medicinals can be safely stored and consumed for only a limited period of time. Generally such fluid medications will safely survive the duration of an acute illness, following which they should be discarded.

Flavoring syrups are sometimes selected because the flavor is historically

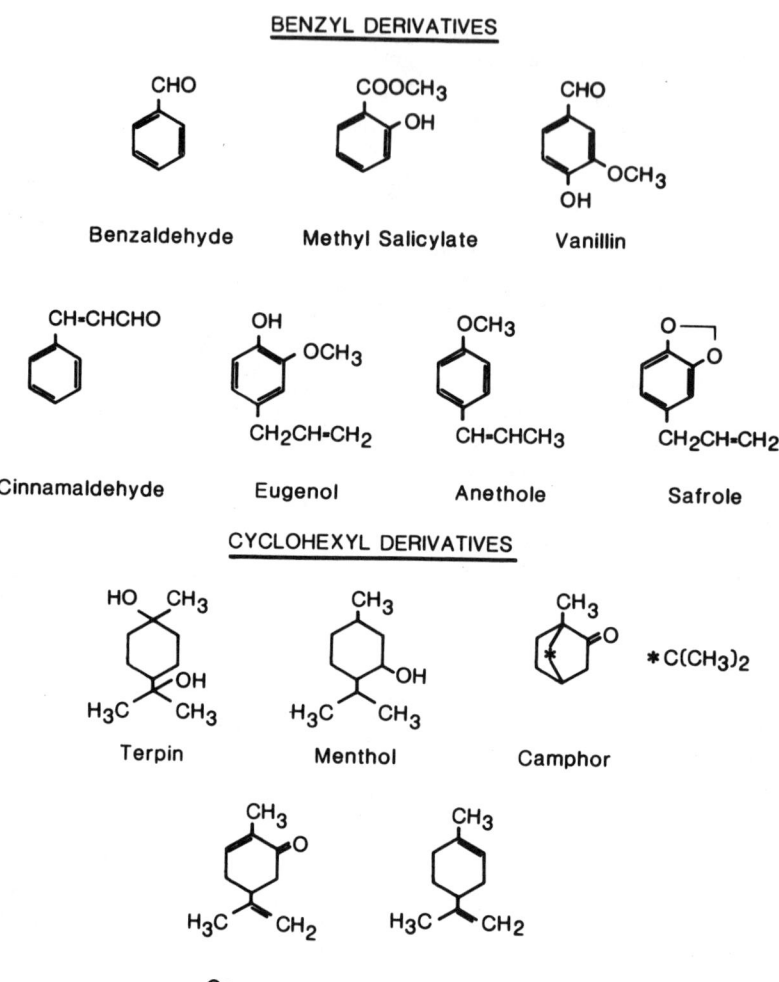

Figure 2 Chemical structures of common flavoring components.

associated with the particular use, and may itself be reputed to have the desired therapeutic effect. Thus, ginger syrup has been associated with laxative products. Its pungent taste is perceived as consistent with this medicinal purpose. Licorice has long been used for coughs, probably because the liquid extract is presumed to have some expectorant action. In some instances there are historic associations of certain flavors with a particular utility even though the presumed efficacy is lacking.

Licorice is prepared from the roots of glycyrrhiza. It has a strong, lingering sweet taste that can counter excessive saltiness. However, its use is limited because it is not a universally admired flavor. It has been the source of purified derivatives with potent pharmacological activity. Some of these may resemble the synthetic congener, carbenoxalone, which is used to hasten the healing of peptic ulcers (34) and has significant adverse effects on potassium and blood pressure changes, suggesting actions analogous to those of mineralocorticoids. However, there are no reports of such effects from licorice used as a flavoring agent.

Cocoa in various guises and derivatives, such as cocoa syrup and chocolate, is one of the most popular flavoring agents in pediatric preparations. It is prepared from the powder obtained from the ripe seeds of *Theobroma cacao*. Hundreds of specific chemical entities have been identified in cocoa (22) and the potential contribution of most of them to various responses to cocoa remains unknown.

The complex flavor sensation responsible for the popularity of roasted cocoa derivatives is probably due to a variety of flavinoids, sugars, and amino acids. Defatted cocoa forms the chocolate base from which chocolate flavor is derived by the addition of other components, particularly vanillin. The NF syrup formula contains 18% cocoa plus vanillin, sodium chloride, the preservative sodium benzoate, and sweeteners (sucrose, glucose, glycerin). Medicinal cocoa is specified to contain less than 12% material extractable in nonpolar solvents, in contrast to "breakfast cocoa," which contains twice as much such material. The tendency to use "cleaner" cocoa preparations in medicinal flavoring than in foods makes adverse reactions less likely. However, they can occur, especially in highly sensitive subjects.

Two types of adverse effects may result from cocoa. Allergic reactions to chocolate are reviewed in more detail in Part III of this volume. Pharmacological reactions induced by cocoa alkaloids are, by and large, sympathomimetic. These alkaloids resemble theophyllin and caffeine in both their chemical structure and effect. About two dozen pyrazine derivatives and nine pyrroles have been identified. In most individuals, the pharmacological response to chocolate in the usual amounts ingested in foods is imperceptible. However, an occasional individual does react sufficiently to make avoidance desirable. Tachycardia and insomnia are probably the most common complaints associated with these alkaloids. There is a theoretical possibility that cocoa flavoring of preparations of aminophyllin, caffeine, or related sympathomimetic agents might influence the physiological disposition (pharmacokinetics) or response to the active drug. Cocoa derivatives should be avoided for 12–14 hr before bronchial challenge tests are administered.

IV. AROMATIC (ESSENTIAL) OILS

This class of flavoring agent consists of materials that in their undiluted form are frequently locally irritating and systemically toxic. The term "aromatic", used to describe these materials, is based on the literal meaning of the word—volatile substances with an aroma (smell)—rather than the chemical term indicating organic compounds with unsaturated cyclic carbon structures. However, many essential oils contain large amounts of chemically aromatic compounds. Cyclohexyl derivatives are also frequently important components of essential oils. Many have short unsaturated aliphatic substitutions of the terpene type (Fig. 2). Free aliphatic terpene compounds are also commonly found as components of these oils.

A few decades ago, when pharmacists compounded prescriptions, they would flavor a bottle of liquid medicine by dipping the tip of a glass rod into a small bottle of the essential oil and then into the bottle with a pint or quart of the liquid medicine. The adequacy of that procedure in imparting the desired flavor reflects the small amount of many essential oils needed for flavoring. Toxic consequences are not expected and rarely observed unless there is accidental ingestion or direct topical application of the concentrated oil itself. There is also recorded evidence of ill effects from inhalation among workers in facilities processing essential oils. While these experiences are helpful in considering the possible nature of adverse effects of essential oils used as excipients in medications, they do not constitute evidence that medications flavored with traces of these oils are dangerous to the consumer. However, immunological sensitization and idiosyncratic reactions remain a possibility.

When the preparation of aromatic materials involves extraction of protein-free lipidic compounds, the likelihood of direct IgE-mediated reactivity is remote. However, there seems to be little doubt that exposure to fragrance materials as commonly marketed may be responsible for a variety of contact sensitivity manifestations, including photosensitivity dermatitis (35).

Some flavoring oils, such as bitter almond, have long been included in lists of materials not recommended for use in foods (36). As long ago as 1850, the toxic potential of oil of bitter almond, especially in liquors and baked goods (ratafia), was recognized and attributed to its hydrocyanic acid content. Even then, a method was suggested that "entirely deprived [oil of bitter almond] of its deadly poisonous properties, although its flavoring quality is not in any way affected" (37).

Essential oils are rarely pure chemical agents. They generally consist of several organic compounds with a low boiling point such as the cyclic derivaties shown in Figure 2 plus a variety of alcohols, aldehydes, ketones, esters, ethers, phenols, terpenes, and other hydrocarbons, sometimes including nitrogen and sulfur derivatives. Their toxicological consequences are likely to be complex, with more than one component involved. On the other hand, it is interesting that the toxic effects of essential oils as a group seem to be similar (38). The chemical structures of some major components of essential oils with important flavor characteristics are compared in Figure 2.

There have been several approaches to describing and grading the toxic potential of aromatic oils. Accidental poisonings in children have been reviewed (39) and toxicity ratings prepared on the basis of mortality (38). Animal studies of toxic effects occurring by percutaneous absorption (36) illustrate the potency of some of these preparations. However, quantitative toxicological data are not available for most essential oils used as excipients. As with fruit flavors, product uniformity and definition leave much to be desired, and isolated clinical reports often confuse idiosyncratic, allergic, and direct or classic toxic reactions.

A great deal of information about the allergic/hypersensitivity potential of the volatile oils has come via their use in perfumes (40). The experience of chemical and dermatologic experts in trying to track down the components of essential oils that are allergenic has been both informative and frustrating. These are reviewed in detail in Part III. Patch test results (40), lists of sensitizing components in perfumes, essential oils, or oil components (41), and detailed studies of particular commercial products (42–44) reflect the clinical complexity of the problem.

In general the "gemisch" that constitutes many essential oils could be associated with not only multiple covalent reactions but also reversible hydrogen bonding that can change antigenicity. Perfume manufacturers frequently store or "age" their products for months to let them "mature" to their full fragrance and particularly to reach a "balanced, stable" status with correspondingly altered antigenicity. Subsequently, when perfume contacts air and light on application, significant chemical changes may rapidly ensue, again providing an opportunity for change in sensitization potential.

Known sensitizers may not show their allergenicity when certain other substances are present in the formulation. Patients with demonstrated cinnamic aldehyde sensitivity have used perfume containing this chemical without reaction and do not react to oils with as much as 85% of the aldehyde (45). Eugenol has been found to block the sensitivity reaction to cinnamic aldehyde in some subjects. Aside from considerations of concentration, the absence of sensitivity reaction could be a consequence of the aldehydes reacting with amines to form a Schiff base, or with alcohol to form a hemiacetal (see Part III).

While one can identify a list of substances in essential oils associated with sensitization reactions, the factors discussed above point out the complexity of trying to do away with such reactions by listing "permitted" and "forbidden" substances.

Essential oils in toothpaste and mouthwashes may be responsible for lesions at the corners of the mouth that are often confused with cheilitis due to vitamin A deficiency. Numerous oils have been held responsible, including clove, eugenol, cinnamon, benzoin, vanilla, orange, lemon, caraway, dill, anise, and menthol (see Part III).

From 1930 to 1950, over 10% of accidental poisoning deaths in British children were attributed to the direct toxicity of volatile oils (39), mostly from household products rather than medicinals. The following is a discussion of reports concerning some specific essential oils of interest as excipients.

1. Oil of Camphor

Camphor is an aliphatic cyclohexyl compound originally derived as the D-isomer from camphor trees, but is now mostly the D-L racimate of synthetic origin (46). It is a ketonic terpene derivative used primarily as a topical agent in liniments and for inhalation. Oil of camphor is the naturally derived product, which contains about 35% camphor plus several other complex natural organic compounds. In contrast, camphorated oil, prepared specifically for use as a liniment, is 20% camphor in a vegetable oil. Spirits of camphor, formerly used orally as a stimulant, is a 10% alcoholic solution of camphor, and is now banned for internal use. Only tincture of camphorated opium (paregoric) is still permitted for oral consumption, although it has largely been replaced by simple tincture of opium without camphor. The toxic consequences of paregoric when taken in excess doses are largely due to the opium rather than the camphor.

Camphor poisoning is manifested by vomiting and central stimulant effects including convulsions and mental changes (47,48). Deaths reported have generally involved doses well in excess of 10 g, although as little as a 2 g dose has been reported to cause discernible toxicity (39,49).

Camphor is not a commonly used flavoring agent today, and the amounts and concentrations used for this purpose are minimal. It is used in topical preparations to give a cooling sensation, and is absorbed through the skin and respiratory tract (38).

Besides the dominant central nervous system effects, camphor also may cause some transient hepatic and renal derangement. Its detoxification by hepatic conjugation with glucuronic acid may be deficient in infants, leading to greater toxicity. Successful detoxification by lipid hemodialysis (50) and particularly by resin hemoperfusion with amberlite XAD-4 has been reported (51).

2. Dill Oil (Oleum Anethi)

Dill oil is a distillate of seeds, stalks, or leaves that darkens with age. It is about 50% carvone (Fig. 2). An acceptable daily intake of carvone is said to be 1 mg/kg/day, although further studies are required to evaluate better its toxic potential (52)

3. Caraway Oil

This preparation from freshly crushed caraway consists mostly of ketones of the carvone type. There are no reports of adverse effects from its use as an excipient.

4. Oil of Cloves

Oil of cloves is about 80% eugenol (Fig. 2), and has long been used topically to control the pain of toothache. When used as a flavoring agent, the dose involved rarely approaches the presumably safe intake level of 2.5 mg/kg. The oral LD_{50} is 2-3 g/kg in rodents (53). The pattern of systemic toxicity is described as closely resembling that of phenol (38,54). Skin sensitivity aspects of eugenol are reviewed in Part III.

5. Oil of Peppermint

This volatile oil from the flowering tops of *Mentha piperita* resembles the oils from other *Mentha* species. It contains esters and free alcoholics of menthol, a cyclohexyl aliphatic compound (Fig. 2), and related structures. There is also a dementhylated preparation of oil of peppermint that still retains its mint flavor.

Chronic consumption of large doses of peppermint candy has been reported to be capable of causing atrial fibrillation (55) and muscle pain described as palindromic rheumatism (56). Minty flavors are associated with a cooling sensation occasionally perceived as burning. However, clinically significant adverse reactions to modestly peppermint flavored materials are not common.

6. Spearmint Oil

This oil is also prepared from a species of mentha (*M. viridis*) and contains primarily carvone. Its toxic potential is presumed to be similar to that of peppermint.

7. Oil of Cinnamon

Oil of cinnamon is composed primarily of cinnamic aldehyde (cinnamal). It is a simple benzyl derivative ($G_6H_5CH=CH-CHO$), which is readily oxidized to cinnamic acid and excreted by conversion to benzoic and hippuric acids. It is therefore presumed to have little systemic toxic potential. However, oil of cinnamon and the aldehyde have been reported to be capable of producing dermatitis (57-59) (see Part III for details).

8. Oil of Wintergreen

This oil, also known as Ol. betulae or sweet birch oil, is probably the purest of the essential oils, being 98% methyl salicylate. It needs to be protected from light, alkaline, and iron salts, and should not be stored in containers (e.g., poly-styrene) with which it may react.

The systemic toxic potential of methyl salicylate had been attributed to its hydrolysis in the stomach to methyl alcohol and salicylic acid. The adverse effects of these two derivatives are well known, and the amounts liberated from a dose of oil of wintergreen can be calculated readily. However, the weight of evidence suggests that hydrolysis occurs primarily in the liver after absorption (60), with little if any ill effect attributable to the liberated methyl group.

There are sporadic reports of systemic intoxication (60-62) and allergic topical sensitivity (55,63,64). Salicylism can occur from topically absorbed methyl salicylate, according to some reports (65).

The ingestion of 0.5 mg/kg/day is considered safe (66), and its use as a flavoring agent involves quantities that are pharmacologically insignificant. Quantities used to flavor toothpaste (a small fraction of 1%) are not likely to be harmful, although enthusiastic ingestors of wintergreen "mint" candies could develop adverse reactions, particularly involving the oropharyngeal mucosa (64).

There are few data to suggest cross-sensitivity among aspirin-intolerant people to topical methyl salicylate or to the many topical preparations that contain salicylic acid as a keratolytic. While there are anecdotal reports of cross-intolerance, these have not been documented by double-blind challenge tests. Lists of salicylate-containing food, drug and plant products have been compiled (56) for patients with apparent salicylate intolerance. The clinical usefulness of such lists is debatable.

9. Oil of Eucalyptus

Oil of eucalyptus or sassafras has had a variety of uses (67) including for flavoring and perfumery. It consists mostly (about 75%) of safrole, a propenyl benzo-dioxole (Fig. 2). It can be severely depressant, with vertigo, ataxia, and coma resulting from ingestion of a dose of several grams. Respiratory symptoms and pupillary changes may also be of central origin. Mild symptoms may occur following a dose of less than 1 g. Severe poisoning has been successfully treated with intravenous mannitol and dialysis (68). Chronic administration of large doses of safrole or its derivatives to animals is hepatotoxic (32), and dehydro-safrole caused malignant esophageal tumors.

10. Rose Oil

The fresh flower of a variety of species of damask rose is used to produce this oil, which contains primarily geraniol and citronellol. It is used in lozenges and dental and topical preparations, commonly in the form of rose water, which is a saturated aqueous solution of the rose oil terpinoids.

Adverse reactions to rose oil have not been reported other than as a possible contributor to cosmetic dermatitis (56, p. 288). Its terpinoids are generally considered harmless at oral doses of 0.5 mg/kg (52).

11. Lavender Oil

This ill-defined material is used to color, flavor, and to cover up unpleasant odors. There are several varieties, both natural and synthetic, that are characterized as containing at least 35% esters calculated as linalyl acetate, and are presumed to be safe orally at dosages of 0.5 mg/kg (52). It is often compounded into alcoholic solutions (tinctures, spirits) with other agents.

12. Nutmeg Oil

The volatile oil distilled from nutmeg or mace (West Indian or East Indian oil) is composed chiefly of terpenes. When used in large doses as a therapeutic agent, it is capable of causing severe and even fatal reactions due largely to central nervous system effects (69,70). Its presumed antidiarrheal utility may not involve a prostaglandin mechanism, as previously proposed (71).

13. Orange Oil

Orange oil prepared from the peel of fresh oranges is used alone or in mixtures with other agents such as lemon, coriander, and anise oils to form Aromatic Elixir or Compound Orange Spirit. Bitter orange peel in a dried form is also used to make a variety of tinctures, syrups, elixirs, and orange flavoring excipients. Orange oil contains over 90% limonene (Fig. 2), a simple terpene derivative also found in the oils of lemon, caraway, and dill. While limonene itself is described as a skin irritant and sensitizer, and sensitiveity to orange peel is recognized clinically, there are no reports of adverse effects to orange-flavored preparations attributed to the flavoring component.

A more strongly flavored and more water-soluble preparation known as terpeneless orange oil is prepared from orange oil by low-pressure treatment or solvent partition. Oral intake of up to 0.5 mg/kg of this oil is considered safe (52).

14. Lemon Oil

Lemon oil is prepared from fresh lemon peel and, like orange oil, consists mainly of limonene. Its uses and safety characteristics are essentially the same as those described above for orange oil. A WHO committee considers 500 μg/kg an acceptable daily intake (72). Its possible role in causing contact dermatitis is discussed in Part III.

15. Oil of Anise

About 90% of anise oil is anethole (Fig. 2), a methoxypropenylbenzene closely resembling safrole chemically. Even though it is also called anise camphor, it is chemically unrelated to camphor itself, which is a fully saturated cyclohexyl derivative. Anethole is quite toxic in animals (36) but considered safe in humans in doses of 2.5 mg/kg (52). Part III discusses reports of oral cavity and skin sensitivity to this agent (73).

In considering the contribution of these and other essential oils used as a flavoring excipients to the consequences of accidental overdose of the final formulation, one is forced to conclude that unrealistic quantities of the flavored formulation would have to be consumed. In contrast, the eessential oil itself, consumed in error as an industrial product or by erroneous prescription or dispensing, could have serious consequences.

The revolting taste of some essential oils in their concentrated form is sometimes considered to be the best protection against accidental ingestion. However, such "protection" is far from complete, particularly in children (39). It is well established that tastes or smells that are strong and revolting to some people can be neutral and even pleasant to others.

V. SYNTHETIC (IMITATION) FLAVORS

This class of flavoring agents has enjoyed a steady increase in popularity in spite of the negative connotation of terms such as "artificial," "synthetic," or "imitation," which are properly applied to them. Compared to natural flavors, their composition is more constant, availability more reliable, stability more predictable, cost generally lower, and incompatibilities more consistent and reliably determined. These characteristics reflecting greater consistency make any toxic potential easier to evaluate and predict. However, synthetic flavors do share problems with natural products concerning the toxic potential of impurities, particularly if the commercial grades used are not as pure as they might be. For both natural and synthetic flavoring agents, "carryover" materials involved in the production process can be significant. Essentially all the derivatives illustrated in Figure 2 are available as synthetics. Their toxic potential has been reviewed. Many unsaturated aliphatic derivatives are frequently used.

It is the common consensus that natural flavors taste better and are safer than the synthetic products. Considering that many of the synthetics have the identical structure as key components of the natural flavors, it is difficult to accept the notion that they are more toxic. It is possible that toxic impurities from the manufacturing process could be carried into the final product. In addition, natural products may contain other components that protect against the toxic potential of the primary agent, and are not present in synthetic preparations. Such conceivable effects are difficult to observe and document. Similar considerations may also apply to the many artificial flavoring formulations that commonly contain 20 or more ingredients.

Some synthetic substances have long been known for their intrinsic merits as flavoring agents rather than being an imitation of a natural flavor. Chloroform, for example, has a sweet, pleasant taste and has been used in aqueous ("chloroform water"), alcoholic ("spirits"), and emulsion formulations. It is, of course, a potent systemic anesthetic and poisonous when taken in adequate dosage, but is generally without pharmacological action when used as an excipient in such formulations.

1. Amyl Butyrate

This ester and the aryl acetates, were used to imitate the flavor of bananas even before they were shown to be components of the natural aroma (22). Synthetic formulations are now frequently augmented by a variety of other esters, citrous oils, and vanillin. The components used are not all contained in natural banana aroma and several components of the natural product remain unidentified. Amyl butyrate is also employed in apricot, pear, plum, and pineapple flavoring.

Esters of butyric acid are readily hydrolyzed by serum esterases (74) that are probably similar or identical to the serum alkaline phosphatases. The resulting simple hydrocarbon acids are essentially all normal components of carbohydrate and fat metabolism, consistent with the absence of reports of side effects. Thus simple butyric acid esters as used for flavoring are apparently not toxic.

2. Vanillin

The popular flavor of vanilla, originally extracted from the vanilla bean, has essentially been replaced by the much cheaper synthetic vanillin. There are still some cooking recipes that insist on the use of material from the tropical bean, but essentially all the vanilla flavoring used as a medicinal excipient is synthetic vanillin. Toxic responses reported are similar to those for eugenol (32).

3. Menthol

Volatile oils from several species of *Mentha* (see discussion of oil of peppermint above) contain menthol in the levorotatory form. Synthetic menthol is prepared as either the levo- or racemic forms. Essentially all toxicological information comes from its use for therapeutic purposes, particularly its vapors, rather than as a flavoring agent. It is often included in formulations for bronchitis and sinusitis and topically for its cooling effect, particularly for localized pain.

Large doses of menthol are directly toxic (38,75,76) but the clinically more important problem in regard to its excipient use is the potential for hypersensitivity reactions, which are discussed in Part III (77,78). Rare systemic allergic reactions are also reported (79).

4. Benzaldehyde

This synthetic material (Fig. 2) has the burning taste and smell of bitter almonds characteristic of the essential oil of almond. An alcoholic spirit is used as an alternative to wild cherry syrup and, in combination with vanillin and orange water, it is prepared as an elixir.

In large doses, benzaldehyde is centrally toxic. Doses of 1 g/kg may be fatal in humans (38). Up to 5 mg/kg/day orally is considered acceptable (66).

5. Newer Synthetic Flavoring Agents

In recent years, newly synthesized molecules have been prepared with properties that blend well with aromas characteristic of fruit flavors. For example, several new allyl (CH_2=CH–CH_3) derivatives (i.e., proprionate, butyrate, and cyclohexyl valerate, and caproate) are described as useful in imitating the aroma of apricot. Such newly synthesized agents may be used only as permitted by regulatory agencies.

Some natural flavors have proved very difficult to imitate synthetically. Common chemically defined flavor ingredients do not blend well with currant flavor, leading experts to resort to mixtures of essential oils in their attempt to produce the currant flavor artificially.

Artificial grape flavor presents a different problem. Grape flavor varies considerably with the grape species and the extent to which the peel is included with the pulp. The flavor of grape juice can be quickly altered on storage unless steps are taken to block the change.

In summary, this review of flavoring agents reveals that they are probably the most complex of all excipients to evaluate scientifically for potential side effects. Fortunately, the side effects attributable to flavoring agents are not severe, unless large amounts of essential oils are ingested.

REFERENCES

1. Martindale. The Extra Parmacopoeia. (J.E.F. Reynolds, ed.), The Pharmaceutical Press, London (1982).
2. Newcomer, A.D. Disaccharidase deficiencies. Mayo Clin. Proc. 48:648–652 (1973).
3. Brunzell, J.D. Use of fructose, xylol or sorbitol as a sweetener in diabetes mellitus. Diabetes Care 1:223 (1978).
4. Life Sciences Res. Office: Dietary sugars in health and disease. III. Sorbital. Federation of American Societies for Experimental Biology, Bethesda, Maryland (1979).
5. Life Sciences Res. Office: Dietary sugars in health and disease. II. Xylitol. Federation of American Societies for Experimental Biology, Bethesda, Maryland (1978).
6. Walters, D.E., Pearlstein, R.A. and Krimmel, C.P. Procedure for preparing models of receptor sites. J. Chem. Ed. 63:869–872 (1986).
7. Ranney, R.E., Opperman, J.A., Muldoon, E. and McMahon, F.G. Comparative metabolism of aspartame in experimental animals and humans. J. Toxicol. Environ. Health 2:441 (1976).

8. Weiner, M. Discussions. *In* Obesity: Causes, Consequences and Treatment. (Lasagna, L., ed.). Medcom Press, New York, pp. 98–100 (1974).

9. Kalkhoff, R.K. and Levin, M.E. The saccharin controversy. Diabetes Care 1:211 (1978).

10. Isselbacher, K.J. and Cole, P. Saccharin—the bitter and sweet. N. Engl. J. Med. 296:1348 (1977).

11. The saccharin question re-examined: An A.D.A. statement. J. Am. Dietet. Assoc. 74:574 (1979).

12. Morrison, A.B. Sugar substitutes. Can. Med. Assoc. J. 120:633 (1979).

13. Cohen, B.L. Relative risks of saccharin and calories ingestion. Science 199:983 (1978).

14. Bauer, J.K. and Horwitz, D.L. New trends in diabetic diets. Compr. Ther. 5(12):12 (1979).

15. Horwitz, D.L. and Bauer, J.K. How do we feed the person with diabetes. Conn. Med. 44:707 (1980).

16. Harper, A.E. Aspartame in sweeteners: Issues and uncertainties. National Academy of Sciences, Washington, D.C. pp. 182–188 (1975).

17. FDA: Aspartame: Commissioner's final decision. Fed. Reg. 46:38285 (1981).

18. Baldwin, R.E. and Kroschgen, B.M. Intensification of fruit flavors by aspartame. J. Food Sci. 44:938 (1979).

19. Novick, N.L. A case of granulomatous panniculitis. Ann. Intern. Med. 102–205 (1985).

20. Novick, N.L. Aspartame-induced granulomatous panniculitis. Ann. Intern. Med. 102:206 (1985).

21. Wurtman, R.J. Aspartame: Possible effect on seizure susceptibility. Lancet 2:1060 (1985).

22. Furia, T.E. and Bellanca, N. *In*: Fenaroli's Handbook of Flavor Ingredients. Second Ed., Vol. 2. CRC Press, Cleveland, p. 597.

23. FDA: Aspartame—decision of the public board of inquiry. Docket No. 75F-0355 (1980).

24. Stegink, L.D., Filer, L.J. and Baker, G.L. Effect of aspartame plus monosodium L-glutamate ingestion on plasma and erythrocyte amino acid levels in normal adult subjects fed a high protein meal. Am. J. Clin. Nutr. 36:1145 (1982).

25. Smith, R.J. Aspartame approved despite risks. Science 213:986 (1981).

26. Johns, D.R. Migraine provoked by aspartame. N. Engl. J. Med. 315:456 (1986).

27. Bradstock, M.E., Serdula, M.K., Marks, J.S., et al. Evaluation of reactions to food additives: The aspartame experience. Am. J. Clin. Nutr. 43:464–469 (1986).

28. Shiffman, S.S., Buckley, C.E., Sampson, H.A., Massey, E.W., Baraniuk, J.N., Follett, J.V. and Warwick, Z.S. Aspartame and susceptibility to headache. N. Engl. J. Med. 317:1181–1185 (1987).

29. Cyclamates Antagonistic to Antibiotic. Anonymous news item: J.G. Wagner reports that absorption of lincomycin hydrochloride drops 75%

when present with sodium or calcium cyclamate. J. Am. Diet. Assoc. 54: 121 (1969).

30. Wagner, J.G. Antibiotic News 5:6 (1968).

31. Adverse reactions to foods. NIH Publication No. 84-2442. AAAI and NIAID Report, July 1984.

32. Hagan, E.C., Jenner, P.M., Jones, W.I., Fitzhugh, O.G., Long, E.L., Browner, J.G. and Webb, W.K. Toxic properties of compounds related to safrole. Toxciol. Appl. Pharmacol. 7:18-24 (1965).

33. Gleason, M.N., Gosselin, R.E., Hodge, H.C. and Smith, R.P. Clinical Toxicology of Commercial Products. Acute poisoning. Ed. 3. William & Wilkins, Baltimore (1969).

34. Baron, J.H. and Sullivan F.M. (Eds.) Carbenoxolone Sodium. Butterworths, London (1979).

35. Addo, H.A., Ferguson, J., Johnson, B.E. and Frain-Bell, W. Relationship between exposure to fragrance materials and persistent light reaction in the photosensitivity dermatitis with actinic reticulois syndrome. Br. J. Dermatol. 107:261-274 (1982).

36. Flavoring Agents in Foods, Report of the Food Standards Committee, Her Magesty's Stationary Office, London (1965).

37. Anonymous. Confectionary, how it becomes poisonous. Am. J. Med. Sci. 23:271-2 (1952).

38. Gosselin, R.E., Smith, R.P. and Hodge, H.C. Clinical Toxicology of Commercial Products. 5th Ed. Williams & Wilkins, Baltimore (1984).

39. Sibert, J.R. Poisoning in children. Br. Med. J. 1:803 (1973).

40. Larsen, W.G. Perfume dermatitis. Arch. Dermatol. 113:623 (1977).

41. Opdyke, D.L. The safety of fragrance ingredients. Br. J. Dermatol. 93: 351 (1975).

42. Goldberg, H.S. Allergic dermatitis from the perfume in Mycolog cream. Arch. Dermatol. 105:896 (1972).

43. Coskey, R.I. and Bryan, H.G. Contact dermatitis due to perfume in Mycolog cream—a letter. Arch. Dermatol. 111:131 (1975).

44. Larsen, W.G. Allergic contact dermatitis to the perfume in Mycolog cream. J. Am. Acad. Dermatol. 1:131 (1979).

45. Fisher, A.A. and Dooms-Goossens, A. The effect of perfume "aging" on the allergenicity of individual perfume ingredients. Contact Derm. 2:155 (1976).

46. The Merck Index. 9th Ed. Merck & Co., Rahway, New Jersey (1976).

47. Skoglund, R.R., Ware, L.L. and Schanberger, M.C. Prolonged seizures due to contact and inhalation exposure to camphor. Clin. Pediatr. 16:901–902 (1977).

48. Trestrail, J.H. and Spartz, M.E. Camphorated and castor oil congestion and its toxic results. Clin. Toxicol. 11:151–158 (1977).

49. Vasey, R.H. and Karayannopocilos, S.J. Camphorated oil. Br. Med. J. 1: 112 (1972).

50. Antman, E., Jacob, G., Volpe, B., Finkel, S. and Savona, M. Camphor overdosage: Therapeutic considerations. N.Y. State J. Med. 78:896-7, (1978).

51. Koppel, C., Tenczer, J., Schirop, T.H. and Ibe, K. Camphor poisoning. Arch. Toxicol. 51:101 (1982).
52. 23rd Report of Joint FAO/WHO Expert Committee on Food Additives. Tech. Rep. Serv. WHO No. 648 (1980).
53. Sober, H.A., Hollander, F. and Sober, E.K. Toxicity of eugenol: determination of LD50 on rats. Proc. Soc. Exp. Biol. Med. 73:148-151 (1950).
54. Lauber, F.U. and Hollander, F. Toxicity of the mucigogue, eugenal administered by stomach tube to dogs. Gastroenterology 15:481-486 (1950).
55. Thomas, J.G. Peppermint fibrillation. Lancet 1:222 (1962).
56. Williams, B. Palindromic rheumatism: A request. Med. J. Austr. 2:390-391 (1972).
57. Fisher, A.A. Dermatitis due to cinnamon and cinnamic aldehyde. Cutis 16: 383 (1975).
58. Kern, A.N. Contact dermatitis from cinnamon. Arch. Dermatol. 64:52 (1951).
59. Noter 4 News. Sunscreen Allergy (cinnamate). Lancet 1:639 (1984).
60. Davison, C., Zimmerman, E.F. and Smith, P.K. On the metabolism and toxicity of methyl salicylate. J. Pharmacol. Exp. Ther. 132:207-211 (1961).
61. Cancelmo, J.J. Methyl salicylate poisoning. J.A.M.A. 136:651 (1948).
62. Adams, J.T., Bigler, J.A. and Green, O.C. A case of methyl salicylate intoxication treated by exchange transfusion. J.A.M.A. 165:1563-1565 (1957).
63. Morgon, J.K. Iatrogenic epidermal sensitivity. Br. J. Clin. Pract. 22:261-264 (1968).
64. Speer, F. Allergy to methyl salicylate. Ann. Allergy 43:36-37 (1979).
65. Arena, J.M. Poisoning. 2nd Ed. Charles C Thomas, Springfield, Illinois (1970).
66. Specifications for the identity and purity of food additives and their toxicological evaluation: some flavouring substances and non-nutritive sweetening agents. Eleventh Report of the Joint FAO/WHO Expert Committee on Food Additives. Tech. Rep. Series WHO No. 383 (1968).
67. Ramaswamy, A.S. Review of eucalyptus oils—constituents, properties and uses of medicine, perfumery and industry. Pharmacist 11:11 (1965).
68. Gurr, F.W. and Scroggie, J.G. Eucalyptus oil poisoning treated by dialysis and mannitol infusion. Aust. Ann. Med. 14:238-249 (1965).
69. Venables, G.S., Evered, D. and Hall, R. Nutmeg poisoning. Br. Med. J. 1:96 (1976).
70. Panayotopoulos, D.J. and Chisholm, D.D. Hallucinogenic effect of nutmeg. Br. Med. J. 1:754 (1970).
71. Dietz, W.H. and Stuart, M.J. Nutmeg and prostaglandin. New Engl. J. Med. 294:503 (1976).
72. 23rd FAO/WHO. Expert Committee on food additives. Tech. Report No. 648 WHO (1980).
73. Lovema, A.B. Report of a case of sensitivity of mucous membranes and the skin to oil of anise. Arch. Dermatol. 37:70 (1983).

74. Shapiro, S., Wroblewski, F., Weiner, M. and Spitzer, J. Ethyl butyante hydrolyzing activity of human serum. Am. J. Clin. Pathol. 20:614 (1950).
75. Luke, E. Addiction to mentholated cigarettes. Lancet 1:110–111 (1962).
76. Highstein, B. and Zeligman, I. Nonthrombocytopenic purpura caused by mentholated cigarettes. J.A.M.A. 146:816 (1951).
77. Papa, C.M. and Shelley, W.B. Menthol hypersensitivity. J.A.M.A. 189:546–548 (1964).
78. Rudzki, E. and Kleniewska, D. The epidemiology of contact dermatitis in Poland. Br. J. Dermatol. 83:543–545 (1970).
79. McGowan, E.M. Methol urticaria. Arch. Dermatol. 94:62–63 (1966).
80. Teeter, J. and Gott, G.H. Sensory transduction: A taste of things to come. Nature 331:298–9 (1988).

9

Adverse Effects: Coloring Agents

I. Purpose of coloring agents   159
II. Composition of coloring agents   161
III. History of regulation of coloring agents in the United States   161
IV. Reactions to specific dyes   162
    References   164

I. PURPOSE OF COLORING AGENTS

The spectrum of purposes for which coloring agents are used is now undergoing careful scrutiny in the face of reawakened concerns about the potential for significant undesirable reactions. As with all other aspects of medicine, there is a need to balance the benefits against the risks. It is therefore necessary to review the purposes served by coloring agents, to be balanced against the risks involved in their use.

The color of medicinals is sometimes looked upon as a matter of esthetics rather than necessity. Prior to the modern pharmaceutical era, if one walked into the back room of a pharmacy and inspected the rows of powdered materials used in the compounding of most prescriptions, one would find the products to be mostly white or gray–brown to off-white. These ingredients were generally weighed, mixed by mortar and pestle, and distributed into powder papers, rolled into pills or inserted into translucent gelatin capsules as individual dose units with no attention to or concern about the color.

On occasion, these medications were dissolved or suspended in water, labeled "shake well before use," again with little concern about color. Many liquids, particularly topical lotions or ointments, had colors characteristic of their contents (calamine lotion, iodine solutions, etc.). Many liquid medications were elixir or syrup extracts of botanical products that frequently had a characteristic color other than white. Flavoring agents, and particularly natural fruit flavors, tended to determine the color of the medicine.

The deliberate addition of a coloring agent sometimes raised suspicions of a fraudulent intent to lead the consumer to look upon the product as something other than what it was. On the other hand adding color, even if only for psychological or esthetic reasons, was believed by many to be a legitimate procedure to enhance the acceptability of a product and to help achieve the desired therapeutic responses. Even in modern times controlled studies have shown that a medication's color can influence therapeutic response.

An ancient and still important purpose of coloring a medicine is to help give a unique identity to the product. Characteristic colors and shapes have simplified the lives of patients, pharmacists, and physician for decades. The triangular dark green tablet of enteric-coated iron sulfate (Feosal) has been known to millions for decades and is promptly recognizable.

In today's environment of polypharmacy, primarily a reflection of necessity rather than overtreatment (1), the patient frequently identifies and takes medications according to their color. The need to take different medications that look the same is a clear invitation to confusion, noncompliance, and errors.

Colors are sometimes added to enhance the purpose of flavoring. A red mint-flavored product, or a green cherry-flavored prescription would be bound to cause confusion and distrust, while the opposite—green mint-flavored prescriptions and red cherry-flavored medicines—is readily accepted.

Some materials are difficult to prepare consistently with a precisely reproducible color and shade. Sometimes perceptible color changes occur on storage, even though sophisticated chemical and biological tests show no significant change in composition. A patient is likely to become concerned if a refilled prescription compared with the remnant of the original appears detectably different. This problem is a prime motivation for manufacturers to control the uniformity of the appearance of their product by the use of coloring agents.

The coloring of liquids is generally achieved by dissolving a coloring agent into the product. Solid formulations can be colored in a variety of ways. The color can be added to the formulation so as to permeate the whole formulation. If the product is a scored tablet, intended to be broken into halves in some instances, this method of coloring is usually essential. On the other hand, capsules or unscored tablets can have their color confined to the coat. Whether a capsule or tablet coating designed to be opaque is considered to contain a coloring agent is a semantic problem of no real importance. The significant fact is the amount and nature of the substance used and ingested, and therefore a potential cause of adverse reactions. The most common opaquing agent in capsules is titanium dioxide, which is presumably unabsorbed and nontoxic in the amounts used for this purpose.

The consequences of beautifying the appearance of products to be ingested without regard for the harmful potential of the agent employed has a long history. Over 100 years ago the medical profession recognized the danger and condemned the use of colorful arsenic and lead salts to decorate fancy baked goods (2). Later the carcinogenic potential of the popular food and drug dye, butter yellow, was recognized and its use prohibited. More recently there has been concern that some "grandfathered" or "GRAS" (generally recognized as safe) coloring agents have not undergone the type of long-term expensive testing for carcinogenesis currently required of new drugs. From the economic point of view, the magnitude of the market and the absence of patent protection is not conducive to the support of such studies by private enterprise. Nevertheless, carcinogenic potential must be considered with reason rather than panic.

Colorants are particular candidates for concern about phototoxicity: becoming toxic only after they are chemically altered by exposure to light (3). Evaluation of sensitivity to colorants is reviewed in Part III and includes patch test techniques (4) (5).

In order to understand better the possible side effects of coloring agents, it will be useful to review briefly their nature and the history of their use.

II. COMPOSITION OF COLORING AGENTS

Coloring agents used in pharmaceuticals fall generally into two classes: *dyes*, a term applied to soluble colored materials that go into true solution, generally in water; and *pigments*, which are colored particulates capable of coloring liquid or solid materials into which they are dispersed. A subclass of pigments are *lakes*, prepared by the tight adsorption or bonding of dyes to otherwise uncolored, insoluble particulate materials such as alumina (6).

Frequent reports in the older literature describe the development of sarcomas from intramuscularly injected pigments. These results are now generally believed to be more a consequence of the particulate nature of material trapped at a local site than an inherent carcinogenic characteristic of its chemical structure. If this concept is accepted, the occurrence of such injection site tumors can be considered irrelevant to the potential carcinogenesis of orally consumed pigments. While the concept is not universally accepted (7,8), the absence of carcinogenesis when the agent is taken by other routes and test modalities makes the significance of local consequences following intramuscular injection of dubious systemic significance.

III. HISTORY OF REGULATION OF COLORING AGENTS
IN THE UNITED STATES

By the late 19th century, synthetic dyes had largely replaced natural dyes, and at the turn of the century about 80 synthetic dyes were in use for various food, medicinal, and cosmetic purposes (9). In 1906, the first Food and Drug laws permitted the use of only seven of these in materials for human consumption: amaranth, erythrosine, indigotine, light green, naphthol yellow, orange 1, and ponceau 3R. Between 1915 and 1930, seven more were added to the list of permitted dyes.

New laws in 1938 redefined coloring agents into three categories and substituted color prefexes and numbers for the common names. The 15 approved colors then existing were subjected to fresh toxicologic evaluation and were declared "harmless and suitable. . ."

In the 1950s a series of reports reopened concerns about potential side effects of coloring agents. Diarrhea was reported in children consuming foods with excessive amounts of orange 1 and red 32. After further chronic animal feeding toxicity studies, these agents and orange 2 were "delisted." Yellow 1, 2, 3, and 4 were also delisted later on the basis of the Delaney Amendment, which introduced the "zero tolerance" concept for any agent causing malignant changes at any dose (see discussion in part 1, Chapter 1). In 1960, another law eased the dose inflexibility that had resulted from the prior court rulings. However, as recently as the end of 1987 courtroom conflicts have yet to be resolved concerning FDA judgements about "de minimis" trivial risks for some coloring agents (orange no. 17, red nos. 8, 9, 19) in the light of the rigid Delaney Clause language about colors that "induce cancer. . . in animals" (10).

IV. REACTIONS TO SPECIFIC DYES

Recent literature suggests that the prime current concern about coloring agents is on behalf of a relatively small but significant number of people who, by one or another mechanism, are hypersensitive to one or another coloring agent and develop significant adverse responses to medications that contain them. Such hypersensitivity may be manifested systemically or topically, and is reviewed in Part III. There is an instructive report of reactions to only the weaker of several strengths of a product marketed with distinctive colors for each strength. The offending dose size was the only one colored yellow, and the yellow dye proved to be responsible for the reaction (11). Had the yellow dye been used for the higher-strength formulation, the observed reactions might have been considered a dose-related side effect.

Subjects who are intolerant to aspirin seem to have an increased likelihood of reacting to dyes (12). An outstanding example discussed in detail in Part III concerns tartrazine. Other suspect colors are also briefly reviewed below.

1. Tartrazine

Tartrazine (FD & C yellow no. 5) is a yellow azo dye that becomes reddish at a higher pH and green when mixed with blue. While the exposure per dose is generally only a fraction of a milligram, it has become a major public health concern. A variety of clinical studies concerning this dye (13–16) and the interpretation of these results are reviewed in Part III.

There is an increasing tendency to avoid its use and to require that its presence be explicitly announced on the label of any product to which it has been added.

2. Carmine

Carmine (natural red 4) is an aluminum lake containing about 50% carminic acid, which is an anthraquinone glycoside. Since it is capable of supporting the growth of microorganisms (*Salmonella* is a particular concern), its sterilization by autoclaving or with 70% alcohol is recommended (17). Its safety is illustrated by its use in doses up to 500 mg as a marker to measure gastrointestinal transit time. A report (18) of asthma in two workers who repeatedly inhaled carmine-containing products is reviewed in Part III.

3. Amaranth

Amaranth (red dye no. 2) (FD & C no. 2) was the most widely used coloring agent in foods, drugs, and cosmetics in the United States before its delisting by the FDA in 1976. Most other countries still permit its use in medicines, food-stuffs, and cosmetics. Although amaranth was noted by Russion investigators to exert toxic effects on various components of the male and female reproductive systems, these findings were not subsequently confirmed by a multicenter study. Fetotoxicity studies in animals showed no effect (19,20). However, in 1976, high doses of FD&C no. 2 were reported to produce cancers in rats, and the agent was officially delisted. This regulation specifically prohibits use of the dye in all new food, drug, and cosmetic products. However, whether high-dose carcinogenic effects in rats can be extrapolated to humans has been a subject of heated debate for the past 10 years in the United States.

4. Eosin

Eosin, used particularly in lipsticks, and discussed in Part III is an example of a product causing reactions that may be due to an impurity (21,22).

5. Erythrosine

Erythrosine is an agent suspected of developing toxic potential after exposure to light, that is, phototoxicity (23). It also has been reported to be capable of causing a modest elevation in the levels of protein-bound iodine in euthyroid subjects (24).

6. Other D&C Colors

D&C red no. 9, discussed in Part III varies in its effects in accordance with differences in methods of manufacture and its content of "subsidiary colors" (25). D&C red no. 17 (26), Ponceau 4R (27), and D&C yellow nos. 10 and 11 (28-37) are all potential "sensitizers" reviewed in detail in Part III.

REFERENCES

1. Weiner, M. The clinical significance of drug interactions. *In* Pharmaco-kinetics, Drug Metabolism and Drug Interactions. (McMahon, F.G., ed.). Futura, New York (1974).

2. Anonymous. Confectionary, how it becomes poisonous. Am. J. Med. Sci. 23:271–272 (1952).

3. Valenzeno, D.P. and Pooler, J.P. Phototoxicity: The neglected factor. J.A.M.A. 242:453–454 (1979).

4. Kozuka, T., Tashiro, M., Sano, S., Fujimoto, K., Nakamura, Y., Hashimoto, S. and Nakaminami, G. Brilliant-lake-red-R as a cause of pigmented contact-dermatitis. Contact Derm. 5:297–304 (1979).

5. Rapport, M.J. Patch testing of color additives. Contact Derm. 6:231–232 (1980).

6. Swartz, C.J. and Cooper, J. Colorants for pharmaceuticals. J. Pharm. Sci. 51:89–99 (1962).

7. Huper, W.C. Carcinogenic studies on water-soluble and insoluble macro-molecular. Arch. Pathol. 67:589–617 (1959).

8. Huper, W.C. Bioassay in polyvinylpyrrolidones with limited molecular weight range. J. Natl. Cancer Inst. 26:229 (1961).

9. Noonan, J. Color additives in food. *In* Handbook of Food Additives (Furia, T.E., ed.). The Chemical Rubber Co., Cleveland, pp. 25–50 (1968).

10. Dickenson's FDA Newsletter. 3, (21):12 (1987).

11. Goetz, C.G. Skin rash associated with sinemet 25/100. N. Engl. J. Med. 309:1387–1388 (1983).

12. Speer, F., Denison, T.R. and Baptist, J.E. Aspirin allergy, Ann. Allergy 46: 123–126 (1983).

13. Speer, D., Denison, T.R. and Baptist, J.E. Aspirin allergy. Ann. Allergy 46: 123–126 (1981).

14. Neuman, I., et al. The danger of "yellow dyes" (tartrazine) to allergic sub-jects. Clin. Allergy 8:65–68 (1978).

15. Lockey, S.D., Sr. Hypersensitivity to tartrazine (FD & C Yellow #5) and other dyes and additives present in foods and pharmaceutical products. Ann. Allergy 38:206–210 (1977).

16. MacCara, M.E. Tartrazine: Potentially hazardous dye in Canadian drugs. Can. Med. Assoc. J. 126:910–914 (1982).

17. Lang, D.J., Kunz, L.J. and Martin, A.R. Carmine as a source of nosocomial salmonellosis. N. Engl. J. Med. 15:276–829 (1967).

18. Burge, P.S., O'Brien, J.M., Harries, M.G. and Pepys, J. Occupational asthma due to inhaled carmine. Clin. Allergy 9:185–189 (1979).

19. Holson, J.F., Gaines, T.B., Schumacher, H.J. and Grammer, M.F. Is red dye no. 2 teratrogenic? A joint government-industry approach to a toxicological problem. Toxicol. Appl. Pharmacol. 33:122 (1975).

20. Mastalski, K., Jenkins, D.H., Plank, J.B., Kinoshits, G.K., Keplinger, M.L. and Calandra, J.C. Teratrologic study in dogs with FD & C red no. 2. Toxicol. Appl. Pharmacol. 33:122–123 (1975).

21. Kalivas, J. A guide to the problem of photosensitivity. J.A.M.A. 209: 1706–1709 (1969).
22. Cronin, E. Contact dermatitis from cosmetics. J. Soc. Cosmet. Chem. 18: 681–691 (1967).
23. Valenzeno, D.P. and Pooler, J.P. Phototoxicity: The neglected factor. J.A.M.A. 242:453–454 (1979).
24. Haas, S. Contamination of protein-bound iodine by pink gelatin capsules colored with erythrosine. Ann. Intern. Med. 7:549–552 (1970).
25. Naganuma, M., Ohtsu, Y., Katsmura, Y., Matsuoku, M. and Mitsui, T. Analysis of subsidiary colors in D & C red No. 9 and its pruification: Development of nonallergenic D & C red No. 9. J. Soc. Cosmet. Chem. 34: 273–284 (1983).
26. Calnan, C.D. Quinazoline yellow dermatitis (D & C yellow 11) in an eye cream. Contact Derm. 7:271 (1981).
27. Myers, C. An unusual measure to prevent an adverse drug reaction. Br. Med. J. 291:450 (1985).
28. Lamson, S.A., Kong, B.M. and DeSalva, S.J. D & C yellow nos. 10 and 11: Delayed contact hypersensitivity in the guinea pig. Contact Derm. 8:200–203 (1982).
29. Weaver, J.E. Dose response relationships in delayed hypersensitivity to quinoline dyes. Contact Derm. 9:309–312 (1983).
30. Rapaport, M.J. Allergy to D & C yellow dye no. 11. Contact Derm. 6: 364–365 (1980).
31. Bjorkner, B. and Magnusson, B. Patch test sensitization to D & C yellow no. 11 and simultaneous reaction to quineline yellow. Contact Derm. 7:1–4 (1981).
32. Kita, S., Kobayashi, T., Kutsuna, H. and Kligman, A.M. Human maximization testing of D & C yellow #10 and yellow #11. Contact Derm. 11:210–213 (1984).
33. Weaver, J.E. Disparate skin allergenicity of 2 quinolone dyes. Contact Derm. 9:526–527 (1983).
34. Palazzolo, M.J. and DiPasquale, L.C. The sensitization potential of D & C yellow no. 11 in guinea pigs. Contact Derm. 9:367–371 (1983).
35. Sato, Y., Kutsuna, M., Kobayshi, T. and Mitsui, T. D & C nos. 10 and 11: Chemical composition analysis and delayed contact hypersensitivity testing in guinea pigs. Contact Derm. 10:30–38 (1984).
36. Rapaport, M.J. Allergy to yellow dyes. Arch. Dermatol. 120:535–536 (1984).
37. Bjorkner, B. and Niklasson, B. Contact allergic reaction to D & C yellow no. 11 and quinoline yellow. Contact Derm. 9:263–268 (1983).

10

Adverse Effects: Other Addition Products

I. Controlled-release and binding agents   167
II. Buffers   169
   A. Phosphate buffers   170
   B. Borate buffers   170
   C. Acetate buffers   171
   D. Citrate buffers   171
   E. Amino acid buffers   171
   F. Barbiturate buffers   172
   G. Tris buffers   172
III. Suspending, emulsifying, and stiffening agents   172
   A. Ionic agents   173
   B. Nonionic agents   174
   C. Tragacanth and acacia   174
   D. Methylcellulose   175
   E. Paraffin   175
   F. Lubricants   175
   G. Fatty alcohols   176
IV. Preservatives   176
   A. Antimicrobials   178
   B. Antioxidants   181
   C. Chelating agents   183
V. Sterilizing agent: ethylene oxide   184
VI. Propellants   184
   References   190

I. CONTROLLED-RELEASE AND BINDING AGENTS

Achieving the controlled release of active ingredients from a formulation is a function of mechanical aspects and materials. Any formulation intended for controlled release that does not function as planned carries a potential for untoward reactions to the active ingredient. The potential consequences of too rapid release are generally apparent from the nature of the drug and the dose. Too slow release from an oral preparation can lead to elimination of the unabsorbed drug in the stool. Mechanisms for controlled release range from implanted devices to simple binding agents or coatings to delay dissolution of injected or orally administered drugs.

There is now a wide spectrum of osmotic devices, including oral tablets with a laser-produced hole through which active ingredient is expelled over a period of time by osmotic pressure. Other systems involve granules, microcapsules, web and pore materials, as well as laminated multicoated tablets and enteric acid-resistant coatings.

Discussion of the mechanical aspects of these formulations is beyond the scope of this text. The prime consideration to be reviewed is the toxic potential of the materials used in controlled-release formulations. These consist mostly of common tableting materials discussed elsewhere, such as stearate esters, cellulose derivatives, talc, and a variety of aliphatic alcohols, polymeric carboxylates, polymeric gels, and copolymeric derivatives and resins.

Microencapsulation techniques are being used with increasing frequency to control the rate and locus of the release and availability for absorption of an active substance. Materials used for enteric tablet coatings (i.e., coatings that will not dissolve in acidic media) serve to protect materials from exposure to gastric juice and delay their bioavailability until they reach the small intestinal tract. These same materials can serve a similar function when used for microencapsulation. Some relatively special substances such as synthetic phospholipids and simple proteins such as prolamins are also used for microencapsulation, as are a variety of phospholipids, particularly phosphatidyl serine and phosphatidyl ethanolamine. Since these substances are notorious procoagulants, there is concern about their use in intravenous formulations. On the other hand, phosphatidylcholine (lecithin) is a key component of current parenteral alimentation formulations that are well tolerated when administered in large intravenous doses. Since these moieties are common components of foods, their oral use is generally presumed to be acceptable.

The cores of controlled-release preparations are sometimes prepared with wax and wax esters or materials made of silicon dioxide. The toxic potential of most of these materials has been discussed. In general, the literature concerning their adverse consequences is limited.

A major problem with some controlled-release intramuscular formulations is local pain. Gelatin has been used as a vehicle for intramuscularly injected materials with the goal of delayed absorption (e.g., Pitkin menstruum) but is rarely the excipient of choice for this purpose. Intravenous gelatin as a plasma expander has a relatively high incidence of side effects compared to other plasma expanders (1), a fact of no relevance to its use as a binding agent by other routes.

Solutions containing 10-25% povidone (PVP, polyvinylpyrrolidine) have been used to delay the absorption and prolong the action of intramuscularly administered drugs. Inflammatory and granulomatous reactions at the injection site of these materials have been reported (2). More disturbing are reports that after repeated injections, this presumably inert material has been found in many organs. In the skin it can cause panniculitis (3) and erythematous and papular lesions (4,5). Elsewhere granulomata (3,6,7) and reticuloendothelial (2) lesions have been reported. Lung lesions following use of PVP-containing hair spray (8) and eye reactions from a PVP-coated intraocular lens (9) have been described.

The carcinogenic potential of synthetic polymers such as PVP has been an important issue in the last two decades. The idea that the physical characteristics of large inert molecules are adequate to produce malignancy, regardless of their chemical nature, has been disputed (10,11). Concerning PVP specifically, there is no doubt that significant tissue reaction can occur (4) but carcinogenesis has not been proved (11,12) despite earlier reports to the contrary (10).

It is noteworthy that there is very little absorption of orally administered PVP (13). Large oral doses administered over prolonged periods in animals seem to have no toxic effects.

II. BUFFERS

The pH of a medicament is often critical to the stability, solubility, and bioavailability of its active ingredients. It may determine whether components of the vessel wall or cap are leached into the solution. Even with solid oral formulations, the influence of the components on the pH of the gastrointestinal milieu into which they dissolve may significantly alter the bioavailability pattern, and therefore the pharmacologic response.

Even before formulation begins, the decision to use a hydrochloride salt rather than the free base, or a sodium or potassium salt rather than a free acid form of the active ingredient is a critical determinant of the pH status of the final product. Salts are generally more soluble in water than the corresponding free acid or base form of active ingredients, and upon dissolution are less likely to result in strongly acidic or basic solutions. However, the nonionic species of a xenobiotic is often more lipid soluble and better absorbed than the ionic salt form. An appropriate balance between adequate water solubility essential for reaching the absorptive surface and adequate concentration of the lipid-soluble moiety to permit absorption is sometimes critical. The kinetics of the ionic/nonionic equilibrium may also be critical and pH can markedly influence these characteristics. Thus the finer adjustment and maintenance of a desired pH often necessitate the inclusion of a buffering agent in the formulation. Potential adverse consequences of buffers in common use will be reviewed.

In general, solutions for intramuscular or subcutaneous injection are more likely to be painful if their pH is not close to that of the tissue into which they are injected. Modest deviation from physiologic pH is more likely to be tolerated in solutions given by intravenous infusion, especially if the deviant pH is due to a low molarity of acid or base and the material is infused slowly. Extremes of pH can induce venous spasm and may disrupt red cells. Consequently, pH adjustment by buffer is an essential aspect of the formulation of parenteral medications.

The use of buffers in oral preparations may raise the semantic problem as to whether they are merely excipients or serve a therapeutic purpose as an active ingredient. Answering that question is really not important as long as it is recognized that there may be beneficial or undesirable consequences following administration of an oral buffer, irrespective of its influence on a particular active ingredient.

In topical preparations, pH is frequently a significant contributor to the response. Intravaginal preparations are almost always acidic, since a pH of about 4 or 5 is essential to the maintenance of normal vaginal flora. Skin preparations that are not slightly on the acid side seem to have a greater likelihood of being irritating.

Some buffers used commonly in the chemical laboratory are not suitable for medicinals. The choice of buffer is generally made on the basis of stability, efficacy in achieving and maintaining the desired pH, and satisfactory clinical tolerance without side effects.

A. Phosphate Buffers

These commonly used buffers usually consist of a balanced ratio of the disodium or potassium salts and the mono- or "acid" phosphate salts. These materials, if consumed in large amounts or over prolonged periods of time, may have significant effects on calcium metabolism. When given parenterally, they can alter plasma calcium levels rapidly and severely with serious consequences (14). Extraskeletal calcification (15) may follow very large and repeated doses by mouth. However, the modest amounts of buffer and the relatively small volume of the usual medicinal formulated with a phosphate buffer could hardly result in significant side effects.

B. Borate Buffers

Boric acid and its salts are used in external preparations only, particularly in topical eye solutions. The toxicity of boric acid when given systemically is well documented (16). Acute poisoning causes vomiting, diarrhea, and central nervous system stimulation followed by depression, renal and cutaneous damage, and circulatory collapse. While these severe consequences are seen acutely only after ingestion of large doses, there is concern that the absorption of small amounts of boric acid over long periods of time may lead to cumulative toxic levels, since excretion of borate is slow. Consequently, topical preparations containing boric acid should not be applied to extensive areas of damaged skin.

C. Acetate Buffers

Since acetate is a prominent normal product of the intermediate metabolism of carbohydrates and fats and is readily oxidized to carbon dioxide and water, its potential for harm is limited to its misuse in excessive concentrations or amounts, particularly in association with cations such as sodium. Thus glacial acetic acid is caustic when administered both topically and systemically, but it is not so used for buffer purposes. If acetic acid/sodium acetate buffer is administered in large quantities, the acetate is metabolized, leaving an excess of sodium that may be harmful in subjects with hepatic, renal, or cardiovascular disease. The use of ammonium acetate avoids this problem, but could be undesirable if there are disturbances of ammonia metabolism associated with hepatic cirrhosis. Ingested ammonium acetate can also be a gastric irritant. None of the above problems are realistic concerns when modest amounts of acetate preparations are used for their buffering effect.

D. Citrate Buffers

Another product of intermediate metabolism used as a buffer is citrate, sometimes combined with orthophosphate as citrophosphate. Citric acid itself is accused of eroding tooth enamel (17). This effect is probably not due to its acidic nature, but to its capacity to complex with and solubilize calcium. In fact citrate solution, carefully adjusted to the desired near-neutral pH, is the most prevalent anticoagulant into which blood is collected for processing and storage in blood banks. Citrate blocks the clotting process by binding ionic calcium. Only when multiple transfusions or other citrate-containing parenterals result in the intravenous administrations of citrate faster than in vivo metabolism is there danger of a clinically significant citrate-induced fall in plasma calcium levels. Such an effect is not seen with the use of oral citrate preparations.

E. Amino Acid Buffers

Natural amino acids such as glycine are effective buffering agents with a low potential for side effects, but with occasional problems of stability. Glycine solutions used as irrigants can, under some circumstances, result in enough absorption to cause local tissue and systemic reactions (18), including hypertension, confusion, and hyponatremia. This has led to the suggestion that urologists use normal saline rather than glycine as an irrigant during transurethral resection and other urosurgical procedures to avoid overhydration (19) and acute renal insufficiency (20).

A variety of proteins, including human serum albumin, serve as excellent buffers when their presence in formulations is practical. The potential for allergic reactions even with human serum albumin (21) is discussed in Part III.

Hydroxylamine (NH_2OH) is also an amino-acid-type buffer. It has the potential to produce methemoglobinemia if given parenterally (22).

F. Barbiturate Buffers

Phenobarbital and barbitones are popular laboratory buffers but are rarely used in medications because they themselves are active sedating drugs. The well-known actions and adverse effects of barbiturates will not be reviewed here. Other common laboratory buffers that are rarely used as medicinal excipients are the phthalate and imidazole buffers.

G. Tris Buffers

These hydroxymethyl amino derivatives buffer in the slightly alkaline (pH 7-9) range and also function as surfactants. Their prime use is in topical preparations. When used in parenteral preparations, they can be irritating to the vein and surrounding tissues, particularly if extravenous extravasation occurs. Tris has been used clinically for the treatment of respiratory acidosis and may be preferable to sodium bicarbonate because it does not induce a sodium burden. However, reduction of blood sugar as well as liver (23) and bladder (24) injury have been reported following intravenous administration. Tris buffers are used primarily in topical preparations and as laboratory buffers. They have been reported to complex with copper so as to interfere with the action of copper-dependent enzymes (25).

III. SUSPENDING, EMULSIFYING, AND STIFFENING AGENTS

Members of this class of excipients are used in both liquid medications and solid dosage forms. During the manufacture of solid formulations it is often necessary to add a very small but important quantity of an active ingredient in a form that will ensure uniform dispersion throughout the batch. As a consequence, a wide variety of agents useful for this purpose find their way into the final solid product. While their potential for harm needs to be considered, only trace quantities are likely to be involved. In general, it is critical to consider the amount involved as well as the nature of the potential side effects of this class of excipients in judging the risk vs. benefit of their use.

Many suspending and emulsifying agents are surfactants that aid in the development of solutions and topical formulations of materials that may otherwise be difficult to prepare in an acceptable form. They are also used as medicinals in aqueous solutions inhaled to hydrate and liquify tenacious bronchopulmonary   secretions and to help clear debris in other areas accessible to topical application. Some are used as spermicides. Their cleansing effects augment their antimicrobial action, which make them useful in mouth washes and as preservatives. Their toxic potential has long been of interest (26).

Surfactants are generally classified as ionic or nonionic. The nonionic agents include tyloxapol, a water-miscible polymer that can withstand antoclaving, and the macrogel ethers. There are few reports of reactions to these agents, although the rapid installation of tyloxapol via aerosol can cause signs of pharyngeal and tracheobronchial irritation (27) and maculopapular rashes have been attributed to its use. The glycols, discussed in detail elsewhere, are also surfactants.

Newer surfactants are under continuing evaluation, particularly with a view toward how their presence influences the absorption of coadministered drugs. When these agents result in increased absorption, a suspicion must be entertained that they may be exerting an adverse effect on the gastrointestinal mucosa. Electron microscopy and chemical analytic techniques are being used to study such effects in animals. They show differences in the effect on the morphology of rectal vs. small intestinal mucosa, suggesting that some surfactants that may create problems in oral preparations might be acceptable in rectal suppository preparations to increase absorption (28). Each instance needs to be examined on its own merits.

A. Ionic Agents

1. Anionic Agents

Bile salts Bile acids are nature's prime intestinal emulsifying agent, and their use as an oral medication to aid in digestion is ancient. In recent years, understanding of the relative role and influence of different bile acids has increased considerably (29), with particular emphasis on concern for cholesterol metabolism and development of gallstones. Repeated daily doses on the order of hundreds of milligrams are perceived as potentially harmful (30), while cholic and deoxycholic acid and their salts are considered safe in doses up to 1.25 mg/kg/day (31). When these agents are used to solubilize material in vaccines, for example, the injected dose is negligible in terms of systemic toxicity.

Sodium lauryl sulfate In the context of medicinal excipients, the sodium salt of the anionic emulsifier, lauryl sulfate, is far more commonly used in liquid formulations, not only to create emulsions but also as a surfactant (see below).

Sodium lauryl sulfate shows a concentration- and time-dependent irritant effect in some subjects (32).

2. Cationic Agents

Cetrimide (cetrimonium bromide) This cationic surfactant is used in relatively high concentrations as a topical antiseptic and in lower concentrations as a preservative, presumably by virtue of its surface tension effects.

As with other quaternary compounds, large systemic doses have potent anticholinergiclike effects including nausea, vomiting, muscle paralysis, CNS depression, and hypotension. Local tissue damage to the esophagus, peritoneum and skin surface may result from use of high concentrations (33–35). Such concentrations of cationic surfactants are not involved in their use as excipients, as contrasted with their therapeutic use.

Skin sensitivity and patch test studies (36) are reviewed in Part III. Comparative studies on mouse skin suggest that sodium lauryl sulfate, an anionic emulsifier/surfactant, is less damaging to skin than cetrimide, while Tween 80 shows essentially no adverse effect in this model (37).

Benzylkonium chloride This agent is a mixture of alkyl benzyl dimethyl ammonium chloride salts that are used as disinfectants. They are quaternary ammonium compounds that have a potential for the same systemic toxicity described for cetrimide if applied systemically in relatively large doses. Preparations with concentrations as low as 0.1% may be irritating to the eye, but 0.01%, the commonly used preservative excipient concentration, apparently does not cause detectable damage (38). Allergic topical reactions (39–42) are reviewed in Part III.

B. Nonionic Agents

This group includes the sorbitans and the sorbitan esters of fatty acids. They are commonly known as poloxamers, Spans, Tweens, sorbesters, and Polawax. They are widely used with few adverse consequences (see Part III).

C. Tragacanth and Acacia

These mucilages or gums from the sap of the botanical family Leguminosae consist of complex glycoprotein polymers and methylated derivatives. Acacia is a calcium, magnesium, and potassium salt of arabic acid, a high-molecular-weight polysaccharide composed of the D-isomer of galactose, glucuronic acid, and other sugars. The capacity of these agents to thicken, suspend, and bind has made them widely useful excipients in oral and topical preparations as well as demulcents for lozenges. While finished formulations can generally be sterilized by autoclaving, tragacanth itself cannot be protected from bacterial contamination by dry heat or radiation without destroying its useful properties. Gassing with ethylene oxide or the addition of preservatives is therefore common practice. The activity of several common preservatives is reduced in the presence of tragacanth (44).

Acacia is not used parenterally (45) but is widely used orally. The nature and relative sensitizing capacity of tragacanth and acacia are reviewed in detail in Part III.

D. Methylcellulose

This methyl ester of cellulose is not hydrolyzed (digested) in the intestine and, like cellulose itself, is not absorbed and therefore not caloric. It is frequently used as an emulsifying agent in liquids, a binding agent in tablets, and as a thickening agent for a variety of creams, jellies, and ophthalmologic preparations as standardized in official compendia (46).

Methylcellulose is essentially inert but, if consumed in large quantities, can be responsible for significant physiological alterations. Most data concerning these alterations are derived from studies concerned with its use as a bulk laxative rather than an excipient. When consumed in multigram doses per day, it can interfere with the absorption of several minerals, including zinc, calcium, magnesium, and phosphate (47), as well as other drugs. The rate of glucose absorption may also be altered in the presence of large amounts of methylcellulose, resulting in altered insulin requirements in insulin-dependent diabetes. While it is laxating to the normal bowel in the presence of adequate hydration, methylcellulose may aggravate intestinal spastic and obstructive diseases, including ulcerative colitis and regional ileitis (48).

All of the above problems are the consequences of doses that are rarely consumed when methylcellulose is used merely as an excipient to achieve the physical characteristics desired in tablets or other formulations consumed in modest quantities.

E. Paraffin

Reactions to petroleum products, including the paraffins are reviewed in Chapter 6. The amounts used as addition products to improve the physical properties of a formulation are not likely to create side effects.

F. Lubricants

The flow characteristics of liquid medications are largely a function of viscosity. Flow control achieved with materials previously discussed is a prime consideration in the art of manufacturing liquid pharmaceuticals. The flow of solids as powders or granular materials is also critical to the manufacture of solid dosage forms. The term lubricant is also applied to materials that enhance the flow of solid formulations through solid dose manufacturing machinery. Such lubricants are often critical to the handling of solid formulations by modern high-speed machinery.

Talc (French chalk) is an excellent solid lubricant. It is finely powdered hydrous magnesium silicate. It has long been used as a dusting powder and filler, particularly because of its lubricating properties when tablet molds and other solid phase pharmaceutical production machinery are used.

While talc is essentially unabsorbed and therefore systemically nontoxic when administered orally, its use has been curtailed because of the consequences of the parenteral abuse of formulations intended for oral administration (49). Severe granulomatous lung lesions result not only from intravenously administered talc but also from "snorting" or snuffing of materials formulated with talc (50).

If talc is inadvertently introduced into peritoneal cavities by way of its use as a lubricant on surgical gloves, it can result in an irritative reaction. At one time it was used to induce a vascular inflammatory reaction of the pericardial sac in the hope of diverting some of the pericardial blood flow supply into ischemic myocardial tissue. Nevertheless, the toxic potential of talc in oral formulations used as intended is very low.

Edible oils, such as hydrogenated vegetable oil, which are essentially triglycerides of stearic and palmitic acids, are used as lubricants in tablet manufacturing. The fatty acids alone are also effective lubricants. Their potential for side effects is very low, even though some of these agents used as ointment bases have been alleged to cause skin reactions (51).

G. Fatty Alcohols

The higher fatty alcohols, such as stearyl alcohol (a solid) and cetyl alcohol (a liquid), are useful emulsifiers and stiffening agents. While skin sensitivity reactions have been reported (52-55) and are reviewed in Part III, these alcohols are not associated with significant problems when used for oral formulations.

IV. PRESERVATIVES

Preservatives in foods and drugs have become a way of life in the modern world. With the unrelenting centralization and specialization of manufacturing, ways had to be found to prevent the deterioration of products in the interval between production and use. Organically or "naturally" produced pharmaceuticals that reach the patient in a standardized, unspoiled manner without additives may be considered the ideal by some, but are essentially an unattainable goal for drugs that need to be produced in the quantities currently required. Even with pure synthetic drugs, stability problems often require the addition of some product to preserve the quality of the drug as it reaches the consumer.

Preservatives have been defined by British regulatory agencies (The Preservatives of Food Regulations, SI 1982, No 15) as "any substance which is capable of inhibiting, retarding or arresting the growth of microorganisms or any deterioration of food by microorganisms or of masking the evidence of any such deterioration." However, the definition goes on specifically to exclude a broad spectrum of additives such as sweeteners, spices, colors, and so on, that might otherwise seem to fit this definition. A precise definition is more difficult to achieve than is the general understanding of the term.

Ideally all additives should be without significant adverse effects. The concentrations of preservatives needed in formulations so as to serve their purpose usually results in negligible potential pharmacologic effects. Some of the reported reactions involve highly specific situations, such as the competitive displacement of bilirubin from albumin in infants with kernicterus or the absorption of bisulfite from peritoneal dialysis solutions.

It is the general perception that the risk of an added preservative is less than the risk of spoilage. Such spoilage is not of concern solely because of loss of product potency but because of the potential dangers of unknown products generated by spoilage. The fungal growths on legumes that produce aflatoxin, an extremely potent carcinogen, are likely to be more dangerous than prevention of the fungal growth with a suitable fungistat or fungicide.

Problems of reactions to preservatives generally arise when a formulation is misused, resulting in greater exposure to the preservative than was anticipated (56) or in a small but significant group of consumers who are intolerant of the agent. When a medication produces a response that is uncharacteristic of the active ingredient, the preservative becomes suspect. Such reactions to parenteral drugs especially call for a review of the pharmacology of the perservative (57, 58). With topical preparations, both primary irritation and hypersensitivity are a concern, particularly the latter (59) since low concentration is no guarantee against its occurrence.

Preservatives will be reviewed under three general classes: those that are primarily antimicrobial, those that interfere with oxidative reactions (antioxidants), and those that bind metals that catalyze undesired reactions, or inhibit metal-dependent enzymes responsible for such reactions (chelating agents). The distinction between these preservative types is often not clear, since both antioxidant action and chelating action could interfere with the growth of microorganisms. The spoilage that accompanies the growth of microorganisms could involve mechanisms that may be inhibited by either antioxidants or chelating agents.

A. Antimicrobials

The addition of these agents to drug products is not presumed to result in sterile preparations but in formulations that will not deteriorate as a result of microbial growth and its consequences. Since they are putative inhibitors of microbial growth, there is concern about their potential for interfering with growth processes in cells of the host. Teratogenicity as a result of systemic exposure of pregnant women to the preservative is a particular concern. An extensive follow-up study of malformation in children of women treated with topical preparations containing a variety of antimicrobial agents during lunar months 1–4 of pregnancy failed to show evidence of such a problem (60). Benzethonium, phenylmercuric acetate, cetalkonium, and cetylpyridinium, each used in several hundred cases, were not associated with a significantly increased risk of malformation.

Besides the agents reviewed in this section as antimicrobial preservatives, the surfactants discussed previously may also have antibacterial action and may be classified as preservatives.

Phenol Phenol is one of the earliest of the preservatives, having been used by Lister with the specific objective of killing microorganisms. Information concerning its side effects has been generated largely from its use as an active ingredient in deodorant soaps and in mouth washes to "kill germs that cause bad breath" rather than as an excipient with preservative function, that is, protection of the formulation from bacterial overgrowth.

Based on laboratory studies, phenol has been considered to be a possible carcinogen. However, it remains an acceptable medicinal ingredient based on long-term innocuous results of clinical experience.

Thymol Thymol is a derivative of phenol, which it resembles in many of its characteristics and uses as a disinfectant and deodorant. It is less toxic, probably because it is less soluble. Nevertheless, it is readily absorbed and can discolor urine (61). It is a local irritant. Unusual exposure to excessive amounts of thymol may occur inadvertently due to improper draining of vaporizers, causing thymol to accumulate to levels sufficiently toxic to cause pulmonary edema (62).

Chloramine The sulfonechloramides, chloramine B and chloramine T, are used as antiseptics in 1 and 2% solutions and for irrigating solutions at 0.1 and 0.2% concentrations. Reported reactions (63,64) are largely related to sensitization, as reviewed in Part III.

Chlorocresol Chlorocresol is used as a preservative at concentrations on the order of 0.1% as a substitute for its more toxic predecessor, phenol. A report that it may be a primary irritant in the eye is based on extrapolation from a severe challenge in an animal model (65). Sensitization reports (66,67) are reviewed in Part III.

Chlorobutanol/Chlorbutol This is used in a 0.5% concentration as a preservative, and also as a mild sedative and topical analgesic in acid solutions. It is unstable in alkali. Exposure to large doses has toxic potential (68,69) and eye irritation has been reported (56). Sensitivity reactions (70-72) are reviewed in Part III.

Sorbic acid This simple acid has both antibacterial and antifungal activity. It is generally used in concentrations of 0.1-0.2% in pharmaceutical formulations, especially those containing nonionic surfactants. It is also used with proteins: enzymes, gelatin for capsules, and with vegetable gums. It is directly irritant to the eye and may be irritating to skin (73-77).

Phenylmercuric nitrate/acetate These preservatives have antibacterial and antifungal properties when used in concentrations between 0.001 and 0.002% in solutions for injection. The acetate is sometimes preferred because of its greater solubility. The nitrate has also been used as a spermicide.

The use of phenylmercuric nitrate in topical eye preparations has been discouraged since the discovery of eye lens changes known as mercurialentis after prolonged use of eye drops containing this preservative (78-81). Concern about absorption of mercury from the vagina and its consequences (60) has resulted in the ruling that intravaginal use of phenylmercuric nitrate as a contraceptive is unsafe (82).

Thimerosal (merthiolate) This once-popular bacteriostatic and fungistatic, used as a preservative as well as a wound antiseptic, has been characterized as creating "a nationwide iatrogenic sensitization" (83,84) (see Part III).

Being a mercurial, thimerosal is subject to the same concerns about chronic mercurial poisoning (85,86) described above for phenylmercuric nitrate. Acute toxicity is a special concern in the perinatal period (87). An unusual reaction was reported to be the consequence of the exothermic interaction between thimerosal and aluminum, resulting in a burn when an aluminum foil diathermy electrode contacted an area prepared for surgery with 0.1% thimerosal in alcohol (88).

Benzyl alcohol Benzyl alcohol in concentrations of about 10% has long been used as a disinfectant, a local anesthetic, and at 1% concentration as an additive to injectables. Prolonged exposure can cause neurotoxicity and intrathecal injection of preparations containing benzyl alcohol has been reported to cause paraplegia (89). In 1982 it was discovered that premature neonates were receiving toxic amounts of benzoic acid and/or benzyl alcohol in bacteriostatic solutions used to flush intravenous catheters (90). These agents are no longer recommended as preservatives for injectables to be administered to neonates, since the infants receive relatively high doses per kilogram and apparently have a low tolerance for these agents (91). Thus, while animal toxicity studies suggest that the usual amounts of benzyl alcohol in preparations used for adults are safe, there are no data to support the same assumption for neonates.

In adults, benzyl alcohol is oxidized to benzoic acid and is readily converted to and excreted as hippuric acid. This metabolic pathway may not be well developed in neonates. When parenteral preparations with benzyl alcohol are heat sterilized, some of the preservative may be converted to the aldehyde if oxygen is not excluded by nitrogen flushing.

Benzyl alcohol has been reported to cause eye irritation (56) and contact allergy (93) in rare instances (see Part III). One report (94) records an inflammatory reaction to a benzyl-alcohol-containing procaine hydrochloride solution used for local anesthesia of the eyelid. No such reaction was noted with similar preparations without benzyl alcohol.

Benzoic acid Benzoic acid and its salts, particularly sodium benzoate, are commonly used as preservatives, and are permitted in food products up to a concentration of 1:1000. Efficacy may be lost in preparations with a pH over 5.

Benzoates are also used as antifungal agents and in relatively large doses for hepatic and renal function tests. While these uses may be interpreted as indicating safety, there are concerns about potential toxicity in neonates (95,96). There is a possibility that the adverse experiences with benzyl alcohol (90) might relate to its metabolic conversion to benzoic acid. The problem in neonates may also involve the ability of benzoic acid to displace bile from albumin-binding sites, a special problem in relation to kernicterus (97).

The benzoates as preservatives have survived long and widespread use with very little evidence of toxic side effects. Sensitivity studies are reviewed in Part III. Several reports (98–101), including a double blind study that failed to differentiate between 500 mg of benzoic acid and a similar dose of lactose (102), bring into question the relationship of benzoates to suspected reactions.

Parabens Parabens are esters (usually methyl or propyl) of para hydroxybenzoate used as antifungal and bactericidal preservatives in pharmaceuticals, in concentrations ranging from 0.1–0.3%, and in foods and cosmetics at lesser concentrations (39). They are often used in combination because their preservative action in formulation had been found to be synergistic (103). They are not generally considered suitable for injectables (104) or ophthalmic solutions since they cause pain and signs of irritation at these sites.

The parabens show a low but distinct incidence of skin sensitization and cross-sensitization with each other (105–108) that is reviewed in Part III.

Germall (imidazolidinyl urea) This agent is described as a new broad-spectrum preservative, suitable for medicinals and cosmetics. Animal studies (31) show it to be of low systemic toxicity by the oral route or when applied to abraded skin. It is neither a primary irritant nor a sensitizer to the skin or eye in concentrations much greater than those used clinically. In a review of commonly used preservatives (77), Germall 115 is described as nontoxic, nonirritating, and relatively nonsensitizing in comparison to the parabens, which are commonly used and considered safe even though they are topically sensitizing for about 1% of the population.

Bronopol Bronopol (BNDP) (1-bromo-2-nitro-1,3 propanediol) is one of several preservatives that generate their antimicrobial effect by the release of formaldehyde (77). It is used primarily in topical preparations and suppositories, but is considered too toxic for oral liquid preparations (109), despite the fact that another formaldehyde-releasing agent, methenamine hippurate, is safely administered as an oral drug for urinary antisepsis. It is effective against a broad spectrum of bacteria, including pseudomonas organisms, but is less active against yeasts and fungi.

It is reasonable that concern about the toxicity of formaldehyde should carry over to products that presumably act by the generation of formaldehyde. Exposure to formaldehyde vapor has been found to cause carcinoma in the nasal cavity of rats (110) but not mice. It has been suggested that epizootic viral infections in rats but not mice may play a role. While a variety of tumor types occurred in the nasal cavities of rats, there was no evidence of a systemic carcinogenic response in other tissues.

The relevance of the these findings to the preservative use of formaldehyde-generating agents is highly questionable. Methenamine hippurate, the systemically administered formaldehyde-generating urinary antimicrobial, shows negative findings in standard empirical carcinogenicity studies. Another formaldehyde-generating preservative, hexamethylenetetramine (HMT), was found to cause subcutaneous sarcomas in rats at the site of repeated injections (111), but studies of high oral doses showed no carcinogenic (112) or teratogenic (113) effects.

The toxicologic characteristics of bronopol have been described by Bryce et al. (114). They conclude that in the concentrations generally used (0.01–0.1%), BNDP is essentially nonirritating although higher concentrations (0.5–1% or higher) are irritating (115). While this study reported no sensitization even by the higher concentrations, other reports reviewed in Part III indicated otherwise (59,77,116).

B. Antioxidants

Nordihydroguairetic acid Nordihydroguairetic acid (NDGA) is a lipid-soluble antioxidant frequently added to oils and fats in topical products in a small fraction of a percent. Reports concerning reactions to NDGA are confined to sensitivity reactions (see Part III).

Butylated hydroxyanisol (BHA) and toluene (BHT) These are phenolic antioxidants used primarily in concentrations up to 0.02% for the preservation of fixed oils (i.e., fats that are liquid at ambient temperatures), fats (solid at ambient temperatures), and vitamin oil concentrates. Studies of BHA in animals showed essentially no teratogenic effects, even at doses as high as 400 mg/kg/day by mouth. However, as little as 50 mg/kg/day resulted in distinct histologic changes in the liver and thyroid of pigs (40). Pending further study, human intake should not exceed 0.5 mg/kg/day, that is, about 25 mg (117).

The phenolic preservatives in a soybean infant formula containing BHA, BHT, and propyl gallate were deemed to be responsible for an episode of methemoglobinemia in infants (118).

Sulfites A group of substances known as sulfiting agents are commonly used as antioxidants and preservatives to prevent microbial spoilage. They include the gas, sulfur dioxide, and the sodium and potassium sulfite, bisulfite, and metabi-sulfite salts. Their chemistry in air and fluids and their intracellular formation and degradation have recently been summarized (119).

Sulfites are commonly found in fruits, vegetables, seafood, beer, and wine as well as medicinal formulations. Very recently (120) the FDA has forbidden their use on raw fruits and vegetables, and packaged materials containing 10 parts per million or more must be labeled accordingly.

The sulfite-type antioxidants are often identified by an E number (European code). Thus SO_2 (sulfur dioxide) is E220, sodium sulfite is E221, sodium bisulfite is E222, and sodium metasulfite E223, potassium metasulfite is E224, and so on. The metabisulfite is commonly used in acidic solutions and syrups, where it breaks down to liberate sulfur dioxide and sulfurous acid. It can cause a variety of clinical problems in intolerant subjects (121). After large oral doses, these breakdown products can cause local gastric irritation, systemic respiratory/circulatory collapse, and central nervous system depression. They undergo fairly rapid metabolic conversion to sulfate, which is readily excreted by the kidney. Major sulfite intolerance problems are detailed in Part III.

Bisulfite absorption from peritoneal dialysis solutions has been reported to be cumulative to the point of central nervous system and cardiovascular toxicity (122). However, other studies (123) suggest that autoclaving dialysis solutions results in a marked reduction of bisulfite content, essentially eliminating the likelihood of a toxic response.

Ethylenediamine Ethylenediamine has been used as a stabilizer, particularly in formulations with aminophyllin and some topical steroids. It has been described as an irritant to the skin and mucous membranes, and is capable of causing serious systemic effects if applied in concentrated solutions. Intolerance to its use in the usual topical formulation is discussed in Part III (124).

Propyl gallate The alkyl gallates are used as antioxidants in formulations with fatty bases. Propyl gallate has been shown not to be a primary irritant, but is a sensitizer as shown by repeated daily patch testing with a 20% solution in ethyl alcohol for more than 2 weeks in humans, and by intradermal injections in guinea pigs (125). This characteristic apparently limits its potential use as a photoprotectant (126).

The gallates were components of a fat preservative used in infant formulations that apparently led to toxicity manifested as methemoglobinemia (118). As a group, some gallates have been described as having catechol-like pharmacologic action when administered in doses of sufficient magnitude. Such action, however, has not been reported in relation to their use in low concentrations as preservatives in fat-based preparations.

C. Chelating Agents

Many reactions responsible for the spoilage of food and instability of medicinal formulations are catalyzed by a trace metal or enzyme that is trace-metal-dependent. Agents that form complexes with such trace metals may block the catalysis or enzyme activity responsible for spoilage and thus serve a preservative function.

A wide variety of agents form complexes with heavy metals but only a few have a sufficiently high metal-binding capacity (i.e., high stability constant) (127,128) to be effective as preservatives in practical, low safe concentrations.

The most commonly used potent chelator is ethylenediamine tetraacetic acid (EDTA, edetate), generally added in the form of the disodium salt, which is highly water-soluble. In spite of its solubility, EDTA is poorly absorbed orally. If administered parenterally, it is essentially unmetabolized and very rapidly excreted by the kidney, mostly as the calcium complex. However, since its affinity for heavier metals is orders of magnitude greater than for calcium, it will bind preferentially to such metals if they are available in spite of the presence of much higher molar concentrations of calcium. Thus parenteral EDTA will enhance the urinary excretion of such metals to the extent that they are available in ionic form. Orally administered EDTA also preferentially binds with iron and trace heavy metals in the gut, thereby interfering with their absorption.

EDTA has essentially no toxicity other than that attributable to the removal of metals. In fact it is used parenterally for that purpose in the diagnosis and treatment of heavy metal poisoning (lead, plutonium) and iron overload (127). It has also been used in topical preparations to block contact sensitivity skin reactions due to the ionic form of allergenic metals such as nickel.

Chronic toxicity studies with large doses of EDTA or related agents have shown significant adverse effects. However, these effects all resemble those of zinc-deficient diets and are prevented by use of zinc supplements (129). In humans the usual daily intake of zinc is 10-20 mg. About 10 mg/day are found in the stool and about 0.4 mg/day in the urine (127). Thus the daily need for absorbed zinc is modest but sufficiently important to create problems if depleted by concurrent administration of large doses of chelating agents. The renal toxicity of large parenteral doses of EDTA both clinically and experimentally is attributed to depletion of zinc and other trace metals (130). Dose-related congenital malformations seen with large doses of dietary EDTA in rats (3% of food) are also completely prevented by dietary zinc supplements (131). In standard toxicity tests, zinc chelates are less toxic than analogous calcium chelates or the free chelating agent (132).

If large doses of disodium EDTA are given orally over prolonged periods, deficiency of calcium and perhaps iron and other metals may result. Administering the EDTA as the calcium complex will avoid calcium depletion. The calcium can be displaced by the heavier metals with stronger stability constants, leading to depletion of those metals. However, EDTA is inefficient in removing metals from strong natural complexes such as iron-transferrin or lead deposited in the complex structure of bone.

Since very little of the orally administered EDTA is absorbed (127,130) and only a fraction of injected or ingested EDTA is eliminated complexed with zinc or other essential trace metals, the amount of EDTA to which the body is exposed as a consequence of its use as a preservative in medication is not likely to induce adverse reactions, including zinc or other metal deficiency. However, should the daily intake of EDTA become excessive, the effect on metal metabolism must be considered (127).

V. STERILIZING AGENT: ETHYLENE OXIDE

This gas is widely used to sterilize instruments and other materials that cannot tolerate steam sterilization. In high concentrations it is severely toxic. The safety concern is not so much with the material that has been treated with ethylene oxide as with the people involved with its handling during the sterilization procedure. There are reports of a high rate of miscarriage and subtle chromosomal changes in the white blood cells of people exposed to the gas. The Occupational Safety and Health Administration (OSHA) has established 1 ppm as the maximum allowable level in air (133). Residual ethylene oxide in sterilized material may cause hemolysis (134) and can be cytotoxic to tissue, at least in culture (135). Products containing chloride ions and polyvinyl chloride previously subjected to gamma radiation may produce toxic reation products on resterilization with ethylene oxide (136). Improper aeration after the use of ethylene oxide sterilization has been held responsible for the leaching of material from ethylene-oxide-sterilized tubing by buffer solutions used in hemodialysis, resulting in anaphylaxis (137,138) and other reactions (137-139) that are discussed further in Part III.

VI. PROPELLANTS

Propellants are materials used to achieve delivery of drugs in the form of aerosols: a fine mist containing an active ingredient. The aerosol product may be two-phase (gas and liquid) or 3-phase (gas, liquid, and suspended solid or liquid) formulation in which the propellant is both a gas and compressed liquid possibly serving as a solvent.

Propellants are excipients in the sense that patients being treated with medications administered by means of propellants are exposed to and may exhibit reactions to the propellants.

By and large, any gas that can be compressed and stored under pressure in a liquified state can be used to propel an active ingredient through the air to the desired site of action. In practice, the technique is used to deliver materials to the skin, other body surfaces, and particularly to the bronchial or alveolar surfaces of the lung. Drugs so delivered may have local (respiratory tract) or systemic effects. Absorption through lung tissue can yield responses resembling intravenous infusion in speed of action. Drugs absorbed by this route do not undergo "first-pass' hepatic or intestinal metabolism. They may therefore have significantly different effects from those seen with the same agent administered orally (140).

Regardless of the chemical nature of the propellant, the mass and mean aerodynamic diameter of the material being propelled and the speed at which it travels determine both the amount and the locus of the agent deposited within the respiratory system. These factors directly influence the bodily response to the agent delivered.

Animal aerosol toxicity experiments provide information of limited value because of the variety of techniques used and differences in anatomical characteristics from species to species (141). The consequences of these variables are superimposed on the intrinsic toxicologic nature of the propellant as a chemical. It is interesting that some reports of the toxicity of substances administered via the lung by aerosol do not even discuss the nature or potential contribution of the propellant to observations of toxicity. For example, in one report a photograph of the system used to aerosolize the product shows that the propellant was difluorodichloromethane but that fact is not mentioned in the discussion of toxicity (142).

Pressure spray delivery of medication was originally accomplished by "atomizers" with hand-squeezed rubber bulbs to create the pressure required to generate a "spray" of the medication. Size and force of the moving particles were poorly controlled and these devices were not useful to deliver medication deep into the lungs (i.e., the respiratory bronchioles and alveoli).

More recently, "aerosol" systems have been developed using a mechanical apparatus in conjunction with a propellant for more uniform delivery of a jet of medication by a more precisely regulated propulsion system. Metered dispensers can readily be designed to produce particles of about 1 μm in mass median aerodynamic diameter that can be carried to the depths of the alveoli (141). However, for clinical purposes most metered dispensers deliver particles ranging in size from 2-5 μm for deposition on small bronchi and bronchioles.

The materials used as propellants are generally substances that are readily compressible and maintained under pressure as liquids in small vessels at ambient temperatures. They are housed in containers fitted with simple trigger mechanisms by which a rapidly moving stream of gas can be released to propel a controlled amount of the active material to the desired impact area. Physical laws and data on the solvent properties of gases under pressure as liquids are important to the selection of propellants and aerosol design (143).

At the time of their introduction a few decades ago, the propellants with these desired characteristics that were most economically feasible were halogenated derivatives of simple aliphatic compounds such as methane and ethane. They were selected largely because they were relatively stable, noninflammable, and odorless.

A drop in temperature is the well-recognized consequence of an expanding gas, and some of these agents (e.g., ethyl chloride) with such coolant properties were originally used to achieve rapid and short-lived topical freezing for local cryosurgery and analgesia. Gases such as CO_2 and N_2 that are intrinsically harmless can also be compressed to liquids and used as propellants, but the pressure and temperature requirements and the degree of cooling achieved limit their utility for common propellant purposes. The use of compressed CO_2 is further limited by its acidity and capacity to form carbonates (143). While nitrogen gas is inert, the formulation pressures necessary for its use are not practical for lightweight portable containers that are now absolute requirements for clinical purposes.

Several of the most frequently used halogenated alkyl derivatives, commonly referred to as fluorocarbons, have come to be known by a simple numbering system used by earlier workers as a more manageable means of identifying various compounds with cumbersome and similar sounding chemical names. Table 1 presents a classification of propellants and some of the commonly used code numbers by which they are identified.

The environmental consequences of the escape of fluorocarbons into the atmosphere have severely restricted the industrial use of some of these agents as refrigerants and for household aerosol products. However, the FDA permits their use for the delivery of essential human medications. Restrictions for their medicinal uses are more germane to potential adverse effects on the individual user. While toxic consequences are particularly disturbing when propellant medications are misused or deliberately abused, adverse consequences may occur even when aerosols are used as intended. Acute central nervous system depression and cardiac arrhythmias may occur and hepatic dysfunction is a concern, particularly with prolonged repeated exposure.

While heating to high temperatures is known to result in the breakdown of some fluorocarbons to highly toxic products such as phosgene, fluorine/chlorine gases, and hydrochloric/hydrofluoric acids, such breakdown does not occur with clinical materials under ordinary conditions of production and clinical use and does not constitute a hazard to patients using products formulated with fluorocarbon propellants.

Because these propellants are gases that are rapidly dispersed and the dose of propellant to which the patient is normally exposed is very small, their use

Table 1 Propellants and Refrigerants

	Code #
Hydrocarbons	
Propane[a]	
Isobutane[a]	
Normal butane[a]	
Flurocarbons	
Methane series	
Trichloromonofluoromethane[a]	11
Dichlorodifluoromethane[a]	12
Monochlorodifluoromethane	22
Ethane series	
Dichlorotetrafluoroethane (Freon)[a]	114, 114a
Monochlorodifluoroethane	142b
Difluoroethane	152a
Trichlorotrifluoroethane	113
Butane series	
Octafluorocyclobutane	C318
Other halocarbons	
Vinyl chloride	
Compressed ambient gases	
Carbon dioxide	
Nitrogen	

[a]Listed as pharmaceutical ingredients in USP-NF XXI (1985).

was initially regarded as having little toxic potential. However, the vapors of some of these agents (e.g., chloroform, which is volatilized from the liquid form at ambient pressures and temperatures) have been known for over a century to cause biologically potent reactions. A report from the Underwriters Laboratories in 1933 (144), supplemented by a favorable histologic study (145) and another publication in 1937 (146), gave reassuring assessments of the general toxicity of fluorocarbons. Even then some chlorocarbons, including chloroform, carbon tetrachloride, and methyl chloride, were already recognized and classified as highly toxic vapors, while others were considered safe. However, in 1950 a study of the consequences of inhalation of numerous halogenated derivatives in rats

(147) was undertaken to determine the safety of their use for anesthesia. Many of these agents were found to cause disturbing pulmonary irritation and increased mortality in rats, A correlation of boiling point with toxicity was reported, that is, the derivatives with lower boiling points were less acutely toxic. No hepatic damage was found. From the data generated, maximum allowable concentrations were suggested for single short human exposures. While the commonly used fluorocarbon 12 (dichlorodifluoromethane) was considered safe, later animal studies of the effect of repeated doses in several species showed that this agent was also capable of inducing interstitial inflammatory lung changes and hepatic necrosis (148). The levels in the inhaled air (about 4 mg/ml) in these experiments were similar to those found in the alveolar gas after use of inhalers with drugs intended to relieve acute asthmatic attacks (149).

An increased fatality rate in young people with asthma was first described in the United Kingdom in 1967. From 1962 to 1967 these rates were as high as 2.2/100,000 compared to a mean annual average rate of 0.45 to 1.22/100,000 between 1867 and 1961. This provoked a brisk controversy about whether the rise in fatality rates was due to higher prevalence of asthma itself or indiscriminate use of medications (150). The initial report concluded that the rise in mortality directly paralleled the excessive use of the pressurized aerosols containing isoproterenol, some of which were formulated in "high-dose" (approximately twice the recommended dose) aerosols. This apparent connection appeared to be substantiated by the subsequent fall in asthma mortality to "preepidemic" levels once the sale of isoproterenol-pressured aerosol preparations was restricted. However, there were inconsistencies when similar comparisons were made in other countries. For example, this relationship was not supported by observations reported from Australia at that time. Other possible toxic interactions were also suspected.

Because of previous toxic changes in animals it was speculated that the hydrocarbon propellant aerosols, either themsleves or in combination with sympathomimetic agents, might be responsible for cardiac arrhythmias and deaths. Although there was much discussion about this hypothesis, firm proof was not established because accurate measurement of various fluorocarbons in the blood of humans only reached peak arterial concentrations of 1.7 μg/ml, a level far below toxic levels. Even volunteers who inhaled one burst of a propellant mixture every 10 min for a total of 6 hr did not have significant toxic levels of these propellants in the blood. For comparison purposes, cardiac sensitization to the development of significant arrhythmias induced by concentrations of 5 μg/kg of intravenous epinephrine only occurred in dogs when the venous blood concentration of fluorocarbons was between 20 and 35 μg/ml. Cardiac sensitization induced by propellants in the monkey does not occur until levels of 20 μg/ml are reached. Thus, the maximum levels found in humans are much lower than the sensitizing levels demonstrated in animals. It was concluded that only extreme abuse of propellant aerosol preparations in humans could lead to sensitizing levels analogous to those that produced cardiac arrhythmias in animals.

In the early 1980s the fatality rate of asthma again increased in specific localities: New Zealand, the United Kingdom, and the United States. Overdosage of neither sympathomimetics nor propellant gases appear to be responsible for this recent increase in the mortality rate due to asthma. The most plausible explanation appears to be that the therapeutic effect of sympathomimetic agents within the aerosol preparation may mask the underlying severity of the disease and thereby prevent the patient from seeking more effective medical treatment. It is now generally thought that propellants contained in aerosol metered-dose dispensers are safe if used in the recommended manner. However, propellants may not be ideal for other household products because of sporadic reports of accidental deaths due to the inhalation of these substances (151). There have also been reports of allergic contact dermatitis in response to propellants (152). It is therefore apparent that care in the selection and use of propellants is certainly warranted (153).

Vinyl chloride toxicity is of interest not only because of this agent's use as a propellant but also because it is the monomer from which plastic polyvinyl chloride is made. Workers exposed to this gas on a long-term basis may acquire a severe systemic illness with features similar to those observed in systemic sclerosis (154). These workers develop soreness and tenderness of the fingertips and Raynaud's phenomenon. They may also develop clubbing, synovial thickening of the proximal interphalangeal joints, hepatic portal fibrosis, splenomegaly, and pulmonary fibrosis (155,156). Some workers have developed varying degrees of acro-osteolysis of the distal phalanges of the fingers as well as erosive and sclerotic changes in the sacroiliac joints. Because of these serious side effects, major efforts have been made to reduce the amount of monomer trapped in the walls of polyvinyl chloride vessels, out of concern that the monomer might leach out into the container contents (see Part II, Chapter 2). The United States Consumer Products Safety Commission has banned the use of vinyl chloride as a propellant for household aerosol products (157).

The propellants involved in more recent reports of adverse effects (158) include monochlorodifluoromethane (fluorocarbon 22) dichlorodifluoromethane (fluorocarbon 12), and dichlorotetrafluoroethane (fluorocarbon 114).

While fluorocarbons are still the chief propellants in medicinal products, simpler hydrocarbons such as isobutane, n-butane, and propane are being used as propellants for many common cosmetic and household products. These products are classified informally on the basis of their flammability limits in air (159). Mixes of compressed liquified gases are also used as propellants (143). There is a recent case report of a life-threatening cardiac dysrhythmia in a previously well child after unintentional exposure to a commercial deodorant containing butane propellants (151). In this instance, at least, the cardiotoxicity appeared to be related to propellant exposure because the butane propellants were demonstrated in the child's serum 2 hr after the initial exposure.

REFERENCES

1. Bing, J. and Mesmer, K. Incidence and severity of anaphylactoid reactions to colloid volume substitutes. Lancet 1:466-9 (1977).
2. Bert, J.M., Balmes, J.L., Cayrol, B., Bali, J.P., Pages, A. and Baldet, P. Case of thesaurismosis due to polyvinyl pyrrolidone (PVP). Semin. Hop. Paris 48:1809 (1972).
3. Kossard, S., Ecker, R.I. and Dicken, C.H. Povidone panniculitis. Arch. Dermatol. 116:704-706 (1980).
4. Thivolet, J., Leung, T.K., Duverne, J., Leung, J. and Volle, M. Ultrastructural morphology and histochemistry (acid phosphatase) of the cutaneous infiltration by polyvinylpyrrolidane. Br. J. Dermatol. 83:66 (1970).
5. Cabanne, F., Chapius, J.L., Duperrat, B. and Putelat, R. L'Infiltration cutanée par la polyvinylpyrrolidane, Ann. anat. Pathol. 11:385 (1966).
6. Gille, J. and Brandau, H. Foreign-body granulation in breast after injection of a polyvinylpyrrolidone containing preparation. Geburtshilfe Frauenheilkd. 35:799 (1975).
7. Soumerai, S. Pseudotumors of the arm following injections of procaine PVP; report of two cases. J. Med Soc. New Jersey 75:407 (1978).
8. Stringer, G.C., Samuel, W.H. and Bonnabeau, R.C. Hypersensitivity pneumonitis following prolonged inhalation of hair spray. J.A.M.A. 238: 888-889 (1977).
9. Junge, J. Cystoid mascular edema association with PVP coating of an intraocular lense. Am. Intraocular. Implant. Soc. J. 6:28-29 (1980).
10. Huper, W.C. Carcinogenic studies on water-soluble and insoluble macromolecular. Arch. Pathol. 67:589-617 (1959).
11. Huper, W.C. Bioassay in polyvinylpyrrolidones with limited molecular weight range. J. Natl. Cancer Inst. 26:229 (1961).
12. Wessel, W., Schoog, M. and Winkler, E. Polyvinylpyrrolidone, its diagnostic, therapeutic and technical application and consequence therof. Arzneim. Forsch. 21:1468 (1971).
13. Burnette, L.W. Proc. Sci. Sect. Toilet Goods Assoc. 38:1 (1962).
14. Shackney, S. and Hasson, J. Precipitious fall in serum calcium hypotension and acute renal failure after IV phosphate therapy for hypercalcemia. Ann. Intern. Med. 66:906 (1967).
15. Casey, R.N., Schmitt, G.W., Kopald, H.H. and Kantrowits, P.A. Massive extraskeletal calcification during phosphate treatment of hypercalcemia. Arch. Intern. Med. 122:150 (1968).
16. Goldbloom, R.B. and Goldbloom A. Boric acid poisoning: Report of 4 cases and a reviw of 109 cases from th world literature. J. Pediatr. 43:631 (1953).

17. Allan, N.D. Enamel erosion with lemon juice. Br. Dent. J. 122:300 (1967).
18. Schultz, R.E., Hanno, P.M., Wein, A.J., Levin, R.M., Pollack, H.M. and Van Arsdalen, K.N. Percutaneous ultrsonic lithotripsy: Choice of irrigant. J. Urol. 130:858–860 (1983).
19. Thomas, D. and Hales, P. Overhydration during transuretheal resection of the prostate using glycine as an irrigating solution. Anesth. Intens. Care 12: 366–9 (1984).
20. Arvieux, C., Peyrin, J.C., Vialtel, P., Naud, G., Fargnoli, J.M. and Gavend, M. Can glycine bladder lavage solution used in urologic surgery be toxic? Apropos of a case of acute renal insufficiency. Therapie 39(5):579–581 (1984).
21. Ring, J. and Messmer, K. Incidence and severity of anaphylactoid reactions to colloid volume substitutes. Lancet 1:466 (1977).
22. Cox, W.W. and Wendel, W.B. The normal sate of reduction of methemoglobin in dogs. J. Biol. Chem. 143:331 (1942).
23. Goldenberg, V.E., Wiegenstein, L. and Hopkins, G.B. Hepatic injury associated with tromethamine. J.A.M.A. 205:81 (1968).
24. Minatsch, M.J., Ohnacker, H. and Goldschmidt, H. Bladder necrosis caused by use of tris-(hydroxymeltry 1)-methl-amino in a newborn infant. J. Urol. III:835 (1974).
25. McPhail, D.B. and Goodman, B. Tris buffer—a case for caution in its use in copper-containing systems. Biochem. J. 221:559 (1984).
26. Eickholt, T.H. and White, W.F. The toxicity and absorption enhancing ability of surfactants. Drug Stand. 28:154–161 (1960).
27. Miller, J.B. Detergent aerosol therapy: A 15 year review of laboratory and clinical tolerance. Clin. Med. 74:37–40 (1967).
28. Tsuchiya, S., Aramaki, Y., Ozawa, S. and Matsumaru, H. Effects of polyoxyethylene cetylether on the absorption of $3'$ -$4'$ dideoxykanamycin B from rat rectum. Int. J. Pharm. 14:279–290 (1983).
29. Smith, B.F. and LaMont, J.T. The pathogenesis of gall stones. Hosp. Pract. 19:93–104 (1984).
30. Low-Beer, T.S. and Pomare, E.W. Can colonic bacterial metabolites predispose to cholesterol gall stones? Br. Med. J. 1:438–440 (1975).
31. 17th Report FAO/WHO #539 (1974).
32. Bruynzeel, D.P., van Ketel, W.G., Scheper, R.J. and von Blomberg-van der Flier, B.M.E. Delayed time course of imitation by sodium lauryl sulfate: Observations on threshold reactions. Contact Derm. 8:236–239 (1982).
33. August, P.J. Cutaneous necrosis due to cetrimide application. Br. Med. J. 1:70 (1975).
34. Gilchrist, D.S. Chemical peritonitis after centrimide washout in hydatid-cyst surgery. Lancet 2:1374 (1979).
35. Inman, J.K. Cetrimide allergy presenting as suspected non-accidental injury. Br. Med. J. 284:385 (1982).
36. Morgan, J.K. Iatrogenic epidermal sensitivity. Br. J. Clin. Pract. 22:261–264 (1968).
37. Landsdown, A.B.G. and Grasso, P. Physio-chemical factors influencing

epidermal damage by surface active agents. Br. J. Dermatol. 86:361–373 (1972).

38. Gasset, A.R., Ishii, Y., Kaufman, H.E. and Miller, T. Cytotoxicity of ophthalmic preservatives. Am. J. Ophthalmol. 78:98–105 (1974).

39. Smith and Dodd, T.R.P. Adverse reactive to pharmaceutical excipients. Adverse Drug React. Acute Pois. Rev. 1:93–142 (1982).

40. Hansen, E.V., Meyer, O. and Olsen, P. Study on toxicity of butylated hydroxyanisole (BHA) in pregnant gilts and their fetuses. Toxicology 23: 79–83 (1982).

41. Padnos, E., Horwitz, I.D. and Wunder, G. Contact dermatitis complicating tracheostomy. Causative role of ageous solution of benzalkomium chloride. Am. J. Dis. Child. 109:90–91 (1965).

42. Shumnes, E. and Levy, E.J. Quaternary ammonium compound contact dermatitis from a deodorant. Arch. Dermatol. 105:91–93 (1972).

43. Anstad, J. Allergic contact dermatitis to Sorbitan monocleate (Span 80). Contact Derm. 8:426 (1982).

44. Eisman, P.C., Cooper, J. and Jaconia, D. Influence of gum tragacanth on the bactericidal activity of preservatives. J. Am. Pharm. Assoc. 46:144 (1957).

45. Bohner, C.B., Sheldon, J.M. and Trents, J.W. Sensitivity to gum acacia, with a report of ten cases of asthma in printers. J. Allergy 12:290 (1941).

46. Methylcellulose. USP XXI. p. 672–673 (1985). Methylcellulose ophthalmic solution. USP XXI. p. 673 (1985). Methylcellulose oral solution. USP (XXI). p. 673 (1985).

47. Ismail-Begi, F., Reinhold, J.G., Faraji, B. and Abadi, P. Effect of cellulose added to diet of low and high fiber content upon the metabolism of calcium, magnesium, zinc and phosphorus by man. J. Nutri. 107:510 (1977).

48. The high-fiber diet: Its effect on the bowel. Med. Lett. 17:93–95 (1975).

49. Walter, B.F., Brownly, W.J. and Roberts, W.C. Self-induced pulmonary granulomatosis. A consequence of I.V. injection of drugs intended for oral use. Chest 78:90–94 (1980).

50. Coooper, C.B., Bai, T.R., Heyderman, E. and Corrin, B. Cellulose granuloma in the lungs of a cocaine sniffer. Br. Med. J. 286:2021–2022 (1983).

51. Hjorth, H. and Trolle-Lassen, C. Skin reactions to ointment bases. Trans. St. Johns Hosp. Dermatol. Soc. 49:127–40 (1963).

52. Shore, R.N. and Shelley, W.B. Contact dermatitis from stearyl alcohol and propylene glycol in fluocinonide cream. Arch. Dermatol. 109:397–399 (1974).

53. Gaul, L.E. Dermatitis from cetyl and stearyl alcohol. Arch. Dermagol. 99: 593 (1969).

54. Pervy, I. and Uhlich, M. Allergie gegen bestandteile medizinischer und kosmetischer externa. Polyathylenglykol, propylenglykol, stearylakohol, hexantriol. Hautarzt 26:252–254 (1975).

55. Hannuksela, M. Allergic and toxic reactions caused by cream bases in dermatological patients. Int. J. Cosmet. Sci. 1:257–263.

56. Turio, S. and King, R.E. (Eds.) Sterile Dosage Forms, 2nd ed. Lea & Febiger Philadelphia, (1979).
57. Dowdy, E.G., Holland, W.C., Yamanaka, I. and Kaya, K. Cardioactive properties of d-tubocurarine with and without preservatives. Anesthesiology 34:256–260 (1971).
58. Schmidt, G.B., Meier, M.A. and Sadove, M.S. Sudden appearance of cardiac arrhythmias after dexamethasone. J.A.M.A. 222:1402–1404 (1972).
59. Marzulli, F.N. and Maibach, H.I. Antimicrobials: Experimental contact sensitization in man. J. Soc. Cosmet. Chem. 24:399–421 (1973).
60. Heinonen, O.P., Slone, D. and Shapiro, S. Birth Defects and Drugs in Pregnancy. Publishing Sciences Group, Littleton, MA, p. 300, (1977).
61. Baran, R.B. and Rowles, B. Factors affecting coloration of urine and feces. J. Am. Pharm. Assoc. NS13:139–140 (1973).
62. Euerby, M.R. and Walker, J.E. HPLC of thymol in halothane BP and halothane vapourizer waste. Br. J. Pharm. Pract. 6:373–374 (1984).
63. Feinberg, S.M. and Watrous, R.M. Atopy to simple chemical compounds—sulfonechloramides. J. Allergy 16:209–220 (1945).
64. Bourne, M.S., Flindt, M.L. and Walker, J.M. Asthma due to industrial use of chloramine. Br. Med. J. 2:10–12 (1979).
65. Davies, M. Rabbit eye irritation from bactericides in soft lens soaking solutions. J. Pharm. Pharmac. 25 (suppl.):134 (1973).
66. Ainley, E.J., Mackie, I.G. and MacArthur, D. Adverse reaction to chloro-cresol-preserved heparin. Lancet 1:705 (1977).
67. Burry, J.N., Kirk, J., Reid, J.G. and Turner, T. Chlorocressol sensitivity. Contact Derm. 1:41–42 (1975).
68. Lebowitz, R.L. Intravesical chemical cauterization and methemoglobi-nemia. Pediatrics 65:630 (1980).
69. Borody, T., Chinwah, P.M., Graham, G.G., Wade, D.N. and Williams, K.M. Chlorobutanol toxicity and dependence. Med. J. Aust. 1:288 (1979).
70. Dux, S., Pitlik, S., Perry, G. and Rosenfeld, J.B. Hypersensitivity reaction to chlorobutol-preserved heparin. Lancet 1:288 (1981).
71. Marsh, B.T. Preservatives in heparin. Lancet 1:860 (1977).
72. Fisher, A.A., Pascher, F. and Kanof, N.B. Allergic contact dermatitis due to ingredients of vehicles. A "vehicle tray" for patch testing. Arch. Dermatol. 104:286–290 (1971).
73. Brown, R. Another case of sorbic acid sensitivity. Contact Derm. 5:268 (1979).
74. Rietschel, R.L. Contact urticaria from synthetic cessia oil and sorbic acid limited to the fece. Contact Derm. 4:347–349 (1978).
75. Saihan, E.M. and Harman, R.M. Contact sensitivity to sorbic acid in "unguentum merck." Br. J. Dermatol. 99:583–584 (1978).
76. Rudzki, E. and Kleniewska, D. The epidemiology of contact dermatitis in Poland. Br. J. Dermatol. 83:543–545 (1970).
77. Fisher, A.A. Cosmetic dermatitis: Part II: Reactions to some commonly used preservatives. Cutis. 26:136–137 (1980).

78. Abrams, J.D. and Majzenou, U. Mercury content of the human lens. Br. J. Ophthalmol. 54:59–61 (1970).
79. Kennedy, R.E., Roca, P.D. and Platt, D.S. Further observations on atypical band keratopathy in glaucoma patients. Tr. Am. Ophthalmol. Soc. 72:107–122 (1974).
80. Abrams, J.D. Iatrogenic mercurialentis. Trans. Ophthalmol. Soc. U.K. 83:263–269 (1963).
81. Winder, A.F., Astbury, N.J., Sheraidah, G.a.K. and Ruben, M. Penetration of mercury from ophthalmic perservatives into the human eye. Lancet 2:237–239 (1980).
82. Lohr, L. The saga of encare oval: An FDA Advisory Panel at work. Am. Pharm. 18 (9):20–24 (1978).
83. Moller, H. Merthiolate allergy: A nationwide latrogenic sensitization. Acta Dermatovener. (Stockh) 57:509–517 (1977).
84. Hasson, H. and Moller, H. Intracutaneous test reactions to tuberculin containing merthiolate as a preservative. Scand. J. Infect. Dis. 3:169–172 (1971).
85. Rohyans, J., Watson, P.D., Wood, G.A. and MacDonald, W.A. Mercury toxicity following merthiolate ear irrigations. J. Pediatr. 104:311–313 (1986).
86. Axton, J.H.M. Six cases of poisoning after a parenteral organic mercurial compound (merthiolate). Postgrad. Med. J. 48:417–421 (1972).
87. Fagan, D.G., Pritchard, J.S., Clarkson, T.W. and Greenwood, M.R. Organ mercury levels in infants with omphaloceles treated with organic mercurial antiseptic. Arch. Dis. Child. 52:962–964 (1977).
88. Jones, H.T. Danger of skin burns from thiomersal. Br. Med. J. 2:504–505 (1972).
89. Saiki, J.H., Thompson, S., Smith, F. and Atkinson, R. Paraplegia following intrathecal chemotherapy. Cancer 29:370–374 (1972).
90. Botstein, P. Neonate toxicity of benzyl alcohol. Am. Soc. Pharmacol. Exper. Therap. meeting 3/29/85.
91. Benzyl alcohol: Toxic agent in neonatal units. Pediatrics 72:356–358 (1983).
92. Kimura, E.T., Darby, T.D., Krause, R.A. and Brondyk, H.D. Parenteral toxicity studies with benzoyl alcohol. Toxicol. Appl. Pharmacol. 18:60–68 (1971).
93. Lazzarini, S. Contact allergy to benzylalcohol and isopropyl palmitate, ingredients of topical corticosteroids. Contact Derm. 8:349 (1980).
94. Alert pharmacists spot product defect. Am. Soc. Hosp. Pharm. Newsletter 9:2, (Sept.) 1976.
95. Edwards, R.C. and Voegeli, C.J. Inadvisability of using caffeine and sodium benzoate in neonates. Am. J. Hosp. Pharm. 41:658, 660 (1984).
96. Green, T.P., Marchessault, R.P. and Freese, D.K. Disposition of sodium begoate in newborn infants with hyperammonemia. J. Pediatr. 102:785–790 (1983).

97. Schiff, D., Chan, G. and Stern, L. Fixed drug combinations and the displacement of bilinibin from albumin. Pediatrics 48:139–141 (1971).

98. Michaelsson, G., Pettersson, L. and Juhlin, L. Purpura caused by food and drug additives. Arch. Dermatol. 109:49–52 (1974).

99. Ros, A.M., Juhlin, L. and Michaelsson, G. A follow-up study of patients with recurrent urticaria and hypersensitivity to aspirin, benzoates and azo dyes. Br. J. Dermatol. 95:19024 (1976).

100. Juhlin, L., Michaelsson, G. and Zetterstrom, O. Urticaria and asthma induced by food and drug additives in patients with aspirin hypersensitivity. J. Allergy Clin. Immunol. 50:92–98 (1972).

101. Meynadier, J.-M., Meynadier, J., Colmas, A., Castelain, P.-Y., Ducombs, G., Chabeau, G., Lacroix, M., Martin, P. and Ngangu, Z. Allergie aux conservateurs. Ann. Dermatol. Venereol. 109:1017–1023 (1982).

102. Lahti, A. and Hannuksela, M. Is benzoic acid really harmful in cases of atopy and urticaria? Lancet 2:1055 (1981).

103. Lorenzetti, O.J. and Wernet, T.C. Topical parabens: Benefits and risks. Dermatologica 154:244–250 (1977).

104. Nagel, J.E., Fuscaldo, J.T. and Fireman, P. Paraben allergy, J.A.M.A. 237: 1594–1595 (1977).

105. Schorr, W.F. Paraben allergy: A cause of intractable dermatitis. J.A.M.A. 204:859–862 (1968).

106. Schorr, W.F. and Mohajerin, A.M. Paraben sensitivity. Arch. Dermatol. 93:721–723 (1966).

107. Schamberg, I.L. Allergic contact dermatitis to methyl and propyl paraben. Arch. Dermatol. 95:626–628 (1967).

108. Epstein, S. Paraben sensitivity. Subtle trouble. Ann. Allergy 26:185–189 (1968).

109. Parker, M.S. Preservatives of fluid oral dosage form. Pharm. J. 222:92 (1979).

110. Swenberg, J.A., Kerns, W.D., Mitchell, R.I., Gralla, E.J. and Pavicor, K.L. Induction of squamous cell carcinomas of the rat nasal cavity by inhalation exposure to formaldehyde vapor. Cancer Res. 40:3398 (1980).

111. Watanabe, F. and Sugimoto, S. Study on the carcinogenicity of aldehyde. 2nd report. Gann 46:365 (1955).

112. Porta, G.D., Colnaghi, M.I. and Parmiani, G. Noncarcinogenicity of HMT in mice and rats. Food Cosmet. Toxicol. 6:707 (1968).

113. Natvig. H., Anderson, J. and Rasmussen, E.W. A contribution to the toxicological evaluation of hexamethylene tetramine. Food Cosmet. Toxicol. 9:491 (1971).

114. Bryce, D.M., Croshaw, B., Hall, J.E., Holland, V.R. and Lessel, B. The activity and safety of the anti-microbial agent broncopol (2-bromo-2-nitropropane-1,3-diol). J. Soc. Cosmet. Chem. 29:3–24 (1978).

115. Maibach, H.I. Dermal sensitization potention of 2-bromo-2 nitropropane-1,3-diol (Bromopol^R). Contact Derm. 3:99 (1977).

116. Storrs, F.J. and Bell. D.E. Allergic contact dermatitis to 2-bromo-nitro-

propane-1,3-diol in a hydrophilic ointment. J. Am. Acad. Dermatol. 8: 157–170 (1983).

117. WHO Technical Report Serv. No. 617 Evaluation of certain food additives—21st report of the joint FAO/WHO Expert Committee on Food Additives. (1978).

118. Nitzan, M. Volovitz, B. and Topper, E. Infantile methemoglobinemia caused by food additives. Clin. Toxicol. 15:273–280 (1979).

119. Stevenson, D.D. and Simon, R.A. Sulfites and asthma. J. Allergy Clin. Immunol. 74:468–472 (1984).

120. Sulfiting agents: Revocation of GRAS status for use on fruits or vegetables intended to be served or sold raw to consumers. Fed. Reg. 51(131): 25021–25026 (1986).

121. Schwartz, H.J. Sensitivity to ingested metabisulfite: Variations in clinical presentation. J. Allergy Clin. Immunol. 71:487 (1983).

122. Halaby, S.F. and Mattocks, A.M. Absorption of sodium bisulfite from peritoneal dialysis solutions. J. Pharm. Sci. 54:52–55 (1965).

123. Wilins, J.E., Jr., Greene, J.A., Jr. and Weller, J.M. Toxicity of intraperitoneal bisulfite. Clin. Pharmacol. Ther. 9:328–332 (1968).

124. Provost, T.T. and Jillson, O.F. Ethylenediamine contact dermatitis. Arch. Dermatol. 96:231–234 (1967).

125. Kahn, G., Phauphak, P. and Claman, H.N. Propyl gallate—contact sensitization and orally-induced tolerance. Arch. Dermatol. 109:506–509 (1974).

126. Kahn, G. and Curry, M.C. Ultraviolet light protection by several new compounds. Arch. Dermatol. 109:510–517 (1974).

127. Weiner, M. The influence of the phsyiologic disposition of chelates on their use in medicine. Ann. N.Y. Acad. Sci. 88:426 (1960).

128. Seven, J.J. and Johnson, L.A. (eds.). Metal Binding in Medicine. J.B. Lippincott, Philadelphia 1960.

129. Sullivan, T.J. The effects of metallic edetates on the growth and formation of rats. Arch. Int. Pharmacodyn. 124:225–236 (1960).

130. Spencer, H. Studies of the effect of chelating agents in man. Ann. N.Y. Acad. Sci. 88:435 (1960).

131. Hurley, L.S. and Swenerton, H. Teratogenic effects of a chelating agent and their prevention by zinc. Science 173:62–63 (1971).

132. Seidel, A., Volf, V. and Catsch, A. Effectiveness of Zn-DTPA in removal of plutonium from rats. Int. J. Radiation Biol. 19:399 (1971).

133. Science News V: 130, 1986.

134. O'Leary, R.K. and Guess, W.L. Toxicological studies on certain medical grade plastics sterilized by ethylene oxide. J. Pharm. Sci. 57:12–17 (1968).

135. Lawrence, W.H., Turner, J.E. and Autian, J. Toxicity of ethylene chlorohydrin. I: Acute toxicity studies. J. Pharm. Sci. 60:568–571 (1971).

136. Boucher, R.M.G. Advances in sterilization techniques. State of the art and recent breakthroughs. Am. J. Hosp. Pharm. 29:661–672 (1972).

137. Poothullil, J. Shimizu, A., Day, R.P. and Dolovich, J. Anaphylaxis from the product(s) of ethylene oxide gas. Ann. Intern. Med. 82:58–60 (1975).

138. Nicholls, A.J. and Platts, M.M. Anaphylactoid reactions due to haemo-dialysis, haemofiltration or membrane plasma separation. Br. Med. J. 285: 1607-1609 (1982).

139. Biro, L., Fischer, A.A. and Price, E. Ethylene oxide burns. Arch. Dermatol. 110:924-925 (1974).

140. Weiner, M. The objectives and timing of drug disposition studies. Drug. Metab. Rev. 4:229-239 (1975).

141. Schlesinger, R.B. Comparative disposition of inhaled aerosols in experimental animals and humans: A review. J. Toxicol. Environ. Health 15: 197-214 (1985).

142. Gerade, H.W. Toxicological studies of hydrocarbon. Arch. Environ. Health 6:329-341 (1963).

143. Martin, E.W. Dispensing of Medication. 7th ed. Mack Publishing (1971).

144. Nuckolla, A.H. Underwriters' Laboratories Report on the Comparative Life, Fire and Explosion Hazards of Common Refrigerants. National Board of Fire Underwriters, Chicago (1933).

145. Yant, W.P. Toxicity of organic fluorides. Am. J. Publ. Health 23:3384 (1933).

146. von Oettingen, W.F. J. Ind. Hyg. Toxicol. Halogenated hydrocarbons: their toxicity and potential dangers. 19:3375 (1937).

147. Lester, D. and Greenberg, L.A. Acute and chronic toxicity of some halogenated derivatives of methane and ethane. Ind. Hyg. Occup. Med. 1:335-344 (1950).

148. Prendergast, J.A., Jones, R.A., Jenkins, L.J. and Siegel, Effects on experimental animals of long-term inhalation of trichloroethylene, carbon tetrachloride, 1,1,1-trichloroethane, dichlorodifluoromethane, and 1,1,-dichloroethylene. J. Toxicol. and Applied Pharmacol. 10:270 (1967).

149. Draffan, G.H., Dollery, C.T., Williams, F.M. and Clare, R.A. Thorax 29: 95 (1947).

150. Speiger, F.E., Doll, R. and Meuf, P. Observation on recent increase in mortality from asthma. Br. Med. J. 1:335-339 (1968).

151. Jefferson, I.G. Accidental death of child playing with deodorant aerosol. Lancet 1:779 (1978).

152. Van Ketel, W.G. Allergic contact dermatitis from propellants in deodorant sprays in combination with allergy to ethyl chloride. Contact Derm. 2: 115-119 (1976).

153. Aviado, D.M. and Drinal, J. Five fluorocarbons for administration of aerosol bronchodilators. J. Clin. Pharmacol. 15:117-129 (1975).

154. Yamakage, A., Ishikawa, H., Saito, Y. and Hattori, A. Occupational scleroderma-like disorder occurring in men engaged in the polymerization of epoxy resins. Dermatologica 161:33-44 (1980).

155. Selikoff, I.J. and Hammond, E.C. Toxicity of vinyl schloride-polyvinyl chloride. Ann. N.Y. Acad. Sci. 246:1-337 (1975).

156. Sucio, I., Prodan, L., Ilea, E., Paduraru, A. and Pascu, L. Clinical manifestations in vinyl chloride poisoning. Ann. N.Y. Acad. Sci. 246:53-69 (1975).

157. Danziger, M. Accidental poisoning by vinyl chloride. Can. Med. Assoc. J. 82:828–830 (1960).
158. Speizer, F.E., Wegman, D.H. and Ramirez, A. N. Palpitation rates associated with fluorocarbon exposure in a hospital setting. Engl. J. Med. 292:624, (1975).
159. Roslaw, M., Belei, A., Smith, D.C., and Aviado, D.M. Toxicity of aerosol propellants in the respiratory and circulatory systems. I.V. Cardiotoxicity in the monkey. Toxicology 2:381 (1974).

Part III
Nonallergic Adverse Effects of Excipients by Class of Excipient

Chapter 11   Allergic Reactions: Bulk Materials   201

Chapter 12   Allergic Reactions: Coatings   223

Chapter 13   Allergic Reactions: Flavoring Agents   231

Chapter 14   Allergic Reactions: Coloring Agents   253

Chapter 15   Allergic Reactions: Other Addition Products   283

11

Allergic Reactions: Bulk Materials

I. Oral   201
  A. Solid formulations   201
  B. Liquid formulations (solvents)   202
II. Topical   206
  A. Solids   206
  B. Liquids (lotions, emulsions, suspensions)   211
III. Parenteral   216
IV. Suppositories   217
V. Miscellaneous Products   218
  A. Topical ophthalmic preparations   218
  B. Topical otic preparations   218
  C. Mouth and throat preparations   218
  D. Vaginal products   218
  References   218

I. ORAL

A. Solid Formulations

The role of bulk excipients in solid oral formulations as causes of human hypersensitivity response is minimal. Although the antigenic properties of microbial polysaccharides have been demonstrated for many years, plant-derived polysaccharides are essentially nonallergenic. Most of the comments on possible allergenicity concern cornstarch. However, critical review of available literature on this subject reveals only a few anecdotal reports of patients experiencing headaches and fatigue after ingestion of cornstarch excipients (1). Even these accounts cannot be taken too seriously because the challenge studies were not performed using a double-blind protocol.

"Allergic" reactivity is sometimes attributed to monosaccharide (glucose, fructose) and/or disaccharide (sucrose, lactose) sugars. This is not altogether unexpected when it is appreciated that simple sugars have a wide range of unique chemical, biological, and metabolic properties and that the effects of these processes may be incorrectly interpreted as allergic reactivity (2). Psseudoallergic reactions occur regularly to one of these agents, lactose, when ingested by susceptible individuals with proven lactase deficiency. Although there is a wide spectrum of response in such individuals, in most cases relatively large amounts of lactose must be ingested before the appearance of abdominal cramps and diarrhea (3).

Methylcellulose is allergically inert by the oral route as are bulk filler inorganic salts, which are discussed in more detail in Part II.

a. Type I–IV immunologic reactivity

None has been reported.

b. Anatomical sites of hypersensitivity reactions

None has been reported.

c. Pseudoallergic responses

Abdominal pain, flatulence, and diarrhea may be mistaken for gastrointestinal allergic symptoms in lactase-deficient individuals. Drug information centers can be consulted to determine whether a preparation contains lactose filler and for recommendations concerning alternative preparations.

B. Liquid Formulations (Solvents)

1. Water

There are no documented instances of allergic reactions to the most common liquid solvents, such as water and simple, colorless, and unflavored syrups.

2. Alcohol

Several types of allergic responses have been observed in patients after ingestion of small amounts of distilled ethanol. Despite the common use of alcohol as a beverage and medicinal antiseptic, primary hypersensitivity responses to alcohol are rare. The majority of documented cases concern patients who develop urticaria shortly after ingestion of small amounts (30 ml) of ethanol (4–8). There is one documented case of anaphylaxis in a young woman who subsequently showed positive prick tests to undiluted ethanol, acetaldehyde, and acetic acid (9). The authors of this communication suggested that skin test results were consistent with the fact that ethanol is metabolized mainly to acetic acid via an acetaldehyde metabolite. Further, they speculated that this particular patient had experienced a previous history of hypersensitivity to vinegar and that this underlying sensitivity was exacerbated by ingestion of alcohol.

The occurrence of an allergic reaction to ethanol must be differentiated from nonspecific reactions that can mimic an immediate-type allergic reaction. In patients receiving disulfiram for the control of chronic alcoholic addiction, the ingestion of ethanol causes skin flushing, headaches, dyspnea, tachycardia, a fall in blood pressure, and general discomfort due to known pharmacologic mechanisms. Similar symptoms may be provoked when ethanol is ingested concurrently with metronidazole, nitrofurantoin, chlorpropamide, sulfonamides, or ketoconazole (10). Cutaneous flushing is a common reaction to alcohol among Asian people. These reactions are unaccompanied by increased levels of plasma histamine after ingestion of ethanol. Thus, the physiological basis of this ethnic difference has not been identified (11). An exaggerated manifestation of such response, including asthma, has been described in several asthmatic Asians who developed vasomotor signs and moderately severe bronchospasm immediately after ingestion of 95% ethanol. This reaction was not inhibited by cromolyn sodium but was partially attentuated by atropine and an H_1 antihistamine, suggesting that the mechanism was nonallergic (12). It should also be noted that chronic ethanol ingestion broadly suppresses the various arms of the human immune defense system. This includes depression of marrow myeloid reserves, which results in neutropenia. There is also convincing in vitro and in vivo evidence that chronic alcohol ingestion depresses the development and expression of cell-mediated immunity (13). Concomitant alcohol ingestion may also interfere with primary antibody responses to new antigens. Acute ingestion of alcohol may also interfere with the interpretation of allergy skin tests (4).

a. Type I. immunologic reactivity

IgE-mediated reactions include acute urticaria and one case of systemic anaphylaxis.

b. Type II and III immunologic reactivity

No reactions have been reported.

c. Type IV immunologic reactivity

One patient developed delayed expression of a fine vesicular eruption after ingestion of ethanol (5). The exact pathogenesis of this reaction was not established but its morphology was consistent with a type IV mediated reaction.

d. Anatomical sites of hypersensitivity reactions: *Cutaneous*: Erythema of face and hands has been described in several patients. The erythema may occur within an hour after ingestion of ethanol and may persist for several hours. In some cases the erythema occurred 8–12 hr after ingestion of alcohol and was accompanied by severe pruritis. The most common cutaneous lesion is urticaria, which may be either localized or generalized. The reaction occurs within 5 or 10 min after ethanol ingestion and persists for about an hour in some of the cases. One must be careful to differentiate alcohol-induced urticaria from urticaria exacerbated by alcohol. The latter is more likely, so the only way that true ethanol-induced urticaria can be documented is by carefully controlled challenge testing. Because it is difficult to conceal the alcohol in an oral challenge test, some investigators have given challenge doses of alcohol through a nasogastric tube. An immediate contact urticaria syndrome has been described in several cases after local contact with ethyl alcohol (14,15). In one of these cases, the contact urticaria reaction was passively transferred by injecting 0.1 ml of the patient's serum into the forearm of a nonsensitive volunteer (15). One cutaneous ethanol reactor developed a fine vesicular eruption on fingers and toes about 12 hr after the ethanol challenge (5).

Respiratory/Systemic: There is only one documented case of systemic anaphylaxis manifested by generalized itching, facial flushing, dizziness, abdominal pain, dyspnea, and collapse after drinking ethanol. Involvement of the respiratory tract was also demonstrated by an oral provocation test performed on this patient (9).

e. Pseudoallergic responses

Nonspecific interactions with drugs have been cited above. As an illustration of alcohol inolerance in Asians, there is one case report of an asthmatic Asian in whom the usual ethnic response was greatly exaggerated, resulting in acute and severe bronchospasm. It should be emphasized that the diagnosis of ethanol-induced urticaria is not easy, because patients with various preexisting allergic conditions may complain that their symptoms are aggravated when they drink alcoholic beverages.

3. Glycerin

In general, allergic reactions to glycerin are extremely rare. A few cases of contact dermatitis have been reported (see the chapter on topical agents) but no reactions after oral ingestion of glycerin-containing liquid preparations have been recorded in the literature.

4. Glycols

Glycols are polyols with a wide variety of uses as industrial solvents and antifreezes. Propylene glycol is a viscous hygroscopic liquid commonly used in the preparation of oral medications. Barbiturates, antihistamines, and vitamins are but a few of the drugs dissolved in propylene glycol. A few immediate-type allergic reactions have been reported after oral ingestion of propylene glycol used as an excipient in liquid preparations (16).

a. Type I immunologic reactivity

Several acute urticarial reactions have been described after ingestion of propylene glycol.

b. Type II and III immunologic reactivity

No reactions have been reported.

c. Type IV immunologic reactivity

Flares of classic epicutaneous (contact dermatitis) reactions have occurred after peroral challenge with propylene glycol (17).

d. Anatomical sites of hypersensitivity reactions: Cutaneous: Acute urticarial lesions have been described in a few patients. Sensitive patients may develop acute exanthematous eruptions within 4 hr of peroral challenge. In some cases this can be so severe that systemic steroid treatment is required for control of the dermatitis.

e. Pseudoallergic responses

Vertigo and other vague subjective symptoms may occur in patients with epicutaneous manifestations after peroral challenge with propylene glycol.

5. Unabsorbed Sugar Alcohols (Polyalcohols)

Mannitol. Although anaphylactoid reactions have been described after mannitol intravenous infusions (see section on parenteral medications), allergic reactions after oral ingestion have not been documented.

Xylitol At one time, intravenous xylitol was used to replenish carbohydrates when the metabolism of glucose was disordered. However, after it was realized that renal and intracerebral calcium oxalate precipitates might be induced by this agent, its use as an intravenous infusion was discontinued (18).

Sorbitol Sorbitol is the most common sweetener in "sugar-free" candies and gums. Smaller amounts are used as drug additives.

a. Type I–IV immunologic reactivity

None has been reported.

b. Anatomical sites of hypersensitivity reactions

None has been documented.

c. Pseudoallergic responses

Sorbitol intolerance is manifested by abdominal pain, bloating, and diarrhea. It has been observed in children ingesting more than 3 g sorbitol in diet candies and in adults using more than 10 g of this substance per day (19,20). These effects of sorbitol are due to its pharmacologic effect as an osmotic laxative.

6. Oils

A variety of oils derived from common foods may be used as excipients in liquid preparations. It has been claimed but not proved that patients with known allergic sensitivity to the protein components in the specific food may also show similar allergic symptoms after ingestion of the respective oil. Since protein allergens are insoluble in oil and the oil extraction process itself excludes these materials, it is highly unlikely that this occurs (21). Indeed, recent prospective investigations proved conclusively that skin tests to peanut oil and soybean oil were completely negative in individuals proven to be sensitive to peanut and soybean proteins (22,23). Consistent with these facts, it is not surprising that documented cases of allergic sensitivity to food oil excipients have not been reported in the literature.

II. TOPICAL

A. Solids

Additives in this category include topical powders and substances that add body and bulk to gels, ointments, and creams.

1. Cornstarch Powder

Cornstarch powder in rubber gloves has been reported to cause contact urticaria (24). Since this adverse effect depends on the concurrent use of rubber gloves, more detailed discussion is included in Chapter 6 of Part III.

2. Petroleum Hydrocarbons

Petrolatums are classified chiefly as natural, artificial, or synthetic. Natural petrolatum is obtained from petroleum distillation residues or from storage tank sediments containing crude petroleum. Artificial petrolatum is a blend of natural hydrocarbon wax (paraffin wax) with paraffin oil. Synthetic petrolatum is produced from synthetic hydrocarbons by cohydrogenation or catalytic polymerization of ethylene. The composition and physical properties of a particular petrolatum depend on the petrolatum stock used as well as the purification methods. White petrolatum is prepared in the same manner as yellow but the purification process is continued until the product is virtually free of the yellow color. Considering the widespread and abundant use of petrolatum, very few cases of sensitivity have been described. Although reactions to both white and yellow petrolatum have been reported, one group of investigators demonstrated that yellow petrolatums are more sensitizing than white, at least when petrolatums of the same brand were compared (25). These workers further showed that the greater sensitizing potential of yellow petrolatum was due to the presence of larger quantities of polycyclic aromatic hydrocarbons such as benzene, naphthalene, and phenanthrene in the yellow variety. However, one possible problem in purifying white petrolatum from naturally occurring yellow petrolatum is that the purification process tends to remove the naturally occurring antioxidants. The finished product will then oxidize on contact with air and light and develop an offensive odor. To prevent this, stabilizers such as butylhydroxytoluene (see Chapter 5), which is itself a sensitizer, may be added to some of the "purified" white petrolatums (26).

a. Type I-III immunologic reactivity

No reactions have been reported.

b. Type IV immunologic reactivity

Contact dermatitis is the chief immunologic reaction induced by either white or yellow petrolatum. Immunologic reactivity can be proved by patch tests, which if performed properly, can differentiate it from other contactant substances as well as irritative responses.

c. Anatomical sites of hypersensitivity reactions

Based on the few case reports available in the literature, contact dermatitis to various petrolatums tends to occur more often on the lower extremities, particularly in patients with leg ulcerations (27,28). This suggests that petrolatum may be completely nonallergenic on healthy skin but may cause eczematous reactions on damaged skin. However, in view of the fact that petrolatums have a certain degree of allergenic sensitization potential, albeit small, it should be noted that petrolatum sensitivity may rarely account for false-positive patch test reactions to substances diluted in it.

d. Pseudoallergic responses

Chronic dermatitis and hyperpigmentation of a black patient's face have been reported (29). This may be more common in South Africa among blacks who use petrolatum as a cosmetic.

3. Glycols

Glycols of varying molecular weights are extensively used as vehicles in topical medications because of their excellent solvent, humectant, and, in some instances, preservative properties. Depending on their concentrations and specific properties, they may act as irritants or true sensitizers. Reactions to these agents in topical medications have been recognized with increased frequency in the past decade.

Propylene glycol is the most frequently used pharmacologic additive in this class of compounds. It has largely replaced glycerine in pharmaceutical preparations and has thus become ubiquitous. Polyethylene glycol is a mixture of glycols. The lower-molecular-weight compounds, ranging from 200 to 700 daltons, are liquids, while the higher weights (1,000-6,000) are solids. Polyethylene glycol of different molecular weights is used extensively as a vehicle for topical medications and suppositories. Polyethylene glycol ointment (USP) is made of solid polyethylene glycol 4,000 (USP) combined with liquid polyethylene glycol 300.

a. Type I immunologic reactivity

Immediate urticarial reactions have been reported in two patients (30). Application of medication containing this ingredient resulted in pruritis, redness, and urticaria within 15 min after application. Reactions in both patients were duplicated after low-molecular-weight polyethylene glycol was rubbed into their skins. Similar tests in normal control volunteers gave negative results. In both cases, the reactions ascribed to contact urticaria reactions were presumed but not proved to be mediated by type I mechanisms.

b. Types II and III immunologic reactivity

No reactions have been reported.

c. Type IV immunologic reactivity

Classic contact dermatitis sensitization has been reported for several of the glycol compounds including polyethylene glycol and propylene glycol. There is considerable divergence of opinion about the proper concentration for the diagnosis of unequivocal sensitization. Some investigators have proposed that patch testing with 2% or lower concentrations of propylene glycol can differentiate allergic from irritative reactions (31). On the other hand, epicutaneous test reactions to higher concentrations (5-10%) may also be indicative of allergic reactivity. One possible way of resolving the problem of suspected allergic sensitization is to confirm the reaction by oral challenge tests. Hypersensitive patients experience widespread exanthematous reactions within a few hours after ingesting as little as 2 ml propylene glycol.

c. Anatomical sites of hypersensitivity reactions: Cutaneous: Contact urticaria is

a rare manifestation of allergic response induced by glycol compounds . It has only been described after local application of medications containing polyethylene glycol (30).

Allergic contact dermatitis is much more frequent and has been induced by both propylene glycol and polyethylene glycol (30,32,33). The prevalence of propylene glycol contact dermatitis worldwide varies from 1.5 to 4.8%. Reports of higher prevalence may include some irritative reactions (34). Some investigators advocate that patch testing with glycol compounds should be performed without occlusion in order to minimize irritancy effects (35).

d. Pseudoallergic responses

One investigative team called attention to the fact that many cases of dermatitis developing after propylene glycol topical use could be due to propylene glycol intolerance rather than true allergic sensitization (34). They described a group of patients who lost dermatologic reactivity rapidly and upon subsequent provocative patch testing showed negative results. They also reported that most propylene-glycol-reactive patients had decreased reactivity within months and eventually did not react at all. They concluded that these patients are not allergenic but have an inadequately characterized form of irritation. Such reactions would therefore fall into the category of pseudoallergy.

4. Lanolin

There is a striking difference of opinion about the frequency of contact allergic sensitization to lanolin. In the past, American dermatologists believed that lanolin allergy was rare. However, European investigators believed that this impression was based on false-negative lanolin patch tests because tests were performed without the proper concentrations of free wool alcohols, which presumably are the main allergens. This controversy is heightened by the fact that lanolin is a complex mixture and the chemicals responsible for lanolin allergy have not been fully identified. Wool alcohols are obviously important, but detergent and antioxidant additives are often added to commercial products.

a. Type IV immunologic reactivity

Allergic contact dermatitis is the primary sensitization phenomenon attributed to lanolin. These reactions are detected by classic patch testing but there is considerable disagreement about how the patch test should be performed and interpreted. In proven cases of lanolin allergy, for example, patch tests with anhydrous lanolin may be negative while similar tests with hydrogenated lanolin or lanolin (wool) alcohols may be markedly positive (36). In contrast, maximization contact sensitivity tests to lanolin or 30% wool alcohols were negative in 25 healthy female volunteers (37). Both European and Japanese investigators determined that the incidence of sensitivity to hydrogenated lanolin was significantly higher than to anhydrous lanolin. Decreased skin sensitivity to the latter preparation was attributed to to the increase in its purity (38). The enhanced sensitization potential to hydrogenated lanolin is postulated to be due to increased concentrations of dihydrocholesterol, other halogenated sterols, saturated alcohols, hydrocarbons, and possible contamination by traces of copper, chromium, and nickel.

b. Anatomical sites of hypersensitivity reactions: *Cutaneous*: Lanolin allergy is more common in older women. Because women have a higher incidence of varicose veins, especially in their latter years, they also have a higher incidence of stasis dermatitis that persists for long periods of time. Thus, it is thought that statistics showing high prevalence of lanolin allergy could be distorted by lanolin reactivity associated with stasis dermatitis. Some investigators have reported that as many as 33% of patients with stasis dermatitis may develop allergy to lanolin. If this high-risk population is excluded, the estimated prevalence of lanolin allergy is between 1 and 2%. Patients with other types of eczema are also at increased risk for lanolin allergy. In contrast, the incidence of lanolin allergy in healthy skin populations is small, at least in reports from the United States (37).

Exaggerated reports of lanolin allergy have been ascribed to several factors. Patients tested with 30% wool alcohols may actually be experiencing false-positive irritant reactions rather than allergic sensitization responses. False-positive reactions may also be due to hyperirritable skin or the "angry back syndrome." False-positive reactions may also be due to unsuspected contaminants of commercial lanolin preparations.

Although lanolin is a relatively infrequent sensitizer, it is always important to consider it as a possible allergen because it is a ubiquitous component of topical medications and lubricating materials.

c. Pseudoallergic reactions

No pseudoallergic reactions have been reported.

5. Isopropyl Myristate

This is a synthetic fatty alcohol that is much less greasy and more resistant to oxidation and hydrolysis than lanolin. Therefore, it may be more acceptable in some topical pharmaceutical preparations. Its sensitizing potential is low but there is a report of six patch-test-positive cases of contact dermatitis (39).

6. Silicates

There is a single case report of an irritant contact dermatitis induced by sodium silicate (40). This patient also exhibited an urticarial reaction 15 min after a scratch test and 24 hr after a patch test with sodium silicate.

7. Beeswax

Purified beeswax (cera alba) may be present in medicated creams and ointments. At one time it was also contained in adhesive plasters but these are no longer widely used. Honey bees use a resinous material known as propolis in building their combs. Propolis is an adhesive, reddish brown substance collected from resinous secretions of trees such as fir, poplar, alder, birch, and willow. It is carried to the hive on the bristles of the hind legs of the bees and mixed with varying amounts of beeswax to varnish and seal the cells of the comb. Most of these resinous impurities are removed in the final purified pharmacologic grade of cera alba.

a. Type IV immunologic reactivity

Contact dermatitis to beeswax was first reported by Schwartz and Peck in an investigation of irritants contained in adhesive plaster (41). The most extensive prospective investigation of contact reactivity to cera alba was conducted by Hjorth and Trolle-Lassen in 2,634 consecutive cases of dermatitis (42). These investigators concluded that purified cera alba was not a contact allergen. In view of this experience, it seems likely that the reactions reported by Schwartz and Peck were due to impurities in their beeswax preparations. A recent study demonstrated that the resinous contactant materials contained in unpurified beeswax cross reacted with balsam of Peru and cinnamic derivatives (transcinnamic acid and cinnamic alcohol aldehyde). The latter chemicals are also components of balsam of Peru and may account for this cross-reactivity. Contact cheilitis and dermatitis have occurred after exposure to propolis in creams, tablets, and oral solutions (43,44).

b. Anatomical sites of hypersensitivity reactions: Cutaneous: The usual cutaneous lesions of contact dermatitis have been described after sensitization to this agent. The hands are most often involved and frequently there is a lichenified and hyperkeratotic eczema of both hands because the cause of the lesion may go unrecognized for months or years. In more severe cases, there may be confluent, papular exanthematous lesions of the facial areas (45).

B. Liquids (Lotions, Emulsions, Suspensions)

1. Aqueous Formulations

There are no known clinically relevant allergic reactions to distilled water used for appropriate pharmacologic purposes. Hyperosmolar solutions administered topically to the nose or bronchial passages may cause direct release of mediators from mast cells in these tissues (46,47). Nasal challenge tests with these solutions may result in nasal obstruction, rhinorrhea, and sneezing. In a similar manner, hyperosmolar solutions administered as an aerosol may cause bronchoconstriction in patients with asthma or underlying bronchial hyperresponsiveness (46).

2. Alcohols

The allergic sensitization potential of alcohols is of a very low order. Despite the fact that various primary and fatty alcohols are used widely in topical preparations, relatively few reports of contact sensitization have appeared in the literature. Individual cases of contact sensitization have been documented, however, after exposure to ethanol, isopropyl alcohol, benzyl alcohol, tertiary butyl alcohol, hydroabietyl alcohol, and stearyl alcohol (48–55). Stearyl alcohol is an 18-carbon aliphatic alcohol present in many topical steroid creams. In one patient who developed contact dermatitis to this fatty alcohol, the cream containing this material was used for over 1 year with no evidence of contact dermatitis. However, an acute dermatitis developed 2 weeks after occlusive dressings were started. This suggested that application of this material in the steroid cream by the occlusion technique increased skin irritation, thereby enhancing sensitization by this agent. Simultaneous use of a potent steroid in this case was not sufficient to mask or inhibit the development of allergic contact dermatitis (53).

a. Type I immunologic reactivity

An alcohol contact urticaria syndrome has occurred after topical sensitization to primary and aliphatic alcohols (54). These reactions can be demonstrated by open patch tests applied for 20 min. In one such case, immediate-type hypersensitivity was confirmed by passive transfer of allergic serum to a nonallergic individual. Reactions after use of topical alcohol are extremely rare.

b. Type IV immunologic reactivity

Classic contact dermatitis has been observed after sensitization by various types of alcohols. These reactions are confirmed by both open and closed patch testing. They can be difficult to differentiate from reactions to perfumes contained in many topical medicinal products. In test procedures designed to predict skin sensitizing potential, 50% aqueous ethanol induced delayed allergic skin reactivity in 6 of 93 human volunteers (55). This study illustrated that maximization tests of this type can identify even weak sensitizers such as ethanol.

c. Anatomical sites of hypersensitivity reactions: *Cutaneous*: The contact urticaria syndrome due to alcohol usually manifests itself in the appearance of local urticarial lesions over the site of the open or closed patch. In more sensitive patients, generalized urticaria has been described and, in a few instances, this has been accompanied by other systemic symptoms such as generalized pruritis and transient drops in blood pressure. Contact dermatitis of the skin occurs over exposed areas in most cases. As with to other types of contact dermatitis, if the offending agent is unrecognized for long periods of time, contact dermatitis may spread locally or may also involve remote areas of the skin.

d. Pseudoallergic reactions

The allergic intolerance syndrome to ethanol has been described above.

3. Oils

Vegetable oils are occasionally used in ointments, liniments, and sometimes as vehicles for contactant allergens used for patch testing. Olive oil and sesame oil are the two most commonly used oils in pharmaceutical preparations. The major components of olive oil have been identified as glycerides of oleic acid, palmitic acid, linoleic acid, stearic acid, and arachidic acid (56). Sesame oil contains similar triglycerides but in different proportions. Two percent of sesame oil is unsaponifiable. This unsaponifiable fraction contains sesamol, sesamolin, and sesamin (57). Olive oil does not contain the same unsaponifiable part. Both of these oils are classified as comparatively safe topical ingredients with extremely low indices of contact sensitivity.

a. Type IV immunologic reactivity

Reports of sensitization to olive and sesame oils are extremely rare. In the case of olive oil, there are only a few documented cases in the world literature. In two major academic centers in Holland, prospective patch testing for 7 years revealed delayed-type hypersensitivity to freshly prepared olive oil in two patients (56). Patch tests in both cases were obtained with fresh and purified olive oil and were strongly positive. There were no cross reactions to other possible cross-reacting topical additives, including sesame oil and arachidic oil. One patient also showed positive patch test results with olive oil prepared more than 6 months earlier. This test was performed because it had been suggested previously that olive oil dermatitis could be due to the aging of olive oil. Both of these patients were also tested with freshly prepared major constituents of olive oil. These tests were all negative, indicating that the major allergen of olive oil has not yet been identified. In contrast, Neering et al. demonstrated positive patch tests to three major ingredients of the unsaponifiable fraction of sesame oil: sesamole, sesamin, and sesamolin (58). Inasmuch as the sesamin concentration of purified oil is about 100 times that of sesamolin, it is postulated that sesamin may be the main inciting contactant allergen of sesame oil.

b. Anatomical sites of hypersensitivity reactions: *Cutaneous*: In most of the reported cases of olive oil dermatitis, olive oil was the major constituent in creams being used primarily for their nonirritative effects by patients with preexisting chronic dermatides. For example, one case occurred in a woman who was being treated for a leg ulcer and another case involved a man whose disseminated dermatitis was being treated with a "nonirritating" topical cream containing 60% olive oil. Thus, sensitization to olive oil appears to occur primarily after application to chronically inflamed skin. Almost all of the reported cases of sesame oil contact dermatitis have also occurred in patients with leg ulcers or previous stasis eczema. These patients had received frequent and prolonged application of sesame oil containing sesamin, and sensitization occurred on the basis of increased susceptibility induced by the chronic inflammatory skin process. When the sesame oil in the liniment used by these patients was replaced by peanut oil, the contact eczema improved rapidly in all cases. This therapeutic observation confirmed the specificity of the contact reaction as well as showing that the substances in the unsaponifiable fraction were responsible for the sensitivity, because peanut oil does not contain unsaponifiable materials.

c. Pseudoallergic reactions

No pseudoallergic reactions have been reported.

4. Glycerin

Glycerin is found in creams, gels, lotions, and lubricating medicinals. It imparts "smoothness" to these products and is an effective humectant or hygroscopic agent. It is stable and relatively nontoxic and nonirritating. Allergic reactions to glycerin are very rare.

a. Type I–IV immunologic reactivity

Contact dermatitis to glycerin has only been described in two patients who were detected in a test program involving several thousand patients. These patients were patch tested with 50% glycerin. One of these patients also gave positive patch tests when tested with 1, 5, and 10% glycerol mixtures in water. Three-plus positive reactions were obtained at the 48 and 72 hr readings (62).

b. Anatomical sites of hypersensitivity reactions: Cutaneous:
One patient developed hand eczema after exposure to a mixture of glycerin (1 part) and 70% ethanol (9 parts) applied on her hands after washing them with soap and water. Another patient developed disseminated dermatitis after using a cream containing 10% glycerin. This patient received an oral challenge with 5 ml of glycerin and developed an eczematous dermatitis within 2 hr. This reaction disappeared on the following day.

c. Pseudoallergic reactions

Topical application of glycerin-containing extracts to the nose and bronchial mucous membrane may cause nonspecific reactions in these tissues. In a prospective study, 21 of 34 patients given a nasal challenge with glycerin-containing solution gave false-positive reactions within 50 min after the nasal test (63). Most of these patients responded to 50% glycerin solution, but five positive reactions were noted after challenge with the 5% glycerin solution. Ten of 27 patients receiving bronchial challenge tests developed significant bronchial obstruction after glycerin applications. Two of these patients gave positive reactions when 5% glycerol solution was inhaled; the remainder responded to 50% glycerin. These studies emphasize the fact that control tests are absolutely essential when glycerin-containing solutions are used for topical testing of the nasal and bronchial systems.

5. Dimethyl Sulfoxide

Dimethyl sulfoxide (DMSO) is a powerful solvent that dissolves most aromatic unsaturated hydrocarbons and organic nitrogen compounds. This property makes it possible to use the skin as an avenue of administration for systemic therapy. The therapeutic uses of topical DMSO are still controversial but it is currently being used experimentally for the treatment of scleroderma (especially for digital ulcerations) and systemically for rheumatoid arthritis. When applied topically it has caused contact urticaria, shortness of breath, facial swelling, gastrointestinal disturbances, headache, nausea, diarrhea, photophobia, and transient disturbances in color vision. Lens opacities have been demonstrated after prolonged administration to animals, but this has not been documented in humans (59).

a. Types I-IV immunologic reactivity

No proven immunologically mediated reactions have been reported.

b. Anatomical sites of hypersensitivity reactions: *Cutaneous*: Topical application of DMSO at high concentrations (80% or greater) will produce tiny follicular papules within 5-15 min. By 20-30 min the papules coalesce into a large single wheal that persists for about 1 hr. Occasionally some normal volunteers will react in a similar fashion to concentrations as low as 20%. Application of DMSO to normal intact skin by means of scratch or intracutaneous tests produce wheals regularly when administered in concentrations of 40% or greater. Intracutaneous injections produce wheals at all concentrations of DMSO (from 10 to 90%). The wheals induced by scratch or intracutaneous tests occur within a few minutes and reach maximum intensity within 20 min. Topical administration of DMSO causes intense pruritis that can be persistent, but the wheals induced by scratch or intracutaneous tests are not accompanied by pruritis (60).

Contact urticaria occurring at remote sites after application of DMSO to the skin is occasionally observed. There have been a few instances of anaphylactoid reactions involving patients presenting with shortness of breath and facial swelling.

Prospective studies in large numbers of volunteers have shown no allergic contact sensitization (61). When patch tests are applied by the occlusion method, the primary irritant effects of DMSO are greatly enhanced, including epidermal vesiculation and erythema. This nonspecific irritant vesicular reaction is impossible to differentiate from contact dermatitis on a morphologic basis alone. DMSO may enhance the contact irritant potential of a drug or additive when such preparations are incorporated into DMSO used as a vehicle (64).

c. Pseudoallergic reactions

Both localized and remote cases of urticaria observed after local applications of DMSO are based on its histamine-releasing properties and have not been shown to be IgE dependent. Similarly, persistent erythematous and vesicular lesions have not been proven to be associated with classic type IV mechanisms. These reactions occur regularly if the skin is treated with DMSO at concentrations of 20-100% and occluded with a bandage or patch test for 2-3 days. Most investigators attribute these reactions to nonspecific irritant effects.

III. PARENTERAL

Bulk additives are generally not found in parenteral preparations. However, there are several notable exceptions to this rule. Mannitol, a hexahydric alcohol, is used in clinical medicine in a variety of situations for its osmotic diuretic properties. Colloid substances such as human serum albumin, dextran, gelatin, and hydroxyethyl starch are used as plasma substitutes. Gelatin preparations and hydroxyethyl starch have not been used in the United States, but dextran and human serum albumin are commonly used as plasma expanders. The latter preparation is now approved by the Food and Drug Administration as a diluent for the preparation of allergy extracts. It prevents denaturation of protein allergenic components by interfering with protein adsorption to glass surfaces. Parenteral administration of iron is possible by using iron–dextran conjugates or a polymer containing sorbitol and gluconic acid. Although these substances must be considered as drugs when they are administered parenterally, some of them are also excipients when they are incorporated into other non-parenteral formulations. The ambivalent status of some of these substances justifies their inclusion in this section.

a. Type I immunologic reactivity

Reactions to normal serum albumin are rare. Allergic patients occasionally exhibit positive prick tests to albumin-containing diluent solutions. Skin test reactivity has been demonstrated in house-dust-sensitive patients tested with mite culture medium containing human serum albumin components derived from human scales used in these cultures (65,66). Thus far, IgE-mediated sensitization has not been documented in systemic reactions occurring after administration of human serum albumin (67).

b. Types II–IV immunologic reactivity

No reactions have been reported.

c. Anatomical sites of hypersensitivity reactions: Cutaneous: Localized urticarial reactions occur after epicutaneous skin tests in a few allergic individuals.

Respiratory/systemic: Anaphylactoid reactions to all the above agents have been reported, but no true IgE-mediated anaphylactic episodes have been documented.

d. Pseudoallergic responses

Anaphylactoid reactions manifested by flushing of the face, shock, respiratory distress, bronchospasm, cyanosis, and pruritic rashes have been described after administration of all the colloid substances. A prospective multicenter study of anaphylactoid reactions to colloid volume substitutes revealed a total of 69 cases of anaphylactoid reactions among 200,906 infusions of colloid volume substitutes (68). The frequency of severe reactions (shock, cardiac and/or respiratory arrest) was 0.0111% for human serum albumin, 0.008% for dextran, 0.006% for hydroxyethyl starch, and 0.038% for gelatin solutions. Prolonged perineal pruritis occurred in four granulocyte donors who received intravenous infusions of a 6% solution of hydroxyethyl starch (69).

Mannitol-induced anaphylactoid reactions have been studied in greater detail. Although a positive scratch test was reported 2 months after an anaphylactoid reaction in a patient receiving this agent for treatment of glaucoma, the possible IgE-dependent nature of this reaction was not confirmed by other immunologic testing (70). In vitro basophil histamine release was studied in another patient who received mannitol before cataract surgery (71). These studies revealed marked hyperresponsiveness to hyperosmolar concentrations of mannitol (>0.1 M). This histamine-releasing ability was markedly enhanced when deuterium oxide (D_2O) was added to the releasing buffer. Under these conditions even low mannitol concentrations (<0.1 M) released significant amounts of histamine from human basophils. Since D_2O is known to augment IgE-dependent release of histamine from human basophils, these experiments suggested that this patient's anaphylactoid reaction could be due to IgE-dependent mechanisms. Thus anaphylactoid reactions to mannitol could be based on either hyperosmolar-dependent histamine release or IgE-dependent mediator release induced by nonhyperosmolar concentrations of mannitol.

Glycols, glycerin, and vegetable oils may be found in parenteral products. More detailed information about allergic reactions to these substances has been presented above.

IV. SUPPOSITORIES

The filler constituents of suppositories may contain glycerides, vegetable oils, mineral oil, polyethylene glycol, cocoa butter, lanolin, petrolatum, beeswax, and glycerin. Topical and systemic reactions to these substances have been discussed above.

V. MISCELLANEOUS PRODUCTS

A. Topical Ophthalmic Preparations

Topical ophthalmic preparations contain a variety of excipients including glycerin, EDTA, polyvinyl alcohol, hydroxymethylcellulose, polyethylene glycol, polysorbate 80, phenylethyl alcohol, glyceryl monostearate, cetyl alcohol, mannitol, white petrolatum, lanolin, various surfactants, ascorbic acid, boric acid, and dextran.

B. Topical Otic Preparations

A variety of filler components are also found in otic preparations. These include glycerin, propylene glycol, cetyl alcohol, and polysorbate.

C. Mouth and Throat Preparations

Mouth and throat preparations (troches, saliva substitutes, lozenges) contain a variety of filler substances, the most important of which are glycerol, sorbitol, sodium carboxymethylcellulose, benzyl alcohol, ethanol, propylene glycol, gelatin, and beeswax.

D. Vaginal Products

Vaginal tablets, suppositories, jellies, creams, and douching materials generally contain the same categories of excipients discussed above. In addition, they may contain wetting agents such as alkyl arylsufonate, sodium lauryl sulfate, and docusate sodium.

REFERENCES

1. Randolph, T.G. Allergy to so-called "inert" ingredients (excipients) of pharmaceutical preparations. Ann. Allergy 8:519–529 (1950).
2. Yudkin, J. Sugar and disease. Nature 239:197–199 (1972).
3. Lieb, J. and Kazienko, D.J. Lactose filler as a cause of "drug-induced" diarrhea. (Letter to the Editor) N. Engl. J. Med. 299:314, (1978).
4. Dees, S.C. An experimental study of the effect of alcohol and alcoholic beverages on allergic reactions. Ann. Allergy 7:185–300 (1949).
5. Drevets, C.C. and Seebohm, P.M. Dermatitis from alcohol. J. Allergy 32(4): 277–282 (1961).
6. Karvonen, J. and Hannuksela, M. Urticaria from alcoholic beverages. Acta Allergol. 31:167–170 (1976).
7. Oermerod, A.D. and Holt, P.J.A. Acute urticaria due to alcohol. Br. J. Dermatol. 108:723–274 (1983).
8. Elphinstone, P.E., Black, A.K. and Greaves, M.W. Alcohol-induced urticaria. J. R. Soc. Med. 78:340–341 (1985).

9. Przybilla, B. and Ring, J. Anaphylaxis to ethanol and sensitisation to acetic acid (Letter to the Editor). Lancet: 1:483 (1983).

10. Magnasco, A.J. and Magnasco, L.D. Interaction of ketoconazole and ethanol. Clin. Pharm. 5:522–523 (1986).

11. Seta, A., Tricomi, S., Goodwin, D.W. et al. Biochemical correlates of ethanol-induced flushing in orientals. J. Stud. Alcohol 39(1):1–11 (1978).

12. Gong, H., Jr., Tashkin, D.P. and Calvarese, B.M. Alcohol-induced bronchospasm in an asthmatic patient. Chest 80(2):167–173 (1981).

13. MacGregor, R.R. Alcohol and immune defense. J.A.M.A. 256(11):1474–1479 (1986).

14. Fisher, A.A. Contact dermatitis. The noneczmatous variety. Cutis 19:409–412 (1977).

15. Rilliet, A., Hunziker, N. and Brun, R. Alcohol contact urticaria syndrome (immediate-type hypersensitivity). Case report. Dermatologica 161:361–364 (1980).

16. Huriez, C., Agache, P. and Martin, P. Allergy to propylene glycol. Rev. Franc. Allerg. 6:200 (1966).

17. Hannuksela, M. and Forstrom, L. Reactions to peroral propylene glycol. Contact Derm. 4:41–45 (1978).

18. Ludwig, B., Schindler, E., Bohl, J., et al. Reno-cerebral oxalosis induced by xylitol. Neuroradiology 26:517–521 (1984).

19. Outbreak of diarrhea linked to dietetic candies—New Hampshire news. N.C. Med. J. 46(2):114 (1985).

20. Jain, N.K., Rosenberg, D.B., Ulahannan, M.J. et al. Sorbitol intolerance in adults. Am. J. Gastroenterol. 80(9):678–681 (1985).

21. Tattrie, N.H. and Yaguchi, M. Protein content of various processed edible oils. J. Inst. Can. Sci. Technol. Aliment. 6:289 (1973).

22. Bush, R.K., Taylor, S.L., Norlee, J.A. et al. Soybean oil is not allergenic to soybean-sensitive individuals. J. Allergy Clin. Immunol. 68(5):372–375 (1981).

23. Taylor, S.L., Busse, W.W., Sachs, M.I. et al. Peanut oil is not allergenic to peanut-sensitive individuals. J. Allergy Clin. Immunol. 68(5):372–375 (1981).

24. Parker, N.E. Pruritis after administration of hetastarch. Br. Med. J. 284:385–386 (1982).

25. Dooms-Goossens, A. and Degreef, H. Contact allergy to petrolatums (II). Attempts to identify the nature of the allergens. Contact Derm. 9:247–256 (1983).

26. Dooms-Goossens, A. and Dooms, M. Contact allergy to petrolatums (III). Allergenicity prediction and pharmacopoeial requirements. Contact Derm. 9:352–359 (1983).

27. Lawrence, C.M. and Smith A.G. Ampliative mediament allergy: Concomitant sensitivity to multiple medicaments including yellow soft paraffin, white soft paraffin, gentian violet and Span 20. Contact Derm. 8:240–245 (1982).

28. Ayadi, M. and Martin P. Contact allergy to petrolatum. Short communications. Contact Derm. 4:62 (1978).
29. Maibach, H. Chronic dermatitis and hyperpigmentation from petrolatum. Contact Derm. 4:62 (1978).
30. Fisher, A.A. Immediate and delayed allergic contact reactions to polyethylene glycol. Contact Derm. 4:135–138 (1978).
31. Hannuksela, M. Allergic and toxic reactions caused by cream bases in dermatological patients. Int. J. Cosmet. Sci. 1:257–263 (1979).
32. Fisher, A.A. Propylene glycol dermatitis. Cutis 21:166–178 (1978).
33. Angelini, G. and Meneghini, C.L. Contact allergy from propylene glycol. Contact Derm. 7:197–198 (1981).
34. Trancik, R.J. and Maibach, H.I. Propylene glycol: Irritation or sensitization? Contact Derm. 8:185–189 (1982).
35. Hannuksela, M., Pirila, V. and Salo, O.P. Skin reactions to propylene glycol. Contact Derm. 1:112–116 (1975).
36. Giorgini, S., Melli, M.C. and Sertoli, A. Comments on the allergenic activity of lanolin. Contact Derm. 9(5):425–426 (1983).
37. Kligman, A.M. Lanolin allergy: Crisis or comedy. Contact Derm. 9:99–107 (1983).
38. Sugai, T. and Higashi, J. Hypersensitivity to hydrogenated lanolin. Contact Derm. 1:146–157 (1975).
39. Calnan, C.D. Isopropyl myristate sensitivity. Contact Derm. Newsletter 2: 38 (1968).
40. Tanaka, T., Miyachi, Y. and Horio, T. Ulcerative contact dermatitis caused by sodium silicate. Arch. Dermatol. 118:518–520 (1982).
41. Schwartz, L. and Peck, S.M. The irritants in adhesive plaster. Public Health Rep. 50:811–819 (1935).
42. Hjorth, N. and Trol'e-Lassen, C. Skin reactions to ointment bases. Trans. St. Johns Hosp. Dermatol. Soc. 49:127–140 (1963).
43. Trevisan, G. and Kokeli, F. Contact dermatitis from propolis: Role of Gastrointestinal absorption. Contact Derm. 16:48 (1987).
44. Young, E. Sensitivity to propolis. Contact Derm. 16:49–50 (1987).
45. Rothenborg, H.W. Occupational dermatitis in beekeeper due to poplar resins in beeswax. Arch. Dermatol. 95:381–384 (1967).
46. Eggleston, P.A. Kagey-Sobotka, A., Schleimer, R.P. et al. Interaction between hyperosmolar and IgE-mediated histamine release from basophils and mast cells. Am. Rev. Respir. Dis. 130:86–91 (1983).
47. Anderson, S.D. Schoeffel, R.E., Follet, R. et al. Sensitivity to heat and water loss at rest and during exercise in asthmatic patients. Eur. J. Respir. Dis. 63:459–471 (1982).
48. Melli, M.C., Giorgini, S. and Sertoli, A. Sensitization from contact with ethyl alcohol. Short communications. Contact Derm. 14(5):315 (1986).
49. Jensen, O. Contact allergy to propylene oxide and isopropyl alcohol in a skin disinfectant swab. Contact Derm. 7:148–150 (1981).

50. Fisher, A.A. Allergic paraben and benzyl alcohol hypersensitivity relationship of the "delayed" and "immediate" varieties. Contact Derm. 1:281–284 (1975).

51. Edwards, E.K., Jr. and Edwards, E.K. Allergic reaction to tertiary butyl alcohol in a sunscreen. Cutis 29(5) 476–478 (1982).

52. Bruze, M. Simultaneous reactions to phenol-formaldehyde resins colophony/hydroabietyl alcohol and balsam of Peru/perfume mixture. Short communications. Contact. Derm. 14(2):119–120 (1986).

53. Shore, R.N. and Shelley, W.B. Contact dermatitis from stearyl alcohol and propylene glycol in fluocinonine cream. Arch. Dermatol. 109:397–399 (1974).

54. Rilliet, A., Hunziker, N. and Brun, R. Alcohol contact urticaria syndrome (immediate-type hypersensitivity). Dermatologica 161:361–364 (1980).

55. Stotts, J. and Ely, W.J. Induction of human skin sensitization to ethanol. Ann. Invest. Dermatol. 69(2):219–222 (1977).

56. Van Joost, T., Sillevis Smitt, J.H. and van Ketel, W.G. Sensitization to olive oil (olea europeae). Contact Derm. 7:309–310 (1981).

57. van Dijk, E., Neering, H. and Vitanyi, B.E.J. Contact hypersensitivity to sesame oil in patients with leg ulcers and eczema. Acta Dermatovener. (Stock.) 53:133–135 (1973).

58. Neering, H., Vitanyi, B.E.J., Malten, K.E. et al. Allergens in sesame oil contact dermatitis. Acta Dermatovener. (Stock.) 53:31–34 (1975).

59. Leake, C.D., Rosenbaum, E.E. and Jacob, S.W. Summary of the New York Academy of Sciences Symposium on the "Biological Actions of Dimethyl Sulfoxide." Ann. N.Y. Acad. Sci. 141:670 (1966).

60. Sulzberger, M.B., Cortese, T.A., Jr., Fishman, L. et al. Some effects of DMSO on human skin *in vivo*. Ann. N.Y. Acad. Sci 141-142:437-450(1967).

61. Kligman, A.M. Topical pharmacology and toxicology of dimethyl sulfoxide. Part I. J.A.M.A. 193:796–804 (1965).

62. Hannuksela, M. Allergic and toxic reactions caused by cream bases in dermatological patients. Int. J. Cosmet. Sci. 1:257 (1979).

63. Haahtela, T. and Lahdensuo, A. Non-specific reactions caused by diluents containing glycerol in nasal and bronchial challenge tests. Clin. Allergy 9:225–227 (1979).

64. Thormann, J. and Wildenhoff, K.E. Contact allergy to idoxuridine. Contact Derm. 6:170 (1980).

65. Voorhorst, R. The human dander atopy. I. The prototype of auto-atopy. Ann. Allergy 39:205–212 (1977).

66. Dandeau, J.P., Fabillon, J. and David, B. Specific house dust allergens are not mythic ones (abstract). J. Allergy Clin. Immunol. 79:132 (1987).

67. Paul, K., Schlesinger, R.G. and Schanfield, M.S. Reaction to albumin (Letter to the Editor) J.A.M.A. 245(3):234 (1981).

68. Ring, J. and Messmer, K. Incidence and severity of anaphylactoid reactions to colloid volume substitutes. Lancet 1:466–469 (1977).

69. Inman, J.K. Pruritis after administration of hetastarch. Br. Med. J. 284:358 (1982).
70. Spaeth, G.L., Spaeth, E.B. and Spaeth, P.G. et al. Anaphylactic reaction to mannitol. Arch. Ophthalmol. 78:583–584 (1967).
71. Findlay, S.R., Kagey-Sobotka, A. and Lichtenstein, L.M. *In vitro* basophil histamine release induced by mannitol in a patient with a mannitol-induced anaphylactoid reaction. J. Allergy Clin. Immunol. 73(5):578–583 (1984).

12

Allergic Reactions: Coloring Agents

I. Capsules   223
II. Tablet coatings   223
   A. Silicone   223
   B. Gluten   225
   C. Shellac   226
   D. Polymers   227
   E. Enteric film formers   227
III. Other substances used for microencapsulation   227
   A. Nonhuman albumin   227
   B. Nonbiodegradable materials   228
   C. Alginates   229
   D. Polyvinylpyrrolidone   229
   References   229

I. CAPSULES

Gelatin is the chief ingredient of capsules. Although gelatin is manufactured from hides, horns, connective tissue, cartilage, and bones of cattle, sheep, goats, and pigs, specific references of allergic responses to this substance in capsules have not been objectively documented even in patients known to be allergic to one of these animals (1). This is in contrast to parenterally administered gelatin, which has a moderately high incidence of anaphylactoid reactions (see Chapter 11). (See note at end of chapter, p. 229).

II. TABLET COATINGS

Some of the typical polymeric coating materials such as cellulose derivatives, gelatin, polyvinyl alcohol, beeswax and waxes have been discussed in the previous chapter.

A. Silicone

As an extensively applied biomaterial in modern medicine, silicone is no longer considered to be inert. Of the millions of artificial implants and prosthetic devices used every year in the United States, a high percentage contain silicone. As a result, silicone-related disease is being observed with increasing frequency. For the most part, adverse reactions are nonimmunologic but scattered case reports suggest that allergic mechanisms may play a minor role. Silicone-induced synovitis and lymphadenopathy occur in about 10% of patients receiving silicone elastomer implants for correction of toe and finger joint abnormalities. Complications of bag-gel implants for mammary augmentation include implant rupture and capsular contractures. "Bleeding" silicone from ruptured bag-gel breast implants may have serious consequences, as evidenced by the fact that acute and chronic pneumonitis may occur (2). Similar pulmonary lesions have been reported in transsexual men after subcutaneous injections of silicone (3). Spallation and migration of silicone from blood pump tubing in patients on hemodialysis have also been reported (4). Granulomatous reactions have been described in soft tissues of the breast and face in patients who received liquid silicone injections. These lesions may be localized near the site of the original injection or as far away as the groin, because silicone gel can migrate through soft tissues. Hematogenous migration is also possible and has been described in patients undergoing cardiopulmonary bypass operations. Silicone microemboli seen in patients after cardiopulmonary bypass surgery are thought to originate from the bubble oxygenators containing silicone as an antifoaming agent.

a. Type I–IV immunologic reactivity

There is one case report of a woman who developed severe erythematous swelling of the mouth, nasolabial folds, and severe periorbital edema 6 weeks after receiving liquid silicone injections for treatment of facial wrinkles (5). A local scratch test with the silicone preparation was negative but all the patient's symptoms worsened within 24 hr. This late response was interpreted as a possible manifestation of Type I allergy. After the wrinkle treatment regime was discontinued, the swollen areas gradually resolved.

No type II or III reactions have been reported.

There is a single case report of a type IV reaction in a woman who developed contact dermatitis 4 weeks after using a sunscreen containing phenyl dimethicone, a mixture of linear siloxane polymers (6). Contact sensitivity was verified by a 2+ positive patch test result.

b. Anatomical sites of hypersensitivity reactions: Cutaneous: The single patient in whom type I mechanisms might be implicated presented with severe periorbital erythematous edema in the various sites of silicone injections on the face. After this acute lesion subsided, the patient did well for the next 6 months but then had a recurrence of symptoms. It is possible that she had used cosmetics containing silicates but not silicone. A skin biopsy taken at the time of recurrence showed fibrosis, sclerosis, and edema. The patient with contact dermatitis presented with a red, vesicular eruption of the face, neck, and arms, where the

sunscreen lotion had been applied. A similar dermatologic response was obtained after direct patch test with the sunscreen lotion itself and a coded patch test containing 2% phenyl dimethicone in petrolatum.

c. Pseudoallergic responses

Bronchoalveolar lavage specimens from patients with either acute pneumonitis (including the adult respiratory distress syndrome) or chronic pneumonitis induced by silicone demonstrate increased numbers of total cells and eosinophils per milliliter of lavage fluid. Levels of neutrophils and alveolar macrophages were also increased. The presence of eosinophils in these bronchial lavage fluids did not appear to be associated with specific immunologic reactivity but with a nonspecific inflammatory response.

It has been suggested that an unusual type of human adjuvant disease may develop in patients receiving silicone implants (7). Four cases of scleroderma have been described after silicone implants (8). Arthritis has also been reported in patients after cosmetic surgery involving silicone.

It is highly unlikely that oral ingestion of trace amounts of silicone used in tablet coatings could ever cause some of the serious allergic and nonallergic tissue reactions described above.

B. Gluten

The presence of gluten in various microencapsulated preparations could exacerbate gluten intolerance under clinical conditions where administration of a substantial number of gluten containing tablets was necessary. There are three types of gluten intolerance: gluten allergy, gluten intolerance associated with celiac disease, and transient gluten intolerance. It should be emphasized that there are no known clinical reports of any of these conditions occurring exclusively after ingestion of tablet formulations containing gluten.

a. Type I immunologic reactivity

IgE-mediated reactions may occur after ingestion of gluten in wheat products or inhalation of gluten contained in various flour dusts by bakery workers (9). Once IgE-dependent sensitization has occurred, exposure to only trace amounts either by ingestion or inhalation may precipitate symptoms. Allergic intolerance to oral gluten may simulate celiac disease in young infants (10). Immunologic studies in bakers and celiac patients have demonstrated gluten-specific IgE antibodies (9). However, the gluten component of wheat was much less likely to induce the formation of specific IgE responses compared to other allergens in wheat.

b. Types II and III immunologic reactivity

There are no reactions reported.

c. Type IV immunologic reactivity

Cell-mediated responses to gluten-derived peptides have been described by several investigators (11,12). These cell-mediated responses occurred only in treated celiac patients (patients on a gluten-free diet) and were not observed in untreated patients.

d. Anatomical sites of hypersensitivity reactions:

Cutaneous: Urticaria and angioedema may occur after ingestion of gluten in various products. Infantile eczema and atopic dermatitis in children and young adults may be exacerbated by various components of wheat. Diagnosis is confirmed by double-blind, controlled, oral challenge with gluten and a corresponding placebo preparation in opaque capsules. Skin testing is sometimes a helpful diagnostic adjunct and a positive radioallergosorbent test to gluten also tends to corroborate the clinical diagnosis.

Respiratory: Inhalation of flour or wheat components under controlled conditions in the laboratory may cause immediate-onset bronchospasm within 10 min of the inhalation challenge. In some cases, a dual response or an isolated late phase asthmatic reaction may occur. This mode of exposure or symptomatic response would not be expected to occur in patients who ingest gluten excipients in pharmaceutical preparations. It is possible that pharmaceutical manufacturing workers exposed to gluten dust could develop this form of occupational asthma.

Gastrointestinal: Infants below the age of 2 are particularly prone to develop diarrhea and loss of appetite as a result of gastrointestinal sensitization to gluten. Inasmuch as these symptoms are nonspecific, it is essential that this type of reaction be differentiated from patients with true celiac disease (10).

e. Pseudoallergic responses

Gluten intolerance frequently occurs in association with celiac disease. Children with this syndrome manifest symptoms of nausea, vomiting, diarrhea, bulky stools, and failure to thrive. The diagnosis can only be confirmed by small intestinal mucosa biopsy, which reveals villous atrophy and a flat mucosa. Avoidance of gluten usually causes dramatic remission of symptoms but anatomical abnormalities of small intestine persist for many years in spite of continued avoidance of gluten.

Transient gluten intolerance is a variant of gluten intolerance associated with celiac disease. This syndrome may occur when a child with gastrointestinal symptoms and an abnormal small intestinal mucosa responds to a gluten-free diet, but subsequently thrives on a normal gluten-containing diet, and after 2 years on such a diet is found to have a normal mucosa (11).

C. Shellac

Shellac is a resinous, waxy protein amorphous substance secreted by an insect (*Laccifer lacca*). It is used as a coating in slow-release tablets. No adverse reactions have been reported after ingestion of such tablets. There is one documented case of contact cheilitis in a woman who used lipstick containing this substance (13).

D. Polymers

Both acidic and basic polymers are used as coating materials. Neither allergic nor pseudoallergic reactions have been reported after ingestion of these compounds. One of the common basic polymers, polylysine, may have histamine-releasing properties under special conditions. This polymer is available in several molecular weight configurations. Only the high-molecular-weight (80,000 daltons or greater) form has histamine-releasing properties in humans, as indexed by positive intracutaneous wheal and flare responses or histamine release from human basophils. Excipient formulations have not been demonstrated to have these properties.

E. Enteric Film Formers

Enteric film formers such as cellulose acetate phthalate (CAP), polyvinyl acetate phthalate (PVAP), hydroxypropylmethyl-cellulose phthalate (HPMCP), and carboxyvinyl polymers (carbomer) are polyelectrolytes containing ionizable carboxyl groups. In the low pH of the stomach, these weak acids are practically nonionized. Allergic reactions to these substances as excipients have not been documented. However, adverse reactions to phthalates have been suspected in other clinical situations. Since dihexylethylphthalate can be readily leached into human blood from soft plastic transfusion containers, it was proposed that freely circulating phthalate could be toxic to various vital organs in humans (14). This hypothesis has never been substantiated or proved, although toxicity to large doses has been demonstrated in rats. In workers who develop asthma after exposure to plastic wrappings containing polyvinyl chloride and adhesive labels containing phthlates, it was postulated that phthalates released during the hot wire fuming process might serve as a chemical cause of asthma (15). However, no evidence of antiphthalate IgE or IgG antibodies was ever found in these workers. Thus, under the most optimal sensitization conditions, allergenicity to phthalates has not been demonstrated.

III. OTHER SUBSTANCES USED FOR MICROENCAPSULATION

A. Nonhuman Albumin

Pharmaceutical grades of albumin contained in oral formulations consist of bovine and egg albumins (16). Egg albumin is used as a coating medium for masking the taste of erythromycin derivatives. The process involves suspending the drug particles in an aqueous solution of egg albumin and then stirring the suspension with a liquid surfactant to form an emulsion. The emulsion is then heated to 50–80°C to coagulate the albumin in the form of microcapsules around the drug. Solid capsules are separated from the suspension and dried. This process denatures the protein and could decrease the likelihood of allergic reactions in patients with prior egg white sensitivity. In any case, there have been no documented cases of allergic reactions to either bovine albumin or egg albumin contained in tablet coatings.

B. Nonbiodegradable Materials

Acrylic polymers such as methylmethacrylate and polymethlymethacrylate are used widely as film formers for microencapsulation. These materials are also used extensively as bone cement for major joint replacement operations (see Chapter 16). The methylmethacrylate monomer is known to be a potent sensitizer in operating room personnel. Contact dermatitis among people who handle this material is not unusual and is thought to be due to the fact that methylmethacrylate is a strong lipid solvent and is able to penetrate rubber gloves (17). Occupational asthma has also been described in operating room personnel. Neither allergic nor toxic symptoms have been reported after oral ingestion of tablets containing acrylic polymers as components of the tablet.

a. Type I immunologic reactivity

IgE-dependent mechanisms have not been demonstrated.

b. Types II and III immunologic reactivity

No reactions have been reported.

c. Type IV immunologic reactivity

Contact dermatitis confirmed by patch tests has been confirmed in workers handling this material. Patch tests are best demonstrated by using monomer methylmethacrylate as the test reagent.

d. Anatomical sites of hypersensitivity reactions: Cutaneous: Classic contact dermatitis has been observed. The lesions occur on the fingers and are typically vesicular at first. Later, as the exposure continues, the dermatitis becomes chronic, fissures appear, and exfoliation develops. In advanced cases, onycholysis may occur.

e. Anatomical sites of hypersensitivity reactions: Respiratory: Occupational asthma has been reported after exposure to methylmethacrylate. It is assumed that the monomer of methylmethacrylate may cause direct irritation to the bronchial mucosa and/or mast cells within the bronchial lumina.

f. Pseudoallergic responses

As discussed above, the asthmatic responses are presently classified as nonimmunologic because antigen-specific mechanisms have not yet been demonstrated.

C. Alginates

Calcium and sodium alginates are complex polymerized polysacchardies that are derived from kelp and are frequently used as film formers for microencapsulation. Adverse reactions to these agents have not been reported. However, it should be noted that immediate-type allergic reactions, including hives, rhinitis, and asthma, have been documented after exposure to natural sources of both green and blue–green algae (18). In addition, contact dermatitis to blue–green algae has been reported in swimmers exposed to fresh water algal blooms (19). Calcium alginate was formerly used as an adjuvant in conjunction with allergy extract immunotherapy (20). Industrially related asthma has occurred in workers involved in the manufacture of alginates from seaweed (21). However, only those employees exposed to raw seaweed dust developed symptoms in contrast to workers exposed exclusively to pure alginate dust, who are asymptomatic.

D. Polyvinylpyrrolidone

Polyvinylpyrrolidone (PVP) is an alcohol-soluble material used in concentrations between 3 and 5%. It is a polymer synthesized by condensation of acetylene with N-vinylpyrrolidone. It is used particularly in multivitamin, chewable formulations. In animals, this compound is a potent histamine-releasing agent. The response is completely inhibited by prior injection of an antihistamine. It should be emphasized that a parenteral dose of 25% PVP solution is required to obtain these reactions in dogs. No clinical side effects have been reported in humans receiving small amounts of PVP in tablets.

NOTE ADDED IN PROOF

Specific IgE antibodies to gelatin proteins with molecular weights in the range of 40-120 kD were recently demonstrated in the serum of a patient who developed contact urtiearia after ingestion of a gelatin-containing candy. These antibodies also exhibited cross-reactivity between colloidal gelatin plasma substitutes, thereby reviving the controversy about the immunologic basis of systemic reactions to intravenous gelatin blood volume expanders (22).

REFERENCES

1. Randolph, T.G. Gelatin as an allergen. J. Lab Clin. Med. 32:1548–1549 (1947).
2. Travis, W.D., Balogh, K. and Abraham, J.L. Silicone granulomas: Report of three cases and review of the literature. Hum. Pathol. 16(1):19–27 (1985).
3. Chastre, J., Brun, P., Soler, P. et al. Acute and latent pneumonitis and subcutaneous injections of silicone in transsexual men. Am. Rev. Respir. Dis. 135:236–240 (1987).

4. Leong, A.S.Y., Disney, A.P.S. and Gove, D.W. Spallation and migration of silicone from blood-pump tubing in patients on hemodialysis. N. Engl. J. Med. 306:135 (1982).

5. Fellner, M.J. and Rukikoff, D. Adverse reaction following silicone injections. Int. J. Dermatol. 18:375–376 (1979).

6. Edwards, E.K. Jr. and Edwards, E.K. Allergic reaction to phenyl dimethicone in a sunscreen (Letter to the Editor). Arch. Dermatol. 120:575–576 (1984).

7. Baldwin, C.M. and Kaplan, E.N. Silicone-induced human adjuvant disease? Ann. Plast. Surg. 10:270 (1983).

8. Kumagai, Y., Abe, C. and Shiokawa, Y. Scleroderma after cosmetic surgery, four cases of human adjuvant disease. Arthritis Rheum. 22:532 (1979).

9. Baldo, B.A. and Wrigley, C.W. IgE antibodies to wheat flour components. Studies with sera from subjects with baker's asthma and coeliac condition. Clin. Allergy 8:109–124 (1978).

10. Jonas, A. Wheat sensitive—but not coeliac. Lancet 2:1047, 1978.

11. Bullen, A.W. and Losowsky, M.S. Cell-mediated immunity to gluten fraction III in adult coeliac disease. Gut 19:126–131 (1978).

12. Holmes, G.K.T., Asquith, P. and Cook, W.T. Cell-mediated immunity to gluten fraction III in adult coeliac disease. Clin. Exp. Immunol. 24:259–265 (1976).

13. Rademaker, M., Kirby, J.D. and White, I.R. Contact cheilitis to shellac, Lanpol 5 and colophony. Contact Derm. 15:307–308 (1986).

14. Jaeger, R.J. and Rubin, R.J. Migration of a phthalate ester plasticizer from polyvinyl chloride blood bags into stored human blood and its localization in human tissues. N. Engl. J. Med. 287:1114–1118 (1972).

15. Brooks, S.M. and Vandervort, R. Polyvinyl chloride film thermal decomposition products as an occupational illness. J. Occup. Med. 19:192–196 (1977).

16. Deasy, P.B. Microencapsulation and related drug process. Core Coating Properties 20:24–25 (1984).

17. Fisher, A.A. Acrylic bone cement sensitization and dermatitis. Cutis 12:333–337 (1973).

18. Bernstein, I.L. and Safferman, R.S. Sensitivity of skin and bronchial mucosa to green algae. J. Allergy 38:166–173 (1966).

19. Cohen, S.G. and Reif, C.B. Cutaneous sensitization to blue-green algae. J. Allergy 24:452 (1953).

20. Georgakis, N.G., Gerardi, A., Popovits, C. et al. The use of alginate adjuvant as a vehicle in the treatment of ragweed pollinosis. Ann. Allergy 25:439–444 (1967).

21. Henderson, A.K., Ranger, A.F., Lloyd, J. et al. Pulmonary hypersensitivity in the alginate industry. Scot. Med. J. 29:90–95 (1984).

22. Wahl, R. and Kleinhaus, D. IgE-mediated allergic reactions to fruit gums and investigation of cross reactivity between gelatine and modified gelatine-containing products. Clin. and Exp. Allergy 19:77-80 (1989).

13

Allergic Reactions: Flavoring Agents

I. Sweetening agents   231
   A. Sugars and other polyalcohols   231
   B. Synthetic sweeteners   231
II. Salts   234
III. Natural flavors from fruits and other botanical sources   234
IV. Essential oils and synthetic derivatives   237
  V. Monosodium glutamate   248
   References   250

I. SWEETENING AGENTS

A. Sugars and Other Polyalcohols

Mono- and disaccharide sugars are nonallergenic. Hyperactive behavioral symptoms have been attributed to glucose but double-blind controlled studies have failed to substantiate a causal effect (1). Malabsorption of sucrose may cause diarrhea, abdominal cramps, and bloating, resulting from the accumulation of hydrogen in the colon. This is due to sucrase/isomaltase deficiency, which is the most frequent primary disacchardiase deficiency of childhood with an autosomal recessive type of inheritance (2). The frequency of this deficiency is 0.2% in the population of North America and 10% among Greenland Eskimos. It is correctable by avoidance of sucrose or addition of fresh baker's yeast as a source of sucrase. Adverse reactions to the polyalcohols, glycerol, sorbitol, and xylitol have been discussed in Part I, Chapter 1.

B. Synthetic Sweeteners

1. Saccharin

Saccharin is the sodium salt of orthosulfobenzimide and can also be classified as an "o-toluene sulfonamide." Although the total number of adverse reactions to saccharin is limited, immunologic mechanisms appear to be involved in most of the cases.

a. Type I immunologic reactivity

Immediate cutaneous, gastrointestinal, and cardiac symptoms have been attributed to IgE-mediated mechanisms (3). In several reports the reactions were confirmed by repeat challenges but not under controlled conditions. Positive skin tests to saccharin have not been demonstrated. However, there is one anecdotal report that 14 or 15 alleged saccharin-sensitive persons exhibited 3+ and 4+ radioallergosorbent reactions to saccharin (4). These results have not been verified or confirmed by other investigators.

b. Type II and III immunologic reactivity

No clinical evidence of these mechanisms exists.

c. Type IV immunologic reactivity

There are anecdotal reports of photosensitization after ingestion of saccharin but these instances have not been documented by objective in vivo or in vitro type IV tests. In addition, none of the cases has been confirmed by controlled photopatch testing so it cannot be assumed that such reactions are based either on phototoxicity or photosensitivity (3).

d. Anatomical sites of hypersensitivity reactions: *Cutaneous*: Urticaria is the major type of cutaneous manifestation. A fine maculopapular rash has been described in several cases. Both urticaria and rash are accompanied by pruritis. In other cases, pityriasislike eczema and edematous prurigolike papules were described. The presumed photoreactive cases exhibited a pruritic, eczematous dermatitis primarily limited to sun-exposed areas of the skin. A number of the cutaneous reactions have occurred in patients with previous history of allergic reactions to sulfonamides, chlorpropamides, and thiazide diuretics.

Photoallergy was suspected as a possible mechanism in these cases based on an incubation period, prior history of sulfonamide ingestion, and the small number of affected patients. Thus the possibility that oral ingestion of sulfonamide or sulfonamidelike agents could exacerbate contact-type eruptions and photosensitivity reactions in saccharin-sensitive individuals must be kept in mind.

e. Anatomical sites of hypersensitivity reactions: *Gastrointestinal*: Nausea and vomiting may occur in saccharin-sensitive patients. Diarrhea has also been observed in several cases of saccharin sensitivity.

f. Anatomical sites of hypersensitivity reactions: *Cardiac*: Tachycardia and premature ventricular systoles have been reported after diagnostic oral challenges in suspected saccharin-sensitive individuals. In several instances, these symptoms were accompanied by a cold sweat.

g. Pseudoallergic responses

Toxic manifestations of saccharin overdose could be mistaken for pseudoallergic reactions. Several cases of generalized edema and nephritic symptoms have occurred in patients ingesting 50 or more tablets of saccharin. In these cases, albuminuria persisted for many years.

2. Aspartame

Aspartame, a dipeptide consisting of L-aspartic acid and the methylester of L-phenylalanine has replaced saccharin as the most extensively used artificial sweetener in both drugs and food. Although it has been approved for use only since 1983, the prevalence of adverse responses appears to be greater than saccharin, as indexed by adverse reports received by the Food and Drug Administration (FDA) and several independent clinical reports (5).

a. Type I–IV immunologic reactivity

Although acute urticarial and angioedema reactions have been documented in several cases after double-blind controlled laboratory challenges to aspartame, no information is currently available about proven immunogenicity or allergenicity of this agent. It has been postulated that amide bonds between aspartame and endogenous body proteins could account for antigenicity but this remains to be demonstrated (5).

b. Anatomical sites of hypersensitivity reactions

Cutaneous urticarial lesions, both acute and chronic, are the chief manifestations of aspartame reactions. In one case, the chronic nature of these reactions was fully established and multiple episodes in this patient were at times accompanied by dyspnea, dysphagia, and, on one occasion, a sensation of a lump in the throat. After double-blind controlled challenges in volunteers, urticarial lesions may occur as early as 90 min and as late as 12 hr after ingestion of aspartame.

c. Pseudoallergic responses

There is one documented case report of granulomatous panniculitis induced by aspartame (6). Although a possible association between migraine headaches and aspartame had been suggested by several anecdotal reports and one unblinded challenge experiment, a subsequent double-blind crossover trial failed to establish this association (7).

3. Cyclamates

The use of cyclamates in all drug products has been banned by the FDA since July, 1970. Prior to that time, there were sporadic reports of photoallergic dermatitis, severe eczema, and pruritis in patients ingesting cyclamate products

(8). The skin lesions were described as erythematous with fine scaling in light-exposed areas of the body and occasionally small edematous papules with lichenification were also observed. Many of these patients showed cross-reactivity to sulfonamides. In all cases, the dermatitis cleared when cyclamates were excluded from the diet. Severe renal tubular acidosis associated with hypophosphatemia occurred in one patient who ingested cyclamate sweetener in unusually large amounts (20 packets, or 4 g) per day (8).

II. SALTS

Neither allergic nor pseudoallergic responses have been reported in association with sodium chloride or potassium chloride used as flavoring agents in drug products. Both sodium chloride and potassium chloride are considered as drugs in their own right and, of course, could cause serious toxic effects if administered improperly by the parenteral route or if ingested in large amounts by the oral route. In addition, oral preparations of these salts contain a variety of excipients that could cause adverse reactions unrelated to the salts themselves.

III. NATURAL FLAVORS FROM FRUITS AND OTHER BOTANICAL SOURCES

Natural flavors are available from a variety of fruit and vegetable sources. Since these are prepared as syrups, they contain both polysaccharides and possible traces of protein constituents that could cause allergic symptoms in subjects with preexisting allergic susceptibility to these ingredients. However, it is essential that adverse reactions to these food derivatives be clearly defined because both immunologic and nonimmunologic factors are often grouped together under the general term of "allergy."

Food hypersensitivity or allergy refers to an immunologic reaction occurring after ingestion of a food or food additive. Such a reaction occurs only in susceptible (atopic) individuals. A small amount of the food elicits the reaction, which can be clearly distinguished from the physiological effects of the food or food additives. An easily recognizable IgE-dependent form of food hypersensitivity is food anaphylaxis which may cause systemic symptoms of varying sensitivity. In contrast, food intolerance is an umbrella term that refers to aberrant physiological response to a food or food additive. It is nonimmunologic and encompasses idiosyncratic, metabolic, pharmacologic, or toxic reactions to food or food additives. Food toxicity is rarely a concern with regard to flavor excipients because such small amounts of the materials are used. Food idiosyncracies are quantitatively abnormal food responses that resemble symptoms of hypersensitivity but do not involve immune mechanisms. For example, an anaphylactic reaction to a food component, metabolite, or additive may occur as a result of nonimmune release of chemical mediators and may mimic the symptoms of IgE-dependent food anaphylaxis. Metabolic reactions occur because of inborn metabolic errors such as lactase or sucrase deficiencies. Finally, an adverse reaction to one of the food-derived flavors could result from a naturally derived or added chemical that produces a druglike or pharmacologic effect in the host. Individual susceptibility to the food flavor sources shown in Table 1 of Chapter 8 (p. 142) is impossible to predict because of the wide range of individual reactivity. However, in general, the prevalence of reactions to legumes, citrus, true nuts, and several of the spice families is significant. Surprisingly, and contrary to popular opinion, immunologic food hypersensitivity to chocolate or cola does not rank high on the list of food reactions.

a. Type I immunologic reactivity

Anaphylactic reactions mediated by IgE-dependent mechanisms may occur after ingestion of any of the food sources listed in Table 1 of Chapter 8 (p. 142). The most frequently implicated foods in this group are peanuts, nuts, seeds, citrus and fruits. Prior ingestion of food may also be implicated in the triggering of exercise-induced anaphylaxis. For unexplained reasons, this reaction is more likely to occur when celery is ingested before exercise (9). This has not yet been reported after ingestion of natural celery flavor, but the possibility must be kept in mind. Other localized manifestations of type I hypersensitivity reactions may occur. The diagnosis of IgE-mediated reactions to foods may be corroborated by direct skin tests, radioallergosorbent tests (RAST), and leukocyte histamine release. The diagnostic reliability of direct skin tests varies widely depending on the potency of allergenic determinants within the food. This constraint also applies to the in vitro tests of RAST and leukocyte histamine release. In the event of a prior history of life-threatening reaction to a specific food, direct skin testing should be avoided.

b. Type II and III immunologic reactivity

It has been proposed that delayed-onset symptoms after food ingestion may be associated with the appearance of circulating food immune complexes. Such complexes could contain either IgE- or IgG-specific antibodies. Circulating immune complexes can be demonstrated regularly after ingestion of dietary antigens, but their clinical association with symptoms of food hypersensitivity has not yet been clearly established (10).

c. Type IV immunologic reactivity

Cell-mediated contact sensitivity may occur with handlers of any of the foods listed in Table 1 of Chapter 8 (p. 142). This has not been a source of concern for drug consumers but could occur in the drug manufacturing industry and in pharmacists preparing formulations with the naturally derived syrups.

d. Anatomical sites of hypersensitivity reactions: Systemic: Although ana-phylactic symptoms induced by food products may involve any organ system, the predemoninant organs are the skin, respiratory tract, gastrointestinal tract, and cardiovascular system. The initial symptoms of anaphylaxis often are pruritus, erythema, widespread urticaria, and angioedema. Later, upper respi-ratory symptoms may occur, there may be a feeling of anxiety, and severe abdominal cramps with vomiting and diarrhea can ensue. Respiratory distress from bronchospasm or laryngospasm may follow and in extreme cases may cause asphyxia. Cardiac arrhythmias may develop and cardiovascular collapse may ultimately lead to death if not treated promptly. Anaphylactic emergencies due to food allergies are life-threatening and should be treated vigorously with antishock measures, respiratory support, epinephrine, vasopressers, steroids, and volume replacement.

e. Anatomical sites of hypersensitivity reactions: Cutaneous: Acute urticaria is common as a result of food allergy. Where exposure to the offending food or additive is prolonged, chronic urticaria may develop. Although the role of speci-fic food allergens or additives has often been doubted in the pathogenesis of atopic dermatitis, recent double-blind crossover trials of possible food allergies in such cases indicate that there is a definite relationship between food hypersen-sitivity and exacerbation of the rash of atopic dermatitis in both children and young adolescents (11). Allergic contact dermatitis may occur in pharmacists or drug employees who handle specific food flavoring materials over prolonged periods of time.

f. Anatomical sites of hypersensitivity reactions: Respiratory: Food allergy may be manifested by acute onset of rhinitis and conjunctivitis or may present with symptoms of chronic nasal stenosis, paroxysmal sneezing, and persistent watery discharge. Wheezing may also be an acute or chronic symptom of food-induced hypersensitivity.

g. Anatomical sites of hypersensitivity reactions: Gastrointestinal: Symptoms of nausea, vomiting, and diarrhea are commonly observed after ingestion of an allergenic food. Gastrointestinal bleeding may occur in infants with proven food allergy. Localized oral and/or pharnygeal pruritus may occur after exposure to certain groups of foods. Melons, bananas, hazel nuts, parsnips, and apples are the most common causes of such reactions.

h. Anatomical sites of hypersensitivity reactions: Cardiovascular: Cardiac ar-rhythmias and sudden cardiovascular collapse are common features of systemic (anaphylactic) reactions to foods. Allergic purpura has been implicated in patients sensitive to legumes and chocolate.

i. Pseudoallergic reactions

Certain foods contain large amounts of histamine or histamine releasers, which may induce direct release of histamine without an intervening immunologic response. Of the natural flavors, strawberry is one. However, it is doubtful whether the amount of histamine carried over into strawberry syrups would be sufficient to cause this type of reaction. A variety of foods contain vasoactive amines and pharmacologically active substances that may induce gastrointestinal and central nervous system symptoms. Chocolate contains considerable amounts of phenylethylamine, a known trigger of headaches. Smaller amounts of vasoactive amines are found in plums, pineapples, avocados, and oranges. Significant amounts of methylxanthines can be found in cola and chocolate flavorings. These agents are known to induce central nervous system stimulation, headache, and abdominal pain in susceptible individuals. Licorice (glycyrrhizinic acid) contains a potent steroidal moiety (glycyrrhetinic acid) with mineralocorticoid activity. Excessive production could produce symptoms resembling hyperaldosteronism. Clinical features of this problem include edema, congestive heart failure, headache, muscular weakness, and myoglobinuria. Administration of licorice causes a significant rise in urinary free cortisol, which is thought to be caused by inhibitin of 11-beta-hydroxysteroid dehydrogenase (12).

It should be emphasized that possible adverse responses induced by either immunologic or nonimmunologic mechanisms induced by natural food flavors are entirely dose dependent. In oral tablet formulations, the proportion of flavoring agents is minor. Trace amounts of flavors contained in these preparations could only be expected to elicit allergic reactions in a very small percentage of consumers who happen to have exquisite allergic susceptibility to the respective flavor. Larger amounts of flavoring agents are used in liquid oral preparations, so that the possibility of observing reactions after ingestion of these formulas is increased. In summary, the overall prevalence of immunologic or nonimmunologic adverse reactions to natural flavors in pharmaceutical preparations is unknown because there has been no systematic survey or study of these reactions.

IV. ESSENTIAL OILS AND SYNTHETIC DERIVATIVES

Essential oils are derived from plant oleoresin fractions, which are the chief sensitizing substances of many plants. Essential oils are derived from flowers (e.g., lavender), leaves (e.g., eucalyptus), bark (e.g., cinnamon), wood (e.g., sandalwood), and peel (e.g., citrus fruits) (13). Essential oils are obtained from plants or plant constituents by distillation and used as both perfume "essences" and flavoring materials. They are volatile, nonsaponifying oils with characteristic odors. There are over 500 essential oil substances, many of which are used as flavoring materials. There are over 5,000 natural and synthetic fragrance materials in current use (14). Among this large group of substances, adverse responses have been reported after exposure to balsams, phenols, aromatic acohols, aldehydes, terpenes, and substituted catechols. Balsams are similar to resins but are secreted following injury to the plant. Balsam of Peru is a viscid fluid extracted from a tree native to El Salvador. It has an odor resembling cinnamon or vanilla and is a complex mixture of resins of unknown composition and simple chemicals including benzyl benzoate, benzyl cinnamate, cinnamic acid, benzoic acid, and vanillin. Other balsams (Tolu, Storax, benzoin, pine, and spruce) are chemically related to balsam of Peru by their content of coniferyl alcohol esters of benzoic acid or cinnamic acid (13,15). Theoretically, any of the essential oils or aromatic chemicals could act as occasional sensitizers but most of the documented adverse responses have been reported after exposure to cinnamon oil, oil of cloves, cinnamic alcohol, cinnamic aldehyde, eugenol, isoeugenol, cassia oil, peppermint oil, menthol, vanillin, Balsam of Peru, and others listed in Table 1.

Essential oils, particularly clove and cinnamon oils, are used extensively in dentistry as mild anesthetics, anodynes, and for flavoring dentrifices and mouth washes. Clove oil and cinnamon oil may cross react with balsam of Peru, which is used in dental cement liquids. Eugenol is the main ingredient in clove oil and is used extensively in periodontal dressings, zinc oxide cement, and impression pastes. Cinnamic aldehyde, one of the major chemicals in cinnamon and cassia oils, is used extensively as a flavoring agent in toothpastes, mouth wash tablets, proprietary ointments, and topical sunscreen preparations.

Several other aldehydes such as phenylacetaldehyde and citral are fragrance chemicals derived from citrus essential oils and are used as fragrances in medicinal preparations (15). Vanillin, a parahydroxybenzaldehyde, can be

Table 1   Partial List of Common Essential Oil Contactants

Jasmin oil

Cananga oil

Ylang-ylang oil

Sandalwood oil

Patchouli oil

Lavender oil

Rose oil Bulgaria

Geranium oil

---

extracted from vanilla but is usually prepared synthetically. It is a common aromatic chemical in topical medicinal preparations (16). The chemical structure of synthetic vanillin closely resembles that of benzoic acid and could account for cross-sensitivity reactions to this chemical as well as balsam of Peru, which also contains benzoic acid. Menthol, a cyclohexyl derivative of oil of peppermint, is used extensively as a flavoring agent or for its cooling effect and distinctive odor in many prescription or over-the-counter medications, toothpastes, mouth washes, nose drops and sprays, chest rubs, douches, cough drops, analgesic balms, vaporized additives, and aerosols (17). A benzyl derivative of methyl salicylate is commonly found in many over-the-counter rubbing compounds.

The widespread use of fragrance materials probably accounts for the relatively high incidence of fragrance sensitivity reactions. Increased sensitization to fragrances probably occurs because fragranced lubricants and therapeutic agents (i.e., Mycolog) are often used for the treatment of dermatitic or inflamed skin (14). The vast majority of sensitivity reactions induced by fragrance materials can be detected by using a perfume screening series (Table 2) (14).

a. Type I immunologic reactivity

There are a number of anecdotal reports of symptoms consistent with type I hypersensitivity reactions occurring after exposure and sensitization to essential oils and their derivatives. The immunologic mechanism of such reactions has not been verified by type I skin and serologic tests. This distinction is emphasized because nonimmunologic contact urticaria has been demonstrated readily after exposure to benzoic acid, sorbic acid, and cinnamic aldehyde (18). There have been several individual case reports of contact urticaria occurring after application of synthetic cassia oil, sorbic acid, balsam of Peru, and ethyl vanillin (19, 20). One of these patients also developed immediate sneezing after sniffing a bottle of synthetic cassia oil that originally had triggered her skin reaction (20). Evidence of clear IgE-mediated mechanisms was not identified in these cases. There is one case report of anaphylactic shock occurring presumably as a result of sensitization to eugenol placed in a pulp cap. This patient required immediate and intensive medical treatment. Unfortunately, immunologic confirmation of a possible type I immunologic reaction was not attempted in this case.

Another immediate-type reaction to eugenol occurred in a patient apparently sensitized to eugenol by repeated exposures in the course of periodontal treatments (21). Within hours after application of eugenol, this patient noted irritation and redness of the oral mucosa and 3 days later experienced sloughing of the oral mucosa, bilateral loss of papillae on the tongue, and ulceration at the vermilion border. In addition, mild facial swelling was noted. Based on the description of this patient's reaction, it is not possible to determine whether this reaction was mediated by humoral antibody or cell-mediated reactivity. Acute episodes of bronchospasm and itching in the ears and throat were experienced

Table 2 Perfume Screening Patch Tests

Common fragrance allergens (for routine screening)	
Cinnamic alcohol	5% petrolatum
Cinnamic aldehyde	1% petrolatum
Hydroxycitronellal	4% petrolatum
Isoeugenol	5% petrolatum
Eugenol	5% petrolatum
Oak moss absolute	5% petrolatum
Musk ambrette	5% petrolatum
Less common fragrance allergens (optional screening)	
Alpha amyl cinnamic alcohol	5% petrolatum
Geraniol	5% petrolatum
Benzyl salicylate	2% petrolatum
Sandalwood oil	2% petrolatum
Anisyl alcohol	5% petrolatum
Benzyl alcohol	5% petrolatum
Coumarin	5% petrolatum
Photoallergen: Musk ambrette	5% petrolatum

by a patient receiving a theophylline preparation (Euphyllin retard) containing vanillin (16). This patient had noted that previous ingestion of vanilla in food products had caused asthma symptoms. These clinical symptoms were documented by double-blind controlled challenge tests. A prick test to vanillin was negative in this patient, so the IgE-dependent nature of her upper respiratory symptoms was not confirmed. This patient coincidentally had experienced aspirin intolerance and it was postulated that the vanillin reaction could be similar to that occurring in patients with aspirin intolerance. In patients previously sensitive to cinnamon or cinnamic aldehyde, the ingestion of substances containing these flavors, including medicinals, may produce urticaria or contact-type eczematous eruptions (22). The immunologic specificity of such reactions has not been established. Several acute urticarial reactions to menthol have been reported (17,23). In two cases, acute symptoms of urticaria, headache, and flushing were reproduced after an oral challenge to menthol. Although skin tests in both cases were not diagnostic, direct in vitro basophil degranulation tests revealed significant degranulation of basophilic leukocytes after challenge with menthol. Although more suggestive than other suspected type I reactions to essential oils, the laboratory results in both of these patients could also be explained on the basis of a nonimmunologic direct histamine release mechanism.

b. Type II and III immunologic reactivity

There is a single report of diffuse necrotizing vasculitis after exposure to balsam of Peru (24). Presumably the pathologic nature of this lesion was consistent with type III mechanisms, but these were not proved.

c. Type IV immunologic reactivity

Classic contact sensitivity has been reported after exposure to numerous flavor and fragrance essential oils and chemicals contained in toothpastes, dentifrices, ointments, creams, lotions, topical sunscreen preparations, mouth washes, and liquid cough preparations. The immunologic basis of these reactions may be confirmed by classic closed patch tests interpreted 24 and 48 hr after application. Detection of contact reactivity to flavors and fragrances requires a high index of suspicion on the part of the consultant. For example, topical ointments or creams may contain a variety of known contactant allergens, some of which may rank much higher in sensitization potential than perfume ingredients (25). If testing does not include aroma or perfume chemicals, their primary importance as contact sensitizers cannot be appreciated.

Contact reactivity has been reported after exposure and sensitization to cinnamon oil, peppermint oil, spearmint oil, oil of anise, star anise oil, oil of cassia, lavender oil, oil of cloves, eugenol, cinnameldehyde, menthol, various balsams (Peru, Tolu, storax, benzoin, pine and spruce), and many perfume

Table 3   Research Institute for Fragrance Materials Testing (Prepared in White Petrolatum

---

a-Amyl cinnamaldehyde, 2%

Amyl salicylate, 5%

Anethole, 1%

Anisic aldehyde, 5%

Benzophenone, 5%

Benzyl acetate extra, 5%

Cinnamic alcohol, 4%

Citronellol, 5%

Coumarin, 5%

Diethylphthalate, 5%

Dimethylphthalate, 5%

Eugenol extra, 5%

Geraniol pure, 5%

Diphenyl oxide, 2%

Geranyl acetate, 2%

Heliotropin extra, 5%

Hydroxycitronellal, 5%

Isoeugenol, 5%

Linalyl synthetic, 5%

Linalyl acetate, 5%

Menthol natural, 5%

Methyl anthranilate, 1%

Phenylethyl alcohol, 5%

ρ-Pinene, 1%

ρ-Pinene, 5%

Terpineol alpha, 5%

Thymol, 1%

---

fragrances (15,17,19,21,22,26-31). Since it is not possible to test for all of the huge number of essential oils and their derivatives, the Research Institute for Fragrance Materials (RIFM) has proposed a test battery of substances listed in Table 3 (32). In addition, because many aromatic substances cross react with balsam of Peru and other balsam products, a special test battery of balsams may be particularly useful for screening purposes (Table 4). Several prospective surveys of patients with contact eczema indicate that contact reactions to balsam of Peru have the highest prevalence among the aroma and fragrance chemicals, ranging from 3 to 5.8% reactions (33,34). However, the prevalence of reactivity to balsam of Peru may be much lower in some countries (33,35). A prospective survey of sensitivity to 35 essential oils among 200 consecutive dermatitis patients has been carried out in Poland, but this may not be relevant to usage patterns of these essential oils in the United States or other western countries (35).

Photoimmunologic skin reactivity has been demonstrated after exposure and photosensitization to musk ambrette and 6-methylcoumarin (36). The ultraviolet spectrum responsible for the reaction is in the longer nonerythema (320-360 nm) wave lengths. Photoallergic reactions are highly specific, as deter-mined by a study in which nitromusk substances (musk tibetene, musk ketone, musk xylol, and musk moskene) did not exhibit photoallergic reactivity when compared to positive reactions induced by the musk ambrette perfume raw material (36). It was therefore suggested that the nitromusk could replace raw musk ambrette as fragrance materials without fear of inciting a photoallergic reaction. Persistent photosensitivity has also been induced by musk ambrette (37). A long-term light reaction may occur in a person who, after becoming photoallergic to a chemical, continues to react to ultraviolet energy for months or years even in the absence of further chemical exposure. Patients with this problem are initially photoallergic to the ultraviolet A spectrum but ultimately become sensitive to the ultraviolet B spectrum as the eruption continues.

Two prevailing theories explain the pathogenesis of this phenomenon. One proposal is that the persistent light reactor initially becomes sensitive to both the hapten and its carrier protein. Eventually, sensitivity to the carrier protein alone leads to a chronic photoeruption. The alternative explanation is that trace amounts of the antigen persist in the skin. thereby causing repetitive stimulation of cutaneous antigen-presenting cells and memory lymphocytes after exposure to the proper ultraviolet spectrum.

The type IV sensitization potential of selected fragrances (clove leaf oil, eugenol, and isoeugenol) in humans has been investigated prospectively by patch tests to these substances in dermatitic and nondermatitic volunteers (38,39). These surveys indicated that these particular fragrances tested at the

Table 4 Peruvian Balsam and Balsam Components (Prepared in White Petrolatum)

Peruvian balsam, 25%

Benzyl cinnamate, 5%

Eugenol, 2%

Methyl cinnamate, 5%

Benzyl benzoate, 5%

Vanillin, 10%

Cinnamic acid, 5%

Cinnamic alcohol, 5%

Cinnamaldehyde, 1%

Benzyl salicylate, 2%

concentrations ordinarily used in a number of consumer products had very low potentials for either eliciting preexisting contact sensitization or inducing new hypersensitivity reactions. The results of these studies also emphasized that both induction and elicitation of allergic contact dermatitis to these substances are dose-dependent and that concentrations below 0.5% prove to be relatively benign.

In evaluating possible contact reactivity induced by certain aldehyde aromatic substances (phenylacetaldehyde, citral, or cinnamic aldehyde), the phenomenon of quenching must be appreciated. Comparative investigations of sensitization induced by individual aldehydes and the essential oil from which the aldehyde was derived revealed that the essential oil in which the aldehyde occurred naturally did not induce sensitization, despite the fact that the aldehyde concentration in the oil was as high as 85%. Thus, it was postulated that other components in the natural oil inhibited or quenched the induction or expression of sensitization. Prospective studies demonstrated that sensitivity induced by phenylacetaldehyde, citral, and cinnamic aldehyde was abolished when alcohols and terpenes were added to the pure aldehyde prior to application of the patch test (40). The mechanism of the quenching phenomenon is at present unclear. One theory holds that quenching agents might interfere with the binding of aldehydes to epsilon amino protein side chains (41). According to this theory, the interference with protein binding to the epsilon amino groups on lysine residues occurs because of Schiff base formation during the curing period. An alternative explanation is that the quenching agent causes interference with binding of the aldehyde to specific tissue receptors, including those within blood vessels (42).

d. Anatomical sites of hypersensitivity reactions: Systemic: There is only one documented case report of anaphylaxis occurring after exposure to a flavored chemical (43). This occurred in a dental patient immediately after application of eugenol to a pulp cap preparation. The patient required immediate and intensive medical treatment which resulted in recovery.

e. Anatomical sites of hypersensitivity reactions: Cutaneous: Acute and chronic urticaria have been reported after oral exposure to several flavor ingredients (18, 21,23). Contact urticaria has also been described after exposure to cinnamaldehyde, cassia oil, balsam of Peru, and ethyl vanillin (18–20,44). Although a few individual cases are suggestive of immunologically mediated urticaria, the majority of cases, especially those induced by cinnamaldehyde, appear to be due to nonimmunologic contact urticaria, which will be discussed in more detail in this section. In patients demonstrating preexistent urticarial reactivity induced by one of the flavor substances, reexposure to that substance in a hidden form (e.g., food such as chocolate confectionary, Coca-Cola, vermouth, and nonalcoholic aperitifs) may cause an acute exacerbation of urticaria. This was reported in a 70-year-old man with preexistent contact sensitivity to balsam of Peru (45). His skin cleared completely after avoiding topical preparations containing balsam of Peru. However, 4 months later, he had an acute exacerbation of facial lesions after consuming large quantities of sweets containing balsam of Peru as a flavoring agent.

Because so many oral preparations and dentifrices contain flavoring agents, the most common contactant reactions involve the lips and oral mucous membranes (46). Rarely, the allergic inflammatory reaction may involve the tongue. The epithelium of the vermilion border of the lips is more susceptible to allergic contact hypersensitivity than the oral mucosa. Thus, the most common lesion seen after exposure to these agents is cheilitis. Angular cheilitis may be the only manifestation of contact reactivity to flavoring agents. Allergic cheilitis may first manifest merely with dryness and fissuring. Later, edema and crusting appear as the patient is reexposed to sensitizing allergens over a prolonged period of time. Contact mucositis may also occur after repeated exposure to periodontal dressings containing flavoring agents (46). Occasionally, contact reactions within the oral cavity can progress to stomatitis, which can be associated with complete sloughing of the oral mucosa, bilateral loss of papillae on the tongue, and ulceration at the vermilion border of the lips. Perioral contact dermatitis may also be observed in such cases.

Classic contact dermatitis of the skin may be induced by topical preparations containing essential oils or fragrance materials. As noted above, such reactions can only be diagnosed if there is a high index of suspicion, because topical preparations contain a variety of drug and excipient materials that also induce allergic contact dermatitis.

Specific intolerance to cinnamaldehyde, carvone, and piperitone has been implicated as a possible cause of orofacial granulomatosis, also known as the Melkersson-Rosenthal syndrome (47). This clinical triad consists of lip/facial swelling, seventh nerve palsy, and a fissured tongue. This swelling is usually localized to the lips and lower half of the face. Initially, the swelling comes and goes but it later becomes chronic. The oral mucosa is thickened and edematous, with the buccal and labial mucosae assuming a corrugated or lobular appearance. Occasionally this condition is accompanied by a characteristic gingival hyperplasia that has a patchy distribution and is more likely to occur in the anterior region of the mouth. Ulceration of the oral mucosa may occur and may range from small, superficial erosions to extensive deep ulcers that heal poorly. This process may be extensive and may progress to demonstrate vertical fissuring and angular cheilitis. Cranial nerve lesions may be a feature of this disorder, with a lower motor neuronal paresis of the facial nerve occurring in about a third of the cases. In nine of these cases, there was evidence of intolerance to flavors. Seven of these patients demonstrated positive patch tests to cinnamaldehyde, piperitone, or carvone. Partial to complete clinical response occurred in eight patients after elimination of suspected contactants. Positive patch tests in these cases suggest that orofacial granulomatosis may be related to some form of cell-mediated allergic response, but further prospective studies will be required to confirm this.

Chronic dermatitis occasionally associated with pseudolymphomatous features (actinic reticuloid) are characteristic features of patients with persistent photosensitivity dermatitis associated with the actinic reticuloid syndrome. These patients have a much higher prevalence of contact hypersensitivity to fragrance substance including oak, moss, jasmine mix, and hydroxycitronellal (48). These patients manifest enhanced susceptibility to phototoxic or photosensitivity reactions induced by a variety of fragrance materials in the environment. The continuous ability of the skin of these patients to react to light may be mediated by specific phototoxic inducer mechanisms leading to altered immunologic reactivity and subsequent phototoxic skin changes.

f. Anatomical sites of hypersensitivity reactions: Respiratory: There is a documented case report of bronchospasm induced by vanillin. This was confirmed by controlled, double-blind challenge tests in an asthmatic patient who also had aspirin intolerance. The mechanism of the reaction in this case was not determined. However, elimination of vanillin-containing pills and foods in this case effectively resolved the patient's symptoms (16).

g. Pseudoallergic responses

Certain flavoring agents, notably cinnamaldehyde and other derivatives of oil of cinnamon, may provoke acute urticarial skin responses 20-60 min after contact with the respective materials. These urticarial responses occur not only in patients suspected of being sensitive to respective flavors but also in the majority of normal control subjects (44). Further in vitro experiments utilizing leukocyte histamine release revealed that cinnamaldehyde has a direct histamine-liberating effect. Similar direct histamine-liberating effects have been observed with higher concentrations of balsam of Peru. Standardized human assays for identifying substances that induce nonimmunologic contact urticaria (NICU) have been developed (18). Panels of control subjects are selected on a basis of a benzoic acid qualification test performed on the area just lateral to the outer canthus of the eye. A grade 1 wheal to this substance qualifies the subject to enter the test panel. Thereafter, the cheek is the site used for routine testing of other substances. The precise site is immediately just above the zygomatic process. Two tests can be carried out on each cheek, enabling four substances to be evaluated at one time. Whealing is graded on a 0-4 scale. Using this test, relatively high whealing scores of NICU have been obtained after testing with neat concentrations of balsam of Peru, cinnamic acid, cinnamic aldehyde, methylsalicylate, and sorbic acid. This test should be a useful way of differentiating between immunologic and nonimmunologic reactivity of topical urticariogens.

As discussed above the only case of acute bronchospasm documented after acute exposure to a flavoring agent (vanillin) could have been a pseudoallergic response similar to those experienced by aspirin intolerant patients. The exact mechanism of such reactions remains to be determined.

Pseudoallergic responses to other flavoring agents (cocoa and peppermint), as characterized by nonimmunologic basophilic histamine release, have been described in penicillin factory workers exposed to cocoa and peppermint additives during the manufacturing process (49).

Gastrointestinal symptoms of pain, nausea, and vomiting have been observed after ingestion of oral antibiotic preparations formulated with tincture of orange, an alcoholic extract of orange peel. Tincture of orange is sometimes used by pharmacists to formulate suspensions for infants when a commercially prepared suspension is not available (50). Recognition of this adverse response is essential if one is to avoid the error of attributing gastrointestinal side effects to the active ingredient.

V. MONOSODIUM GLUTAMATE

This substance is a meaty flavoring agent used chiefly in foods but it also has been used occasionally to flavor pharmaceuticals such as oral liver extracts or protein preparations. For unexplained reasons, some susceptible individuals experience a symptom complex described variously as burning, warmth, pressure, chest tightness, sweating, nausea, and numbness and tingling confined to the face, neck, upper chest, shoulders, and upper arms after ingestion of monosodium glutamate (MSG) in amounts or concentrations in excess of the amount ordinarily used to enhance flavor. Sometimes these sensations were accompanied by chest pain and severe frontal headache. Monosodium L-glutamate has been identified as the offending constituent because the D-isomer causes no reaction. Some investigators have been able to confirm the diagnosis by means of double-blind provocative tests, while others have been unable to do so (51-53). One group of investigators noted that sodium content of a typical Chinese restaurant meal is approximately 225 mEq. They postulated that patient discomfort might be related to the large sodium content (54). However, the amount of MSG used to flavor pharmaceuticals would not approximate this order of magnitude. In the positive double-blind control studies, 1.5-2 g MSG was required to provoke symptoms. A small dose (200 mg) did not provoke a reaction. The mechanism of these reactions is unexplained. It has been suggested that MSG competes with GABA (gamma-amino-butyric acid), a neurotransmitter, thereby causing paresthesias (51).

In a recent clinical investigation of 32 patients suspected of having the MSG syndrome, 13 subjects developed asthma after challenge in a single-blind, placebo-controlled fashion with increasing doses of MSG from 0.5 to 5.0 g (55). Seven patients developed asthma and other MSG symptoms 1-2 hr after ingestion of the MSG challenge. Six patients developed asthma with classic MSG symptoms 6-12 hr after ingestion of the MSG challenge dose. These studies appeared to confirm that MSG is capable of provoking asthma. The asthma induced by MSG in several of these patients was severe enough to require intubation and treatment for respiratory insufficiency (55). The mechanism of asthma in association with the other classical symptoms of the MSG syndrome suggests a peripheral neuroexcitatory effect including stimulation of irritant lung receptors. However, since delayed asthmatic reactions in several patients were not associated with the other neuroexcitatory symptoms, it was postulated that late-onset asthma in these patients could be due to central nervous system mediation of lung reflexes.

There is one reported case of recurrent angioedema of the face and extremities occurring after ingestion of MSG. These symptoms were reproduced during a double-blind oral challenge protocol. In a graded challenge, MSG alone produced angioedema in this patient 16 hr after ingestion of at least 250 mg of MSG. Placebo alone produced no response (52).

There is a single report of a patient with symptoms and signs of orofacial granulomatosis aggravated by exposure to several food additives, one of which was MSG (56). Double-blind challenge in this patient produced a marked reaction to MSG. The mechanism of this association has not been established.

A suggested single-blind challenge protocol for confirming adverse reactions to MSG is presented in Table 5. The recommended challenge dose in this protocol is 10 times less than that recommended for patients with a history of MSG intolerance or asthma after ingestion of larger amounts of the substance in Chinese restaurants. (55). The lower-dose challenge schedule is recommended because the amount of this amino acid used as an excipient is much lower than that used for food flavoring. Prior to this test, patients should exclude all dietary contact with MSG for 5 days. If the patient has asthma, the morning theophylline dose should be omitted. Inhaled beta$_2$ agonist drugs should not be given for at least 3 hr before the first challenge. All challenges are given in the morning after an overnight fast. Patients should be observed closely at hourly intervals, at which time vital signs and pulmonary function parameters (e.g., FEV_1 or peak expiratory flow rate) should be recorded. A challenge is considered positive if the symptoms of the MSG syndrome are reproduced and/or if there is a fall in the FEV_1 or peak expiratory flow rate $\geq$ 20% from baseline tests done on the challenge day and the lowest recorded pulmonary function test was $\geq$20% lower than that recorded on the control day. Because of the greater possibility of delayed reactions induced by MSG, only one test dose should be administered

Table 5   Suggested Single-Blind Challenge Protocol for
Monosodium Glutamate (MSG) Reactions

Challenge day	Placebo[a] (mg)	MSG (mg)
1	50	—
2	250	—
3	500	—
4		50
5		250
6		500

[a]The order of placebo (methylcellulose) or MSG administration
 is determined by random selection.

on each day. All patients should be observed for 10-12 hr after the challenge dose.

REFERENCES

1. Kruesi, M.J.P. and Rapoport, J.L. Diet and human behavior: How much do they affect each other? Am. Rev. Nutr. 6:113-130 (1986).
2. Harms, H.K., Bertele-Harms, R.M. and Bruer-Kleis, D. Enzyme-substitution therapy with the yeast *Saccharomyces cerevisiae* in congenital sucrase-isomaltase deficiency. N. Engl. J. Med. 316(21):1306-1309 (1987).
3. Gordon, H.H. Untoward reactions to saccharin. Cutis 10:77-81 (1972).
4. Gordon, H.H. Photosensitivity to saccharin. Letter to the Editor. J. Am. Acad. Dermatol. 8(4):565 (1983).
5. Kulczycki, A. Jr. Aspartame-induced urticaria. Brief Reports. Ann. Intern. Med. 104:207-208(1986).
6. Novick, N.L. Aspartame-induced granulomatous panniculitis. Ann. Intern. Med. 102:206-207 (1985).
7. Schiffman, S.S., Buckley, C.E., III, Sampson, H.A. et al. Aspartame and susceptibility to headache. N. Engl. J. Med. 317:1181-1185 (1987).
8. Yong, J.M. and Sanderson, K.V. Photosensitive dermatitis and renal tubular acidosis after ingestion of calcium cyclamate. Lancet 2:1273 (1969).
9. Kidd, J.M. III, Cohen, S.H., Sosman, A.J. et al. Food-dependent exercise-induced anaphylaxis. J. Allergy Clin. Immunol. 71:407-411 (1983).
10. Husby, S., Oxelius, V.A., Teisner, B. et al. Humoral immunity to dietary antigens in healthy adults. Occurrence, isotype and IgG subclass distribution of serum antibodies to protein antigens. Int. Arch. Allergy Appl. Immunol. 77:416 (1985).
11. Sampson, H.A. Role of immediate food hypersensitivity in the pathogenesis of atopic dermatitis. J. Allergy Clin. Immunol. 71:473-480 (1983).
12. Stewart, P.M., Valentino, R., Wallace, A.M. et al. Mineralocorticoid activity of liquorice: 11-beta-hydroxysteroid dehydrogenase deficiency comes of age. Lancet 2:821-824(1987).
13. Fisher, A.A. Contact Dermatitis, 2nd ed. Lea and Febiger, Philadelphia, pp. 244-247 (1973).
14. Larsen, W.G. Perfume dermatitis. J. Am. Acad. Dermatol. 12(1):1-9 (1985).
15. Fregert, S. and Rorsman, H. Hypersensitivity to balsam of pine and spruce. Arch. Dermatol. 87:693-695 (1963).
16. van Assendelft, A.H.W. Bronchospasm induced by vanillin and lactose. Eur. J. Respir. Dis. 65:468-472 (1984).
17. Papa, C.M. and Shelley, W.B. Menthol hypersensitivity. J.A.M.A. 189(7):546-548 (1964).
18. Gollhausen, R. and Kligman, A.M. Human assay for identifying substances which induce non-allergic contact urticaria: the NICU-test. Contact Derm. 13:98-106 (1985).

19. Rudzki, E. and Grzywa, Z. Immediate reactions to balsam of Peru, cassia oil and ethyl vanillin. Short communications. Contact Derm. 2(6):360-361 (1976).

20. Rietschel, R.L. Contact urticaria from synthetic cassia oil and sorbic acid limited to the face. Contact Derm. 4:347-349 (1978).

21. Barkin, M.E., Boyd, J.P. and Cohen, S. Acute allergic reaction to eugenol. Oral Surg. 441-442 (1984).

22. Fisher, A.A. Dermatitis due to cinnamon and cinnamic aldehyde. Cutis 16: 383-388 (1975).

23. McGowan, E.M. Menthol urticaria. Arch Dermatol. 94:62-63 (1966).

24. Fisher, A.A. Erythema multiforme-like eruptions due to topical medications: Part II. Cutis 37(3):158-161 (1986).

25. Goldberg, H.S. Allergic contact dermatitis from the perfume in Mycolog cream. Arch. Dermatol. 105:896-897 (1972).

26. Grattan, C.E.H. and Peachey, R.D. Contact sensitization to toothpaste flavouring. J. R. Coll. Gen. Pract. 35:498, 1985.

27. Calnan, C.D. Cinnamon dermatitis from an ointment. Contact Derm. 2: 167-170 (1976).

28. Collins, R.W. and Mitchell, J.C. Aroma chemicals. Reference sources for perfume and flavour ingredients with special reference to cinnamic aldehyde. Contact Derm. 1:43-47 (1975).

29. Rudzki, E. and Grzywa, Z. Sensitizing and irritating properties of star anise oil. Contact Derm. 2:305-308 (1976).

30. Brandao, F.M. Occupational allergy to lavender oil. Short communications. Contact, Derm. 15(4):249-250 (1986).

31. Loveman, A.B. Stomatitis venenata. Report of a case of sensitivity to the mucous membranes and the skin to oil of anise. Arch. Dermatol. Syphilol. 37:70-81 (1938).

32. Larsen, W.G. Perfume dermatitis. A study of 20 patients. Arch. Dermatol. 113:623-626 (1977).

33. Mitchell, J.C. Contact hypersensitivity to some perfume materials. Contact Derm. 1:196-199 (1975).

34. Rudzki, E. and Kleniewska, D. The epidemiology of contact dermatitis in Poland. Br. J. Dermatol. 83:543-545 (1970).

35. Rudzki, E., Grzywa, Z. and Bruo, W.S. Sensitivity to 35 essential oils. Contact Derm. 2:196-200 (1976).

36. Parker, R.D., Buehler, E.V. and Newmann, E.A. Phototoxicity, photoallergy and contact sensitization of nitro musk perfume raw materials. Contact Derm. 14:103-109 (1986).

37. Zugerman, C. Persistent photosensitivity caused by musk ambrette. Arch. Dermatol. 117:432-434 (1981).

38. Rothenstein, A.S., Booman, K.A., Dorsky, J. et al. Eugenol and clove leaf oil: A survey of consumer patch-test sensitization. Fd. Chem. Toxicol. 21 (6):727-733 (1983).

39. Thompson, G.R., Booman, K.A., Dorsky, J. et al. Isoeugenol: A survey of

consumer patch-test sensitization. Fd. Chem. Toxicol. 21(6):735–740 (1983).

40. Opdyke, D.L.J. Inhibition of sensitization reactions induced by certain aldehydes. Fd. Cosmet. Toxicol. 14:197–198 (1976).

41. Majeti, V.A. and Suskind, R.R. Mechanism of cinnamaldehyde sensitization. Contact Derm. 3:16–18 (1977).

42. Guin, J.D., Meyer, B.N., Drake, R.D. et al. The effects of quenching agents on contact urticaria caused by cinnamic aldehyde. J. Am. Acad. Dermatol. 10(1):45–51 (1984).

43. McCarter, R.F. An unusual allergy. Midwest Dent. 42:20 (1966).

44. Nater, J.P., DeJong, C.J.M., Baar, A.J. et al. Contact urticarial skin responses to cinnamaldehyde. Contact Derm. 3:151–154 (1977).

45. Bedello, P.G., Goitre, M. and Cane, D. Contact dermatitis and flare from food flavouring agents. Short communications. Contact Derm. 8(2):143–144 (1982).

46. Kozam, G. and Mantell, F.M. The effect of eugenol on oral mucous membranes. J. Dent. Res. 57:954–957 (1978).

47. Patton, D.W., Ferguson, M.M., Forsyth, A. et al. Oro-facial granulomatosis: A possible allergic basis. Br. J. Oral Maxillofac. Surg. 23:235–242 (1985).

48. Addo, H.A., Ferguson, J., Johnson, B.E. et al. The relationship between exposure to fragrance materials and persistent light reaction in the photosensitivity dermatitis with actinic reticuloid syndrome. Br. J. Dermatol. 107:261–274 (1982).

49. Moller, N.E., Skov, P.S. and Norn, S. Allergic and pseudo-allergic reactions caused by penicillins, cocoa and peppermint additives to penicillin factory workers examined by basophil histamine release. Acta Pharmacol. Toxicol. 55:139–144 (1984).

50. Napke, E. and Stevens, D.G.H. Excipients and additives: Hidden hazards in drug products and in product substitution. Can. Med. Assoc. J. 131:1449–1452 (1984).

51. Ratner, D., Eshel, E. and Shoshani, E. Adverse effects of monosodium glutamate: A diagnostic problem. Isr. J. Med. Sci. 20:252–253 (1984).

52. Squire, E.N. Jr. Angio-oedema and monosodium glutamate. Lancet 1:988, 1987.

53. Kwok, R.H.M. Chinese-restaurant syndrome. N. Engl. J. Med. 278:796 (1968).

54. Smith, S.J., Markandu, N.D., Rotellar, C. et al. A new or old Chinese restaurant syndrome. Br. Med. J. 285:1205 (1982).

55. Allen, D.H., Delohery, J. and Baker, B. Monosodium L-glutamate-induced asthma. J. Allergy Clin. Immunol. 80:53–537 (1987).

56. Sweatman, M.C., Tasker, R., Warner, J.O. et al. Oro-facial granulomatosis. Response to elemental diet and provocation by food additives. Clin. Allergy 16:331–338 (1986).

14

Allergic Reactions: Coloring Agents

I. Background   253
   A. Certified drug colorants   253
   B. Noncertifiable colorants   254
II. Azo dyes   257
III. Xanthene dyes   275
IV. Triphenylmethane dyes   277
V. Indigoid dyes   277
VI. Quinoline dyes   277
VII. FDA Certification-exempt dyes   278
   References   278

I. BACKGROUND

A. Certified Drug Colorants

After the food and cosmetic industries, the pharmaceutical industry ranks third in use of colorants. Since the majority of these substances have been coded by the Food and Drug Administration (FDA), it is necessary to review the regulatory nomenclature. The abbreviated term, FD&C, refers to colors certifiable for use in coloring foods, drugs, and cosmetics. Certification by the FDA requires that an appropriate sample of each manufacturer's batch of product be submitted to the FDA Color Certification Branch along with the requested certification in order to determine if it conforms to the specifications assigned to it. In general, only synthetic organic colorants are subject to certification, while natural organic and inorganic colorants (e.g., caramel and titanium dioxide) are not. From the regulatory point of view, the status of each individual colorant may be either "listed" or "provisional." Listed dye additives have been sufficiently evaluated to ensure human safety, while provisional colorants that have not been considered unsafe up to the present time require further detailed, long-term studies before becoming eligible for "listed" status.

    Colorants used in drugs also have other official designations. D&C colors are those dyes and pigments considered to be safe in drugs and cosmetics when applied locally to mucous membranes or when given by the oral route. EXT D&C colors are colorants not certifiable for use in oral products but considered to be safe for use in externally applied products. The latter listing specifically excludes colorants that may have oral toxicity.

In general, certified colors are cheaper, brighter, more uniform, and better characterized than noncertified color additives. They are available as "primary" colors and as admixtures with other certified colors to form "secondary" colors (1).

Although most of the certifiable drug colorants are derived from petroleum, their chemical structures are variable and can be classified in several main categories: azo colors with one or more azo (-N=N-) bonds; xanthenes; triphenylmethanes; indigoids; quinolines; and anthraquinones. To gain a global perspective of the most commonly used FD&C certified colorants in the pharmaceutical industry, refer to Table 1, which lists some of the most commonly used drug colorants according to total pounds consumed per year. It should be noted that FD&C red #2 was the leading dye on this list before it was delisted in 1977. FD&C violet #1 was also on this list prior to its delisting in 1974. Other provisional FD&C dyes approved for oral drug products include yellow nos. 33, 34, 37; red nos. 8, 19, 22; and orange no. 5. Coloring agents approved for external use only include FD&C red dye no. 4, 17, 31, 34, 39; yellow nos. 7, 8; blue nos. 4, 6, 9; green nos. 5, 6, 8; violet no. 2; and orange no. 4.

B. Noncertifiable Colorants

A number of noncertifiable colorants are also used in the pharmaceutical industry. Most of these are derived from natural sources but a notable exception is canthaxanthin, which is a synthetically produced carotenoid color additive (Table 2).

Several dyes are used primarily as medicinal or diagnostic agents. For example, the use of neutral red treatment for recurrent herpes simplex infections may result in eczematous contact dermatitis of the involved area (2-4). This potential complication is now moot because of the demonstrated carcinogenicity of this dye. Evans blue, an azo-type dye used to outline lymphatics prior to the injection of a contrast medium in performing lymphangiography, may also cause allergic contact dermatitis (5,6). Several triphenylmethane dyes used as diagnostic or therapeutic modalities have also been implicated as causes of severe allergic reactions. Patent blue, commonly used to visualize the lymphatic vessels prior to lymphography, may cause immediate-type hypersensitivity reactions including nonfatal anaphylaxis (7,8). Contact sensitization to other therapeutic dyes (gentian violet, brilliant green, and malachite green) has also been reported in 11 patients with eczema localized to the legs. The immunologic specificity of these reactions was confirmed by patch tests (9). However, none of these dyes are

Table 1 Most Commonly Used FD&C Certifiable Colorants in Pharmaceutical Industrial Listed According to Pounds of Usage in 1967

FD&C listing	Chemical classification	Common name	Permitted use	FDA status
Yellow no. 5	Azo (pyrazolone)	Tartrazine	Ingestion	Listed
Yellow no. 6	Azo	Sunset yellow	Ingestion	Provisional
Red no. 3	Xanthene	Erythrosine	Ingestion	Listed
Blue no. 1	Triphenylmethane	Brilliant blue	Ingestion	Listed
Red no. 4	Azo	Ponceau SX	External	Listed
Blue no. 2	Indigoid	Indigo carmine	Ingestion, sutures	Provisional
Green no. 3	Triphenylmethane	Fast green	Ingestion	Provisional

Adapted from Ref. 1.

Table 2 Representative Natural and Synthetic Drug Colorants Exempt from FDA Certification

Name	FDA name	Source	Used to color
Canthaxanthin	Orange 8	Synthetic carotene	Oil, aqueous solutions; gelatin capsules
Caramel	Same	Heat processed carbohydrates	Cough syrups; placebo solutions
Cochineal extract (carmine)	Carminic acid (anthraquinone)	Insects (coccus cacti)	Pill coatings
Titanium oxide	Same	Crystalline anatase	Capsule and pill coatings
Potassium sodium copper chlorophyllin (chlorophyllin-copper complex)	Same	Alfalfa chlorophyll	Dentrifices

used as coloring ingredients in drug products. The following discussion of individual colorant excipients will focus only on those dyes and pigments used as excipients in the drug industry.

II. AZO DYES

1. Tartrazine

Tartrazine (FD&C yellow no. 5) is one of the most commonly used colorants in drugs. It is classified as an azo dye but is unique in that it also has a pyrazolone structure (Fig. 1). The list of drugs containing this dye is extensive and even includes antiallergic and antiasthmatic medications (10,11). Moreover, by the mid-1970s, the number of possible adverse experiences due to this agent far outweighed any other drug excipient in common usage. In 1980, the FDA issued new regulations that required listing of this dye on package labeling by all manufacturers. The requirement applies to all prescription or over-the-counter oral, rectal, vaginal, or nasal products. After this regulation became effective, many manufacturers reformulated their products either to remove tartrazine or to replace it with another dye. Since the list of tartrazine-containing medications is constantly changing, it should be noted that publications of such data prior to 1981 are often incorrect. Table 3 lists tartrazine-containing drugs compiled

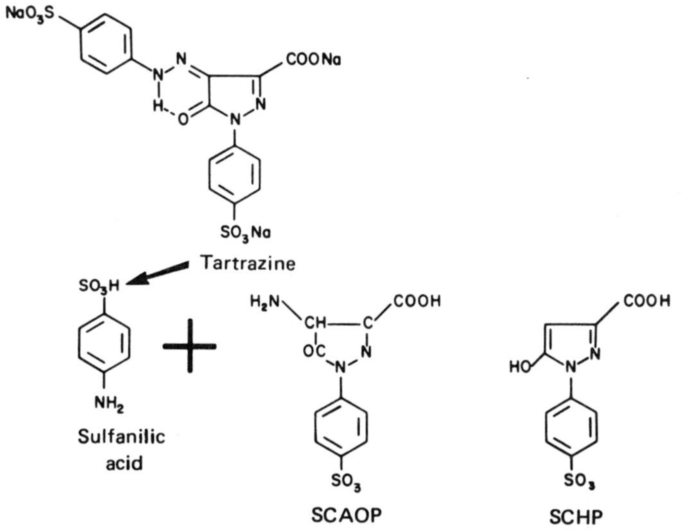

Figure 1 Chemical structures of tartrazine, sulfanilic acid, a tartrazine metabolite, 1-sulfophenyl-3-carboxy-4 amino-5 oxypyrazole (SCAOP), and an analog of the tartrazine metabolite, 1-sulfophenyl-3 carboxy-5-hydroxypyrazole (SCHP).

Table 3   Tartrazine-Containing Drugs

Alto Pharmaceuticals, Inc.
  Akne Kaps
  Akne Oral Kapsulets
  Bifed Capsules
  D'Alpha-E Capsules
  Zinc-220 Capsules

Amfre-Grant, Inc. (Ormont Drug & Chemical Co.)
  Corovas Capsules
  GGI Expectorant
  Kloride Elixir
  Laud Iron Folic Tablets
  Multifluor Tablets
  Primar Tablets
  Venthera Tablets

Arco Pharmaceuticals, Inc.
  Mega-B tablets
  Megadose tablets

Armour Pharmaceutical Company
  Nicolar tablets

Beecham Laboratories
  Conar-A Suspension
  Cotrol-D Tablets
  Hycal (lime) Liquid
  Livitamin Prenatal Tablets

Beutlich, Inc.
  Mevatinic-C Tablets

Boehringer Ingelheim, Ltd.
  Dulcolax Tablets 5 mg
  Persantine Tablets 25 mg
  Preludin Endurets 75 mg
  Serentil Tablets 10 mg, 25 mg, 100 mg
  Torecan Tablets 10 mg

Century Pharmaceuticals, Inc.
  CP-2 Yellow Tablets
  Vita Tot (yellow tablet only)

CIBA Pharmaceutical Company
  Apresazide Capsules 100/50[a]
  Apresoline Tablets 10 mg,[a] 100 mg[a]
  Dianabol Tablets 2.5 mg,[a]
  Forhistal Lontabs 2.5 mg[a]
  Ismelin Tablets 10 mg[a]
  Metandren 10 mg Linguets, 25 mg tablets[a]

Serpasil-Apresoline Tablets #1,[a] #2[a]
Serpasil-Esidrix Tablets #1,[a] #2[a]

Circle Pharmaceuticals, Inc.
  Circavite T Tablets
  Tusquelin Cough Syrup

Delco Chemical Company, Inc. (Lemmon Co.)
  Delcobese Capsules 5 mg, 15 mg
  Delcobese Time Release Capsules 20 mg
  Delcobese Tablets 20 mg
  Delcozine Capsules

Dome Laboratories (Miles Labs, Inc.)
  Lithane Tablets 300 mg

Dorsey Laboratories
  Bellergal-S Tablets
  Tussaminic Tablets

Dow Pharmaceuticals
  Neocholan Tablets
  Novahistine LP Tablets
  Quide Tablets 10 mg, 25 mg

Doyle Pharmaceutical Company
  Meritene Powder and Liquid: egg nog
  Dietene Powder and Liquid: vanilla
  Citrotein Powder and Liquid: orange
  Precision LR Diet: lemon, lime and orange
  Precision High Nitrogen Diet: citrus
  Precision Isotonic Diet: orange

Ferndale Laboratories, Inc.
  Bellkatal Tablets
  Benase Tablets
  Doss 300 Capsules
  Fernhist Tablets
  Flavitab Tablets
  Niapent Elixir
  Super Doss Tablets
  Tin-Co-Green Soap

Fisons Corporation
  Intal Capsules[b]
  Vitron-C-Plus Tablets

Fleet, C. B. Company, Inc.
  Phospho-soda, regular and flavored

Flint Laboratories
  Choloxin Tablets 2 mg, 6 mg
  Synthroid Tablets 100 ug, 300 ug

Table 3 (Continued)

GEIGY Pharmaceuticals
  Butazolidin Tablets 100 mg
  Butazolidin -Alka Capsules[a]
  Tofranil Tablets 10 mg,[a] 25 mg,[a] 50 mg[a]
  Tofranil-PM Capsules 100 mg,[a] 125 mg[a]
  PBZ Tablets 25 mg[a]
  PBZ Lontabs 50 mg[a]

Glaxo, Inc. (formerly Meyer Labs.)
  Athemol-N Tablets

Guardian Chemical Corporation
  pHos-pHaid Tablets 0.5 g
  sugar-coated: 0.5 g
  enteric-coated: 0.25 g

Hoechst-Roussel Pharmaceuticals, Inc.
  Doxinate Capsules 60 mg,[a] 240 mg[a]
  Duadacin Capsules[a]
  Festalan Tablets
  Lasix Oral Solution

Hoyt Laboratories (Colgate-Palmolive Co.)
  Phos-Flur Oral RInse/Supplement, lime flavored

Inwood Laboratories, Inc.
  Nitrobon Capsules, 2.5 mg,[b] 6.5 mg[a]

Knoll Pharmaceutical Company
  Dilaudid Cough Syrup
  Dilaudid Tablets 1 mg, 2 mg, 4 mg
  Theokin Tablets
  Vita-Metrazol Tablets

Lannett Company, Inc.
  Brompheniramine maleate Tablets[a]
  Obalan Tablets[a]
  Trichlormethiazide Tablets[a]

Lemmon Pharmacal Company
  Belap Tablets
  Dexampex Tablets 5 mg, capsules 15 mg
  Diacin capsules
  Dipav capsules
  Dralserp Tablets
  Dralzine Tablets
  Glucoron with B_{12} Tablets
  KEFF Tablets (lemon and lime flavors only)
  Laverin Tablets
  Mepriam Tablets

Neosorb Plus Tablets
Neospect Tablets
Neutralox Tablets
Phentermine HCl Capsules 30 mg (red/yellow)
Phenylpropanolamine HCl Tablets 25 mg
Pyradyne Compound Tablets
S.B.P. Plus Tablets
Statobex Tablets and Capsules
Statobex G Tablets

Marion Laboratories, Inc.
Pretts Tablets
Triten Tablets 2.5 mg

Mayrand, Inc.
Hydrotensin-50 Tablets
Hydrotensin-Plus Tablets

McNeil Laboratories, Inc.
Butibel Elixir
Buticaps Capsules 15 mg,[a] 30 mg, 50 mg
Butigetic Tablets
Butisol Sodium Elixir
Butisol Sodium Tablets 30 mg, 50 mg
Clistin RA Tablets 12 mg
Clistin-D Tablets
Clistin-D Expectorant Syrup
Grifulvin V Suspension
Haldol Tablets 1 mg, 5 mg, 10 mg
Intensin Capsules
Paraflex Tablets
Parafon Forte Tablets
Tolectin DS Capsules
Tylenol Extra-Strength Adult Liquid
Tylenol with Codeine Elixir

Mead Johnson Pharmaceutical Division
Cytoxan Tablets 25 mg, 50 mg
Deapril-ST Tablets 1 mg
Estrace Tablets 2 mg
Megace Tablets 20 mg, 40 mg
Ovcon-35, 28-day regimen
Ovcon-50, 21-day and 28-day regimen
Questran Powder
Sustacal Fortified pudding, vanilla

Merrell Dow Pharmaceuticals
AVC Suppositories[b]
AVC/Dienestrol Suppositories[b]
Cantil Tablets

Table 3 (Continued)

Cantil with Phenobarbital Tablets
Cēpacol Mouthwash/Gargle and Concentrate
Cēpacol Throat Lozenges and Anesthetic Troches
Cotussis Syrup
Decapryn Syrup
Decapryn Tablets 12.5 mg
DV Suppositories
Hiprex Tablets 1 g
Metahydrin Tablets 2 mg, 4 mg
Metatensin Tablets 2 mg
Norpramin Tablets 25 mg, 50 mg, 75 mg, 100 mg
Orenzyme Tablets
Orenzyme Bitabs
Sedadrops
TACE Capsules 12 mg,[b] 25 mg,[b] 72 mg[b]

MK Laboratories, Inc.
Ampicillin capsules 250 mg, 500 mg
Conjugated estrogens tablets 0.3 mg, 0.625 mg, 1.25 mg
Hydralazine HCl 25 mg

O'Neal, Jones & Feldman, Inc.
Sulfaloid Tablets and Suspension

Ortho Pharmaceutical Corporation
Ortho-Novum 1/50 Tablets, 21-day and 28-day regimens

Panray Pharmaceuticals (Ormont Drug and Chemical Co.)
Hexavitamin Tablets
Panahist Tablets
Pan-Kloride Elixir
Rid-A-Col Tablets
Theralets Tablets
Theralets M Tablets
Triasyn B Tablets

Parke, Davis & Company (Warner-Lambert)
Alophen Pills
Cascara Sagrada Extract Filmseals
Euthroid Tablets 0.5 gr, 1 gr, 3 gr
Ferrous Sulfate Filmseals 325 mg
Paladac with Minerals
Panteric Filmseals 325 mg
Thera-Combex HP Kapseals

Pennwalt Corporation
Adapin Capsules 10 mg, 25 mg, 50 mg, 100 mg
Zaroxolyn Tablets 10 mg

Pfipharmecs (Pfizer, Inc.)
  Obron-6 Tablets[a]
  Roeribec Tablets[a]
  Viterra Original Formulation Tablets

Philips Roxane Laboratories
  Chlordiazepoxide HCl Capsules 10 mg
  Dovamide Capsules
  Guaiahist Tablets
  Theophylline Elixir

Riker Laboratories
  Dorbantyl Capsules[b]
  Dorbantyl Forte Capsules[b]
  Rauwiloid Tablets 2 mg
  Veriloid Tablets 2 mg

Robins, A. H., Company, Inc.
  Adabee Tablets
  Adabee with Mineral Tablets
  Allbee with C Capsules
  Exna Tablets
  Tybatran Capsules 250 mg, 350 mg
  Z-Bec Tablets

Roche Laboratories
  Taractan Tablets 10 mg, 25 mg, 50 mg, 100 mg

Sandoz Pharmaceuticals
  Belladenal-S Tablets
  Sansert Tablets[a]

Saron Pharmacal Corporation
  Fem-H Tablets 1.25 mg, 0.625 mg, 0.3 mg
  Gevizol Tablets
  Mega Vita Tablets

Schering Corporation
  Cod Liver Oil Concentrate Tablets
  Demazin Syrup
  Estinyl Tablets 0.02 mg
  Gitaligin Tablets 0.5 mg
  Naquival Tablets
  Permitil Chronotabs 1 mg
  Rela Tablets

Searle Laboratories
  Comfolax Capsules
  Comfolax-plus Capsules
  Pro-Banthine with Dartal Tablets

Table 3 (Continued)

Smith, Kline & French Laboratories
  Compazine Tablets and Spansule Capsules[a]
  Dexedrine Elixir, Spansule, and Tablets
  Eskatrol Spansule Capsule[a]
  SK-Ampicillin Capsules[a]
  SK-Dexamethasone Tablets 0.5 mg[a]
  SK-Diphenydramine Capsules [a]
  SK-Potassium Chloride Liquid[a]
  SK-Triamcinolone Tablets
  Thorazine Tablets[a]
  Tuss-Ornade Liquid[a]

Squibb, E. R.
  Calcium Phosphate and Vitamin D Tablets
  Cephradine Capsules 250 mg
  Dirocide Syrup
  Dirocide Tablets 50 mg, 100 mg, 200 mg, 300 mg
  Engran-HP Tablets
  Esterified Estrogens Tablets 1.25 mg
  Ethril Tablets 500 mg
  Feramel Tablets
  Hydrea Capsules 500 mg
  Ipodate Sodium Capsules
  Kenacort Tablets 8 mg
  Multiple Vitamin with Iron Tablets
  Mycostatin Oral Tablets
  Naturetin Tablets 2.5 mg, 5 mg, 10 mg
  Naturetin with K Tablets 2.5 mg, 5 mg
  Nydrazid Injection
  Ora-Testryl Tablets 5 mg
  Pentids Syrup 250 mg/5ml
  Pentids "400" for Syrup 250 mg/5 ml
  Pentids "800" Tablets
  Princillin Capsules 125 mg
  Prolixin Capsules 2.5 mg, 5 mg, 10 mg
  Pronestyl Capsules 250 mg, 375 mg, 500 mg
  Pronestyl Tablets 250 mg, 375 mg, 500 mg
  Raudixin Tablets 50 mg, 100 mg
  Rautrax Tablets
  Rautrax-N ss Tablets
  Rauzide Tablets
  Spec-T Cough Suppressant Troches
  Spec-T Decongestant Troches
  Theragran Tablets
  Theragran Hematinic Tablets

Veetids Suspension 250 mg/5 ml
Veetids Tablets 250 mg
Vesprin Tablets 25 mg, 50 mg
Vitamin A Capsules 10,000 IU
Vitamin B Complex with B_{12} (yellow)
Vitamin B Complex with B_{12} (Novogran), orange–red only
Vitamin E Chewable Tablets 200 IU, 400 IU

Stuart Pharmaceuticals
  Bucladin-S Tablets
  Ferancee Tablets
  Ferancee-HP Tablets[a]
  Mylanta-II Tablets
  Probec-T Tablets
  Soribtrate Tablets 5 mg[a] and 10 mg[a] oral, 5 mg[a] and 10 mg[a] chewable, 40 mg SA
  Stuart Prenatal with Folic Acid Tablets
  Stuartinic tablets[a]
  Stuartnatal 1+1 tablets[a]

Tutag Pharmaceuticals, Inc. (Reid-Provident)
  Aquatag Tablets 25 mg, 50 mg
  Sprx-2 Tablets[a]
  Tora Tablets 8 mg[a]

Ulmer Pharmacal Company
  Kler-ro Liquid Detergent
  Pheneen Sanitzer

Upjohn Company
  Alphadrol Tablets 1.5 mg
  Cebetinic Tablets
  Cleocin Capsules 75 mg, 150 mg
  Didrex Tablets 25 mg
  Diostate D Tablets 325 mg
  Ferrous Sulfate Tablets 325 mg
  Halotestin Tablets 2 mg, 5 mg, 10 mg
  Maolate Tablets 400 mg
  Medrol Tablets 24 mg
  Micronase Tablets 5 mg, 10 mg
  P–A–C Compound Tablets, green
  P–A–C Compound Capsules
  P–A–C Compound with Codeine 15 mg Tablets
  P–A–C Compound with Codeine 30 mg Capsules
  Panmycin Tablets 250 mg, 500 mg
  Panmycin Capsules 250 mg
  Pensyn Capsules 250 mg, 500 mg
  Phenobarbital and Belladonna Tablets No. 1, No. 2
  Phenolax Wafers

Table 3 (Continued)

Pyrroxate with Codeine Capsules 15 mg
Pyrroxate Tablets
Reserpoid Tablets 0.25 mg
Super D Perles
Unicap Tablets and Capsules
Unicap M Tablets
Unicap T Tablets
Uracil Mustard Capsules 1 mg

USV Laboratories (USV Pharmaceutical Corp.)
Aquasol E Capsules[a]
C–B Vone Tablets[a]
Duo-C.V.P. Tablets[a]
Vi-Aquamin Forte Tablets
Voranil Tablets

Wallace Laboratories
Avazyme 20 Tablets
Barbidonna No. 2 Tablets
Covanamine Tablets
Covangesic Liquid
Covangesic Tablets
Dainite K Tablets
Deprol Tablets
Ephed-Organidin Elixir
Maltsupex Filmtabs
Miltrate Tablets 20 mg
Rynatuss Pediatric Suspension
Ryna-Tussadine Expectorant Tablets

Webcon Pharmaceuticals (Alcon Labs.)
Aquachloral Suppositories 15 gr
WANS No. 2 Supprettes

Western Research Laboratories, Inc.
Ammonium chloride tablets 7.5 gr
Chlordiazepoxide HCl capsules 5 mg, 10 mg, 25 mg
Chlorpromazine HCl tablets 10 mg,[a] 25 mg,[a] 50 mg,[a] 100 mg,[a] 200 mg[a]
Copper gluconate tablets
Digitalis leaf tablets
EFA tablets
Elekap Capsules
Ferrous gluconate tablets
Ferrous sulfate tablets
Hemaferrin Tablets
Laxative Tablets
Lec-Kelp Capsules

Levo thyroxine tablets 0.3 mg, 0.4 mg
Obezine Tablets, yellow and green only
Placebo tablets
Placebo capsules
Pyridamide Tablets
Sodium phenobarbital tablets 0.25 gr
Wes-B/C Capsules
Weslax Tablets
Westvite Tablets

Wyeth Laboratories
A–M–T Tablets
Bicillin Tablets, 200,000 U
Equanil Wyseals
Equanitrate Tablets 20 mg
Ovrette Tablets
Polymagma Plain Tablets
Proketazine Tablets 12.5 mg, 25 mg, 50 mg
Purodigin Tablets 0.15 mg
Serax Tablets 15 mg
Sparine Syrup 10 mg/5 ml
Sparine Tablets 10 mg, 25 mg, 200 mg

Zenith Laboratories, Inc.
Chlorpromazine tablets 10 mg, 25 mg, 50 mg, 100 mg, 200 mg
Chlorzoxazone 250 mg with APAP 300 mg
Decongestant TD II
Dextroamphetamine tablets 5 mg, 10 mg
Dimenhydrinate tablets 50 mg
Ferrous sulfate tablets
Hydralazine HCl tablets 10 mg
Hydrochlorothiazide 25 mg with reserpine tablets 0.125 mg
Hydrochlorothiazide 50 mg with reserpine tablets 0.125 mg
Isosorbide SL tablets 2.5 mg
Meclizine tablets 25 mg
Oxyphenbutazone
PETN tablets 10 mg, 20 mg
Phendimetrazine tablets 35 mg
Phentermine capsules 30 mg
Phentermine tablets 8 mg
Thera M Ten
Tridihexethyl chloride with meprobamate 200 mg
Zenivite, M

---

[a]These products are undergoing reformation to delete tartrazine dye.
[b]Only the capsule shell contains the tartrazine dye.

by pharmaceutical scientists who took these factors into account (11). This survey also ascertained that a sizable number of drug manufacturers no longer include tartrazine in their products (Table 4).

Adverse reactions to tartrazine were first documented in 1959 (12). This report described the occurrence of urticaria in three patients who used steroid tablets (dexamethasone) containing this dye. In the next three decades, there were many documented adverse reactions including anaphylactoid reactions, generalized urticaria, angioedema, rhinitis, bronchial asthma, "allergic purpura," contact dermatitis, and purported aggravation of hyperkinesis in hyperactive children. Apart from contact dermatitis, immunologic mechanisms were not demonstrated in the majority of cases and alternative nonimmunologic mechanisms were suggested as early as 1968 in an investigation that demonstrated that 7.5% of aspirin-intolerant patients were also intolerant to tartrazine (13). This report catalyzed a large series of uncontrolled and controlled clinical investigations concerning possible cross-reactivity between tartrazine and aspirin in aspirin-intolerant patients. These studies revealed an extraordinary range of tartrazine intolerance from 7.5 to 63%. Part of this discrepancy can be attributed to uncontrolled observations.

Double-blind, controlled oral challenge tests with tartrazine revealed a high percentage (25%) of positive reactions after challenge with placebo, even in patients with very suggestive histories of adverse reactions to tartrazine (14). Objective confirmation of suspected tartrazine reactivity by double-blind challenge varies between 25 and 40% (14,15). Variability of tartrazine reactivity in prospectively controlled studies may be explained by different methods of interpretation (i.e., combining all symptoms rather than classifying urticaria/angioedema apart from bronchial hyperreactivity) or actual differences between children and adults. In general, corroboration of tartrazine intolerance by double-blind oral challenges has been easier to demonstrate in children than adults with either acute or chronic urticaria (15,16). Results of a recent report cast considerable doubt on earlier studies purporting that tartrazine is responsible for continued provocation of chronic urticaria (16,17).

With regard to tartrazine-induced bronchoconstriction, interpretation and integration of available documented data are even more complex. One of the largest studies that investigated the prevalence of tartrazine sensitivity in asthmatic patients concluded that 25% of aspirin-intolerant patients exhibited a positive tartrazine challenge test while no reactions were encountered in aspirin-tolerant patients (18). In this study, bronchodilators were withheld for 6–12 hr before double-blind oral challenges were begun. Another independent study demonstrated significant differences in tartrazine challenge results depending on whether bronchodilators were withheld or continued during the provocation experiment. Tartrazine-positive challenges in aspirin-intolerant patients could be completely abrogated by continuing the use of bronchodilators throughout the

Table 4   Manufacturers of Tartrazine-Free Products

Alcon Laboratories, Inc.	Geriatric Pharmaceutical Corp.
American Critical Care	Gilbert Laboratories
Astra Pharmaceutical Products, Inc.	Glenbrook Laboratories
Ayerst Laboratories	Herbert Laboratories
Barnes-Hind Pharmaceuticals, Inc.	Holland-Rantos Co., Inc.
Beach Pharmaceuticals	Hollister Stier Laboratories
Becton Dickinson Immunodiagnostics (see Hynson, Westcott & Dunning)	Hynson, Westcott & Dunning (Becton Dickinson)
Berlex Laboratories, Inc.	Ives Laboratories, Inc.
Bird Corp. (3M)	Johnson & Johnson Health Care Division
Boots Pharmaceuticals, Inc.	
Bowman Pharmaceuticals, Inc.	Kenwood Laboratories, Inc. (Ethical Pharmaceuticals)
Breon Laboratories, Inc.	Key Pharmaceuticals, Inc.
Bristol Laboratories	Kremers-Urban Co.
Bristol-Myers Products	Laser, Inc.
Brown Pharmaceutical Co.	Lederle Laboratories
Brunswick Laboratories (Div. Beatrice Scientific Co.)	Eli Lilly & Co.
Burroughs Wellcome Co.	Mallinckrodt, Inc.
Burton, Parson & Co., Inc.	Medics Pharmaceutical Corp.
Campbell Laboratories, Inc.	Merck, Sharpe & Dohme
Carnrick Laboratories, Inc.	Metro Pharmacal Co.
Central Pharmaceuticals, Inc.	Miller Pharmacal
Cetylite Industries, Inc.	Misemer Pharmaceuticals, Inc.
Comatic Laboratories, Inc.	Mission Pharmacal Co.
Cutter Laboratories, Inc.	Nion Corp.
Dermik Laboratories, Inc.	Norgine Laboratories, Inc.
Dooner, Laboratories, Inc.	Organon Pharmaceuticals, Inc.
Elkins-Sinns, Inc.	Owen Laboratories
Endo Laboratories, Inc.	Person & Covey, Inc.
Everett Laboratories, Inc.	Pfizer Laboratories
Fleming & Co.	Pharmacia, Inc.
Fluoritab Corp.	Polythress, William P. & Co., Inc. (Ethical Pharmaceuticals)
Forest Laboratories, Inc.	
Frye Co., Inc.	Purdue Frederick Co.

Table 4 (Continued)

Rexar Pharmacal Corp. (Obetrol Pharmaceuticals)	Star Pharmaceuticals, Inc.
	Steri-Med, Inc.
Roerig, J. B. & Co. (Pfizer)	Syntex Laboratories, Inc.
Rorer, William H., Inc.	Walker, Corp. & Co., Inc.
Rowell Laboratories, Inc.	Winthrop Laboratories
Rystan Co., Inc.	Vale Chemical Co., Inc.
Savage Laboratories (Byk-Gulden, Inc.)	Viobin Corp. (A. H. Robins)
Serono Laboratories, Inc.	

course of the challenge procedure. Although it is possible that continuation of bronchodilators in this study merely blocked the target organ response to tartrazine, the investigators of this study suggested that a positive tartrazine reaction obtained in patients in whom bronchodilators were withheld could represent a false-positive asthmatic response in a group of bronchodilator-dependent patients with unstable airways (19). This would most likely be the case in aspirin-sensitive asthmatic subjects who frequently rely on chronic intensive treatment for control of symptoms. The controversy about tartrazine positive reactions in various asthmatic subpopulations has not yet been resolved. Despite this unresolved question, the vast majority of positive tartrazine reactions appear to be associated with pre-existing intolerance to aspirin and nonsteroidal antiinflammatory agents. There are, however, several documented exceptions to this general rule (20,21).

Since the definition of a positive tartrazine reaction depends upon the conditions of controlled challenge testing, the precise prevalence of tartrazine intolerance in unknown. However, the FDA estimates that the number of tartrazine-intolerant persons in the United States ranges between 50,000 and 100,000 (22).

There is no uniform agreement about the amount of tartrazine needed to provoke a positive reaction. Positive responses have been elicited to doses as low as 0.85 μg and as high as 25 mg. Most investigators have advised a modified dose–response assay that usually consists of two or three graduated doses of the dye. These challenge tests should be performed with due precautions because severe reactions have been observed after doses as small as 1.5–5 mg. A suggested oral challenge protocol to tartrazine is shown in Table 5.

a. Type I immunologic reactivity

Although there have been several well-documented cases of anaphylactoid symptoms, objective proof of IgE-mediated mechanisms is not convincing

(20,21,23). A direct prick test was positive in one case but this was not confirmed by passive transfer or radioallergosorbent tests (RAST) (23). To demonstrate possible immune mechanisms, extensive skin window techniques were performed in another patient who presented with angioedema/asthma (24). This patient's symptoms were confirmed by a double-blind placebo-controlled oral challenge test. Direct skin tests were negative. A skin window test showed an eosinophilia of 8% after tartrazine was applied to the scraped area, while a concurrent saline control was negative. Passive transfer of the patient's serum to a nonallergic volunteer prior to the skin window procedure revealed a marked eosinophilia of 44% at the site of the tartrazine application. The passively transferable eosinophilic response in this skin window was suggestive of an immunologic reaction but not conclusive: the patient's serum could have contained nonspecific eosinophilochemotactic factors. More complete immunologic evaluation utilizing a battery of IgE dependent in vitro tests (monkey PCA, leukocyte histamine release, and RAST) and antigenic determinants consisting of intact tartrazine and its azo metabolite, phenylsulphonic pyrazolone, coupled to human serum albumin revealed no evidence of immune responses in a group of 11 patients whose clinical reactivity to tartrazine was confirmed by double-blind oral challenge tests (14). Another group of investigators also studied 16 tartrazine-intolerant patients for possible antitartrazyl-specific IgE antibodies (25). This investigation failed to show evidence of specific IgE antibodies. Specific IgE antibodies to tartrazine and sulfanilic acid–HSA conjugates were reported in five patients suspected of showing immediate hypersensitivity to tartrazine. However, the significance of this report is in doubt because double-blind oral challenge tests were not performed (26). The presence of specific antitartrazine IgD antibodies was noted in the sera of patients with histories of tartrazine reactions but it was not clear whether these suspected reactions were confirmed by double-blind challenge tests (27). Subsequent studies failed to detect significant levels of IgD antibodies in patients with positive tartrazine

Table 5 Suggested Double-Blind Dose–Response Challenge Protocol for Tartrazine on Two Separate Days[a]

Time (hr)	0	½	1	1½
Dose (mg)	Placebo or 10	Placebo or 25	Placebo or 100	Placebo or 200

[a]The order of placebo or tartrazine is determined by random selection.

challenge tests (14). The failure to detect IgE-specific antibodies in proven tartrazine-intolerant patients cannot be attributed to an immunologic artifact or failure to prepare the proper hapten protein conjugate, because other azo-reactive dyes have induced IgE-mediated sensitization (28,29).

b. Type II and III immunologic reactivity

No reactions have been documented.

c. Type IV immunologic reactivity

Induction or natural occurrence of type IV contact sensitization to FD&C yellow dye no. 5 is difficult to demonstrate. Induction of sensitization to tartrazine was attempted by the modified Draize-Shelanki-Jordan technique, which uses 10 24-hr induction periods followed by two challenge 48-hr patches every week after the induction schedule is completed (30). Fifty subjects were tested by this technique with a 20% concentration of tartrazine aqueous solution. Neither sensitization nor irritant reactions were observed in any of the subjects during both induction and challenge periods. A single case of contact sensitization proven by a positive patch test has been reported (31).

d. Anatomical sites of hypersensitivity reactions: Systemic: Several life-threatening anaphylactic episodes have been recorded (20,23). One of these cases presented with hypotension, syncopy, bronchospasm, and a moderate urticarial reaction. These symptoms occurred after use of a generic theophylline preparation. Another case of anaphylaxis was described after exposure to an enema containing both FD&C no. 5 and FD&C no. 6. No fatal anaplyactic reactions have been reported.

e. Anatomical sites of hypersensitivity reactions: Cutaneous: The most common manifestation of tartrazine reactivity is urticaria, either acute or chronic. This is often accompanied by angioedema of the face or other parts of the body. Although tartrazine reactivity was initially suggested as an important cause of chronic idiopathic urticaria, recent studies have not justified these earlier suggestions (16,32). Several patients have experienced allergic purpura induced by tartrazine (33). In some of these cases, the purpuric reaction was exhibited only within a thurfyl nicotinate test area, while in others the purpuric reaction was easily visible after administration of the dye. Although purpura was originally described as a hypersensitivity phenomenon, a nonimmunologic mechanism must also be considered because it has been determined that tartrazine and its sulphophenyl metabolite can inhibit platelet-induced aggregation, an effect particularly pronounced in atopic individuals (34). There is an interesting account of persistent tartrazine-induced rash and eosinophilia appearing in a patient with oliguric renal failure (35). Resolution of symptoms and eosinophilia occurred only after recovery of renal function, suggesting that the pyrazolone tartrazine metabolite, which is excreted via the kidneys, may have been involved in this patient's prolonged adverse reaction. Allergic contact dermatitis is extremely rare, presumably because the contact allergenic potential of this compound is weak.

f. Anatomical sites of hypersensitivity reactions: Respiratory: Asthma is a very common manifestation of tartrazine intolerance. It usually occurs in patients with preexisting aspirin intolerance. As discussed above, the overall prevalence of tartrazine-induced asthma among aspirin-intolerant patients is probably greatly exaggerated. However, once this occurs in individual patients, future contacts with tartrazine must be scrupulously avoided.

g. Pseudoallergic reactions

Inasmuch as immunologic mechanisms have not been demonstrated, both cutaneous and respiratory syndromes elicited by exposure to tartrazine should be classified as pseudoallergic reactions. A suggested mechanism involves the possible role of tartrazine as a cyclooxygenase inhibitor. If this was the case, tartrazine could be instrumental in redirecting the metabolism of arachidonic acid so as to favor increased production of lipooxygenase-mediated leukotrienes. An unconfirmed in vitro study of leukocytes and polyps from aspirin-intolerant subjects demonstrated that tartrazine exhibited direct histamine-releasing properties in a concentration-dependent manner in both of these assay methods. Moreover, tartrazine also released significant amounts of slow-reacting substance from polyps of aspirin-intolerance patients (36). The dose-dependent nature of direct histamine release induced by tartrazine was substantiated by in vitro investigation of mediator release from rat peritoneal mast cells (37). This study showed disparate effects of tartrazine in releasing histamine from rat mast cells. Enhancement of histamine release induced by calcium ionophore was obtained from cells preincubated with 10^{-3} M and 10^{-4} M tartrazine. In contrast, there was a marked inhibition of compound-48/80-induced histamine release in the presence of 10^{-5}–10^{-2} M tartrazine. This inhibition was proportional to the concentration of tartrazine present during incubation and not to the preincubation concentration. The latter effect would suggest a surface membrane effect such as inhibition of receptor binding while the enhancing effects at lower concentrations of tartrazine in the calcium ionophore system suggest a direct biochemical action (37).

The most publicized—and controversial—pseudoallergic effect of tartrazine concerns its possible role in the accentuation of hyperkinesis in hyperactive children. The literature on this subject is too extensive for in depth analysis here. However, selected aspects of the controversy will be summarized.

Hyperkinesis, also known as the attention deficit disorder, involves a combination of hyperactivity, impulsivity, distractibility, and excitability, which may involve between 5 and 10% of American schoolchildren. In 1975, Dr. Benjamin Feingold proposed that the hyperactive syndrome could be controlled by a tartrazine- and preservative-free diet (38). Among several clinical studies that subsequently evaluated these results, it was determined that the Feingold diet could help only a small number of children with hyperkinesis (39,40). These studies also revealed that decreases in hyperreactivity were not observed consistently after removal of tartrazine. It was also learned that challenges with ultrahigh doses of tartrazine in susceptible children could produce a pharmacologiclike effect that depressed learning in specific test situations (41). However, the doses used to obtain these results were up to 150 mg, which the FDA estimates to be at the 90th percentile for daily consumption of artificial dyes by children 5-12 years of age. It is highly unlikely that any child, or adult for that matter, could ingest that much tartrazine in a drug preparation.

2. Sunset Yellow

Compared to the documentation of adverse responses to tartrazine, adverse reports involving sunset yellow (FD&C yellow no. 6) are sparse. There are only scattered individual case reports about possible hyperreactivity to sunset yellow, and in about half of these cases objective proof is lacking. A prospective survey of tartrazine hypersensitivity in patients with urticaria revealed that 60% of the patients reacting to tartrazine also reacted to other azo dyes including sunset yellow (17). This suggested but did not prove a possible cross-reactivity between tartrazine and other azo dyes. In another survey of patients with recurrent urticaria and angioneurotic edema of more than 4 months' duration, it was demonstrated that symptoms improved after elimination of sunset yellow as well as other azo dyes (32). Exposure to sunset yellow in an enema was also documented in one case of life-threatening anaphylaxis, but the enema also contained tartrazine so it was not possible to tell whether one or both of these dyes could be implicated as the actual anaphylactogen(s) (20). Finally, severe upper gastrointestinal symptoms of indigestion, retching, belching, pain, and vomiting were experienced by a 53-year-old woman after ingestion of a tablet containing sunset yellow (42). After use of the drug was discontinued and she was rechalleged with sunset yellow, her symptoms were reproduced in full. No further attempts were made to determine whether this reaction could have an immunologic basis.

3. Miscellaneous

There are scattered adverse reports about other azo FD&C dyes. An anaphylactic episode and several recurrent urticarial syndromes were ascribed to amaranth (FD&C Red No. 2) before it was withdrawn from the market (43,44). A positive bronchoprovocation response was obtained in one patient after double-blinded control challenge with FD&C red dye no. 4 (Ponceau SX) (19). Allergic contact dermatitis after exposure to FD&C red no. 36 was reported in a woman reacting to a cosmetic preparation (45). A similar sensitivity reaction has been induced by FD&C red dye no. 17. Although D&C red dye nos. 36 and 17 are both commonly found in lipsticks, they are also approved for use in externally applied drugs and therefore cross-reactions are possible. However, FD&C-approved azo dyes should not be compared or equated with other azo dyes used primarily for cosmetics (e.g., brilliant lake red) or azo textile dyes (e.g., disperse yellow no. 3). The possibility of cross-reactivity between these various agents has not been scientifically tested.

III. XANTHENE DYES

Because documented instances of adverse reactions to dyes in this category are sparse, they will be considered collectively. Members of the xanthene group include erythrosine (FD&C red no. 3), rhodamine (FD&C red no. 19), eosin Y (FD&C red no. 22), and uranine (FD&C yellow no. 8). Fluoran/xanthene dyes consist of the parent compound, fluorescein (FD&C yellow no. 7) and several halogenated analogs (dibromofluorescein: FD&C orange no. 5; diiodofluorescein: FD&C orange no. 10; tetrabromofluorescein: FD&C red no. 21; and tetrabromotetrachlorofluorescein: FD&C Red No. 27). Xanthenes and fluorans are derivatives of sodium fluorescein, which fluoresces when exposed to light at a wavelength of 3,600–4,000 Å (ultraviolet) (46). Activation of energy releases a gold–green or chartreuse light. As a result of this unique property, fluorescein has been used as a diagnostic marker for viable tissue. It is used extensively to test viability of arterialized flaps, examination of the bowel for ischemia, for retinal perfusion, and as a topical agent to detect corneal lacerations. The recommended intravenous dose varies between 15 and 30 mg/kg. Other xanthene/fluoran derivatives of sodium fluorescein are used in much smaller doses when ingested in the form of drugs or when used in topical medications.

a. Type I immunologic reactivity

The most authoritative report of adverse reactions to sodium fluorescein was compiled by the Fluorescein Angiography Complication Survey (FACS) in 1986 (47). Acute-onset urticaria is a frequent adverse reaction, occurring in approximately 0.5% of patients. There are several case reports of severe systemic reactions including anaphylaxis and cardiac arrest. There are two documented deaths, presumably secondary to anaphylaxis. The overall prevalence of anaphylaxis is estimated to be 0.2% (46). Although the descriptive nature of these acute reactions is suggestive of an IgE-mediated reaction, actual proof of such a mechanism has not been obtained by either direct skin test or demonstration of a specific immunologic response. Therefore, the inclusion of these reactions under type I immune responses is tentative; these reactions might be more properly termed "pseudoallergic" until antigen–antibody reactions have been proved. None of the other xanthene/fluoran derivatives of sodium fluorescein have elicited anaphylactoid symptoms.

b. Type II and III immunologic reactivity

No reactions have been reported.

c. Type IV immunologic reactivity

Several fluorans are potent photosensitizers. The most representative examples of this particular sensitizing property are erythrosine and eosin (48–51). As an example of how potent the photosensitizating potential of erythrosine is, at a concentration of less than 1 μmol/L, it can destroy conduction of action potentials in a lobster nerve axon in less than 5 sec of illumination. This would be comparable to the effects of full-intensity sunlight (48). However, the property of photosensitization is chemically specific because the photosensitizing potency of sodium fluorescein is virtually nonexistent (48).

d. Anatomical sites of hypersensitivity reactions: Systemic: Acute urticaria, angioedema, syncopy and shock, and the full-blown clinical picture of anaphylaxis have been reported after intravenous injections of sodium fluorescein. However, these reactions occurred after injection of relatively large doses of the dye and life-threatening reactions of this type have not been observed after xanthine/fluoran dyes used at the concentrations in most drug preparations.

e. Anatomical sites of hypersensitivity reactions: Cutaneous: Urticaria and angioedema have been reported after exposure to sodium fluorescein. Photosensitization reactions are characterized by erythroderma and desquamation. In one instance, complete alopecia occurred (49). Histopathologic examination of these skin lesions revealed either psoriasislike parakeratosis or spongiosis.

f. Anatomical sites of hypersensitivity reactions: Respiratory: Recrudescence of asthma was demonstrated in one patient with a history of chronic, perennial asthma by use of a double-blind and controlled oral challenge test with erythrosine (19). This single documented case stands in stark contrast to a much larger number of asthma cases associated with exposure to azo FD&C-approved dyes.

g. Pseudoallergic responses

Erythrosine apparently contains enough iodine to cause elevation of the protein-bound iodine (PBI) to hyperthroid levels. This was reported in a patient who ingested lithium carbonate capsules coated with this agent (50). Radioactive iodine (RAI) uptake was also depressed in this patient.

As discussed above, it is not clear whether anaphylacotid or asthmatic reactions occurring after xanthine/fluoran dyes should be classified as truly allergic or as pseudoallergic reactions (46,47).

IV. TRIPHENYLMETHANE DYES

Among the most commonly used FD&C certified dyes are FD&C blue no. 2 (brilliant blue) and FD&C green no. 3 (fast green). The incidence of adverse responses or sensitization to triphenylmethane dyes is unknown because they are not routinely tested in suspected dye reactions. Only indirect evidence about their potential sensitization properties can be inferred by comparing their contact sensitization potentials with those of triphenylmethane therapeutic dyes such as gentian violet, brilliant green, and malachite green (52). The total number of contact sensitization episodes reported after exposure to this group of dyes is low and most of the cases have occurred only after the dyes have been used to treat underlying skin diseases such as eczema or ulcers of the leg. Thus it can be generally assumed that triphenylmethane dyes are weak sensitizers. In support of this it was noted that none among 45 perennial asthmatic patients exhibited a bronchoconstrictive response after double-blind control challenge tests with brilliant blue (FD&C blue dye no. 1) (19). There is one case report of an erythema-multiforme-like skin rash occurring after oral challenge with FD&C green no. 3 (53).

V. INDIGOID DYES

Indigo carmine is the sole representative of this dye class among the most common FD&C dyes. It is used as a colorant for some ingested drugs and for nylon sutures. When injected intravenously, it undergoes rapid renal excretion and is therefore useful to the urologist in delineating ureteral orifices during cystoscopy. Hypersensitivity reactions to this agent have not been documented. However, the intravenous use of indigo carmine has produced severe headache, acute pulmonary edema with cardiac arrest, and hypertension because of transient alpha-adrenergic stimulation (46). None of these reactions are thought to have an immunologic basis.

VI. QUINOLINE DYES

The two major prototypes in this dye category are FD&C yellow No. 10 (quinoline yellow) and FD&C yellow No. 11 (quinoline yellow SS). Both are certified and used widely in a variety of topical pharmaceutical formulations. In 1977, 8.16 tons of FD&C yellow no. 10 dye and 2.23 tons of FD&C yellow no. 11 dye were used in the United States. Since the use of both of these dyes is largely limited to dermatologic preparations, the only noteworthy adverse reaction to these dyes, is allergic contact sensitization. Despite the chemical similarity in these dyes, several prospective studies did not reveal significant clinical cross-reactivity (54-56). Moreover, the sensitizing potential of FD&C yellow no. 11 was far greater than that of D&C yellow no. 10, as demonstrated by a study in which 15 subjects of a panel of 56 (27%) were sensitized to D&C yellow no.11 by repeat insult patch testing technique (56). Another prospective clinical investigation revealed that concentrations as high as 1,000 ppm of quinoline yellow did not induce allergic contact hypersensitivity, while concentrations between 10 and 20 ppm of FD&C yellow dye no. 11 induced delayed hyperreactivity readily in human volunteers (54). Despite the differences between the predictive sensitizing potentials of these external yellow dyes, isolated case reports have documented that quinoline yellow may be a primary sensitizing agent (57). One case report indicated that quinoline yellow and D&C yellow no. 11 may cross-react under certain conditions (58). The final word about cross-reactivity awaits future research. Such studies are necessary in view of the fact that related agents such as iodochlorhydroxyquin, chloroquine, and oxolinic acid are used widely throughout the world as drugs (59).

VII. FDA CERTIFICATION-EXEMPT DYES

This category of dyes (Table 2) is remarkably free of hypersensitivity reactions. Carmine used as a lip salve caused allergic cheilitis in three patients, all of whom demonstrated positive patch tests to carmine(60). Two workers developed occupational asthma after exposure to carmine (61). Both of these exhibited dual asthmatic responses after controlled inhalation challenge to carmine. Oral challenge with carmine provoked gastrointestinal symptoms in one of these patients and asthma in both of them. Prick tests and precipitin analysis were negative in both workers and a RAST test was negative in one patient. Thus immunologically mediated mechanisms in these two workers were not demonstrated. Hypersensitivity reactions to some of the other major FDA-exempt drugs including canthaxanthin, caramel, and titanium oxide have not been reported.

REFERENCES

1. Marmion, D.M. Handbook of U.S. Colorants for Foods, Drugs and Cosmetics, 2nd ed. John Wiley and Sons, New York, 1984.
2. Mitchell, J.C. and Stewart, W.D. Allergic contact dermatitis from neutral red applied for herpes simplex. Arch. Dermatol. 108:689 (1973).
3. Goldenberg, R.L. and Nelson, K. Dermatitis from neutral red therapy of herpes genitalis. Obstet. Gynecol. 46:359–360 (1975).
4. Conant, M. Allergic contact dermatitis due to neutral red. Arch. Dermatol. 109:735 (1974).
5. Guill, M.A. and Odom, R.B. Evans blue dermatitis. Arch. Dermatol. 115:1071–1073 (1979).
6. Lupton, G.P. and Odom, R.B. Dermatitis associated with Evans blue dye. Contact Derm. 6:425–429 (1980).

7. Kalimo, K. and Saarni, H. Immediate reactions to patent blue dye. Contact Derm. 7:171–172 (1981).

8. Kopp, W.L. Anaphylaxis from Alphazurine 2G during lympography. J.A.M.A. 198:200–2001 (1966).

9. Bielicky, T. and Novak, M. Contact-group sensitization to triphenylmethane dyes. Gentian violet, brilliant green and malachite green. Arch. Dermatol. 100:540–543 (1969).

10. Tse, C.S. and Bernstein, I.L. Adverse reactions to tartrazine. Hospital Form. 17(12):1625–1637 (1982).

11. Lee, M., Gentry, A.F. Schwartz, R. et al. Tartrazine-containing drugs. Drug Intell. Clin. Pharm. 15:782–788 (1981).

12. Chaffee, F.H. and Settipane, G.A. Asthma caused by FD&C approved dyes. J. Allergy 40:65–72 (1967).

13. Samter, M. and Beers, R.F. Intolerance to aspirin. Clinical studies and consideration of its pathogenesis. Ann. Intern. Med. 68:975–983 (1968).

14. Bernstein, I.L., Gallagher, J.S., Johnson, H. et al. Immunologic and non-immunologic factors in adverse reactions to tartrazine. Proceedings, 4th FDA Science Symposium (Asher, I.M. eds.). U.S. Govt. Printing Office, Washington, D.C., pp. 258–260 (1980).

15. Supramaniam, G. and Warner, J.O. Artificial food additive intolerance in patients with angio-edema and urticaria. Lancet 2:907–909 (1986).

16. Stevenson, D.D., Simon, R.A., Lumry, W.R., et al. Adverse reactions to tartrazine. J. Allergy Clin. Immunol 78:182–191 (1986).

17. Michaelsson, G. and Juhlin, L. Urticaria induced by perservatives and dye additives in food and drugs. Br. J. Dermatol. 88:525–532 (1973).

18. Spector, S.L., Wangaard, C.H. and Farr, R.S. Aspirin and concomitant idiosyncrasies in adult asthmatic patients. J. Allergy Clin. Immunol. 64:500 (1979).

19. Weber, R.W., Hoffman, M., Raine, D.A. Jr. et al. Incidence of bronchoconstriction due to aspirin, azo dyes, non-azo dyes, and preservatives in a population of perennial asthmatics. J. Allergy Clin. Immunol. 64:32–37 (1979).

20. Desmond, R.E. and Trautlein, J.J. Tartrazine (FD&C Yellow #5) anaphylaxis: A case report. Ann. Allergy 46:81–82 (1981).

21. Zlotlow, M.J. and Settipane, G.A. Allergic potential of food additives: A report of a case of tartrazine sensitivity without aspirin intolerance. Am. J. Clin. Nutrition 30:1023–1025 (1977).

22. Yellow No. 5 (tartrazine) labelling on drugs to be required. FDA Drug Bull. 9(3):18 (1979).

23. Trautlein, J.J. and Mann, W.J. Anaphylactic shock caused by yellow dye (FD&C #5 and FD&C #6) in an enema (case report). Ann. Allergy 41:28–29 (1978).

24. Chafee, F.H. and Settipane, G.A. Asthma caused by FD&C approved dyes. J. Allergy 40:65–72 (1967).

25. Weltman, J.K., Szaro, R.P. and Settipane, G.A. An analysis of the role of IgE in intolerance to aspirin and tartrazine. Allergy 34:273–281 (1978).

26. Guerin, B., Hewitt, B. and Brighton, W.D. Prospective testing for allergenicity. *In* Immunotoxicology. (Gibson, G.G., Hubbard, R., and Parke, D.V. eds). Academic Press, London, pp 457–462 (1983).

27. Weliky, N. and Heiner, D.C. Hypersensitivity to chemicals. Correlation of tartrazine hypersensitivity with characteristic serum IgD and IgE immune response patterns. Clin. Allergy 10:375–394 (1980).

28. Alanko, K., Keskinen, H., Bjorkstein, F. et al. Immediate-type hypersensitivity to reactive dyes. Clin. Allergy 8:25–31 (1978).

29. Lagmar, L., Welinder, H. and Dahlquist, I. Immunoglobulin E antibodies against a reactive dye–a case report. Scand. J. Work Environ. Health 12: 221-222 (1986).

30. Rapaport, M. Allergy to yellow dyes. Arch. Dermatol. 120:535–536 (1984).

31. Roeleveld, C.G. and van Ketel, W.G. Positive patch test to the azo-dye tartrazine. Contact Derm. 2:180 (1976).

32. Ros, A.M., Juhlin, L. and Michaelsson, G. A follow-up study of patients with recurrent urticaria and hypersensitivity to aspirin, benzoates and azo dyes. Br. J. Dermatol. 95:19–24 (1976).

33. Michaelsson, G., Pettersson, L. and Juhlin, L. Purpura caused by food and drug additives. Arch. Dermatol. 109:49–52 (1974).

34. Gallagher, J.S., Splansky, G.L., and Bernstein, I.L. Inhibition of platelet aggregation by tartrazine and a pyrazolone analogue in normal and allergic individuals. Clin. Allergy 10:683–690 (1980).

35. Brettle, R.P., Curtis, L., Pinching, A.J. et al. Tartrazine sensitivity in renal failure. Lancet 1: Jan. 26:167 (1979).

36. Hedman, S.E. and Andersson, R.G.G. Release of biological mediators by tartrazine from human leukocytes and polyps. Acta Pharmacol. Toxicol. 52:153–154 (1983).

37. Safford, R.J. and Goodwin, B.F.J. The effect of tartrazine on histamine release from rat peritoneal mast cells. Int. J. Immunopharmacal. 6(3): 233–240 (1984).

38. Feingold, B.F. Why Your Child is Hyperactive. Random House, New York (1975).

39. Conners, C.K. Address to the National Advisory Committee on Hyperkinesis and Food Additives. The Nutrition Foundation, Inc., New York, January (1979).

40. Weiss, B., William, J.H., Margen, S. et al. Food dyes impair performance of hyperactive children on a laboratory learning test. Science 198:1274 (1977).

41. Weiss, B., Williams, J.H., Margen, S. et al. Behavioral responses to artificial food colors. Science 207:1487–1488 (1980).

42. Jenkins, P., Michelson, R. and Emerson, P.A. Adverse drug reaction to sunset-yellow in rifampicin/isoniazid tablet. Lancet 2:385 (1982).

43. Lockey, S.D. Sr. Hypersensitivity to tartrazine (FD&A Yellow No. 5) and other dyes and additives present in foods and pharmaceutical products. Ann. Allergy 38:206–210 (1977).

44. Speer, F., Denison, T.R. and Baptist, J.E. Aspirin allergy. Ann. Allergy 46: 123–126 (1981).
45. English, J.S.C. and White, I.R. Dermatitis from D & C Red no. 36. Contact Derm. 13:335 (1985).
46. Flewellen, E.G. Hazards of intravenous indigo carmine, fluorescein and methylene blue. Texas Med. 76:49–51 (1980).
47. Yannuzzi, L.A., Rohrer, K.T., Tindel, L.J. et al. Fluorescein angiography complication survey. Ophthalmology 93:611–617 (1986).
48. Valenzeno, D.P. and Pooler, J.P. Phototoxicity. The neglected factor. J.A.M.A. 242(5):453–454 (1979).
49. Castelain, P.Y. and Piriou, A. Photosensitization eczema with positive erythrosine test. Contact Derm. 4(5):305 (1978).
50. Haas, S. Contamination of protein-bound iodine by pink gelatin capsules colored with erythrosine. Ann. Intern. Med. 72:549–552 (1970).
51. Kalivas, J. A guide to the problem of photosensitivity. J.A.M.A. 209:1706–1709 (1969).
52. Bielicky, T. and Novak, M. Contact-group sensitization to triphenylmethane dyes. Gentian violet, brilliant green and malachite green. Arch. Dermatol. 100:540–543 (1969).
53. Grater, W.C. Hypersensitive skin reactions to FD&C dyes. Cutis 17:1163–1165 (1976).
54. Weaver, J.E. Dose response relationships in delayed hypersensitivity to quinoline dyes. Contact Derm. 9:309–312 (1983).
55. Weaver, J.E. Disparate skin allergenicity of 2 quinoline dyes. Short communications. Contact Derm. 9(6):526–527 (1983).
56. Rapaport, M. Allergy to yellow dyes. Arch. Dermatol. 120:535 (1984).
57. Bjorkner, B. and Magnusson, B. Patch test sensitization to D & C yellow No. 11 and simultaneous reaction to quinoline yellow. Contact Derm. 7:1–4 (1981).
58. Bjorkner, B. and Nilasson, B. Contract allergic reaction to D & C Yellow No. 11 and quinoline yellow. Contact Derm. 9:263–268 (1983).
59. Fisher, A.A. Allergic reactions to D & C yellow No. 11 dye. Cutis 34:344–350 (1984).
60. Sarkany, I., Meara, R.H. and Everall, J. Cheilitis due to carmine in lip salve. Trans. Ann. Rep. St. John's Hosp. Dermatol. Soc. 46:39 (1961).
61. Burge, P.S., O'Brien, I.M., Harries, M.G. et al. Occupational asthma due to inhaled carmine. Clin. Allergy 9:185–189 (1979).

15

Allergic Reactions: Other Addition Products

I. Controlled release and binding agents   283
II. Buffers   289
III. Suspending emulsifying, and stiffening agents   289
   A. Anionic agents   289
   B. Nonanionic, amphoteric, and polypeptide emulsifiers and
      detergents   290
   C. Cationic agents   292
   D. Vegetable gums   293
   E. Methylcellulose   295
   F. Paraffin products   295
   G. Lubricants   295
   H. Fatty alcohols   296
IV. Preservatives   296
   A. Antimicrobials   296
V. Antioxidants   312
   A. Nordihydroguaiaretic acid, butylated hydroxyanisole, butylated
      hydroxytoluene, gallic acid esters and alpha-tocopherol   312
   B. Sulfites   314
VI. Stabilizers: Ethylenediamine   320
VII. Chelating agents   323
VIII. Sterilizing agents   324
IX. Propellants   328
   References   329

I. CONTROLLED RELEASE AND BINDING AGENTS

The rapidly evolving technology of drug delivery systems has expanded the number and function of excipients. Table 1 is a partial compilation of nearly "inert" substances used in a variety of manufacturing processes as film formers for microencapsulation, slow release and enteric coatings, expandable hydrocolloids, buccal adhesives, osmotic dispensers, implant delivery systems, skin adhesives, and transdermal diffusion devices. It also includes many materials

Table 1 Summary of Selected Nontoxic Adverse Reactions of Commonly Used Biomaterials Contained In Slow Release and Microencapsulation Products

Substance	Immune responses	Other adverse reactions	Exposure		Chapter in text
			Route	Source	
Adipic acid	NE	Asthma	Inhaled	Antibiotic	15
Acid anydrides					
Acetic	Type I (urticaria/angioedema)	NE	Ingestion	Aspirin	15
Citric	NE	NE	—	—	15
Dicarboxylic	NE	NE	—	—	15
Maleic	NE	NE	—	—	15
Acrylic monomers	Type IV (contact dermatitis)	NE	Skin	Bone cement	16
Acrylic polymers	NE	Foreign body	Hip implant	Bone cement	16
Agar	NE	NE	—	—	15
Albumin					
Hen	NE	NE	Ingestion	Tablet film	15
Human	Type I (wheal/flare)	Anaphylactoid	Injection	Biologics	13
Alginates	NE	Asthma	Inhalation	Seaweed	12
Casein	NE	NE	—	—	15
Cellulose					
Methyl	Type I (wheal/flare)	NE	Ingestion	Penicillin	15
Carboxymethyl	Type IV (contact)	NE	Skin	Glove powder	15
Collagen (bovine)	Type I (urticaria)	NE	Injection	Implant (Skin substitute)	16
Dextran	NE	Anaphylactoid	Injection	Plasma expander	11

Agent	Hypersensitivity type	Other reaction	Route	Source/Use	Ref.
Ethylenediamine	Type IV (contact dermatitis)	NE	Skin	Topicals	15
Ethylene–vinyl acetate copolymers	NE	NE	Skin	Topicals	15
Gelatin	NE	Anaphylactoid	Ingestion, injection	Animals	12
Gluten	NE	NE	Ingestion	Wheat	12
Pectin	NE	NE	Ingestion	Apples	15
Phthlates (esters of phthalic acid)	NE	NE	Ingestion	Phthalic acid	15
Polyamides	NE	NE	Ingestion	Synthetic	15
Polyester	NE	NE	Ingestion	Synthetic	15
Polyethylene glycol	Type I (urticaria); Type IV (contact dermatitis)	Intolerance	Skin	Topicals	11
Polyaminoacids	NE	NE	Ingestion	Synthetic	15
Polycarbonates	NE	NE	Ingestion	Synthetic	15
Polyvinyl chloride	Type III (necrotizing dermatitis), Type IV (contact dermatitis)	NE	Intravenous Skin	Dialysis Topicals	15
Polyvinylpyrrolidone	NE	NE	Ingestion	Capsules	12
Epoxy resins	NE	NE	Skin	Topical devices	15
Shellac	NE	NE	Ingestion	Capsules	15
Siloxanes and silicone	Type I (urticaria);	Pneumonia	Systemic	Implants	12
Starch	Type IV (contact dermatitis)	Peritonitis	Skin	Topical (rubber gloves)	16
Stearates and stearic acid	Type I, IV (contact urticaria)	NE	Skin	Sun screen	15

Table 1 (Continued)

Substance	Immune responses	Other adverse reactions	Exposure Route	Source	Chapter in text
Triethylenetetramine	Type IV (contact dermatitis)	NE	Skin	Topicals	15
Vegetable gums					
Acacia					
Tragacanth	Type I (urticaria and asthma)	NE	Ingestion	Tablets	15
Karaya	Type IV (contact dermatitis)		Skin	Topicals	
Guar					
Vegetable oils	Type IV (contact dermatitis)	NE	Skin	Topicals	11
Waxes	Type IV (contact dermatitis)	NE	Skin	Topical	11
Zinc dithiocarbamate	Type IV contact dermatitis	NE	Skin	Topicals	15

NE, not established.

used as excipients in traditional drug manufacturing formulas. Table 1 also indicates specific sections where these agents have been discussed elsewhere in this book.

Adverse clinical experiences with the remaining substances in this list have either been rare or nonexistent. Whatever information is available about this miscellaneous group of excipients will be included in this section. Some of these reactions have been described only after sensitization and/or exposure by non-drug-related routes, so their capacities to cause adverse reactions as medicinal excipients must be considered hypothetical.

Adipic acid is a bicarboxylic acid used as a general additive for its buffer and neutralizing power. The diagnosis of occupational asthma was confirmed by a controlled challenge test to a 1% solution of adipic acid in one patient (1). Several acid anhydride compounds (citric, dicarboxylic, and maleic) may be incorporated into some of these products. Acid anhydride compounds are highly reactive chemicals and are known to combine readily with body proteins. For example, specific IgE antibodies to o-acetylsalicylic anhydride, a contaminant of commercial aspirin, were demonstrated in patients with the urticaria/angioedema type of aspirin intolerance (2). A variety of allergic reactions have been observed after exposure to a number of other acid anhydride compounds (phthalic anhydride, trimellitic anhydride, himic anhydride, tetrachlorophthalic anhydride, and hexahydrophthalic anhydride) required in the manufacturing and curing of epoxy resins, alkyl resins, polyester resins, plasticizers, and vinyl resins (3). Cross-reactivity between the pharmaceutical and occupational acid anhydride compounds has not been demonstrated. Acrylic polymer resins are not sensitizing but acrylic monomers such as methyl, ethyl, and butyl esters of methacrylic acid are potent sensitizers both in humans and animals(4). Exposure to the monomeric acrylates during the acrylate resin curing process may cause allergic contact dermatitis (5).

Plant hydrocolloids such as agar and alginates are derived from algal sources. The former agent is nonsensitizing. Alginates are discussed in more detail in Chapter 12. Egg albumin is one of the components in the tablet film of one brand of erythromycin. Although allergic reactions have not been ascribed to this ingredient, immunologically induced responses to oral erythromycin are not infrequent. In such cases, use of the drug is discontinued on the assumption that the clinical reaction was drug induced. Possible allergy to the egg albumin excipient in the film of the tablet has not yet been investigated. Casein, a natural protein constituent of milk, has a very low sensitizing potential when ingested in the form of food and has not presented problems as a drug additive. Synthetic cellulose derivatives have wide applications in medicinals. They are used as demulcents, colloid laxatives, and as suspending agents in ophthalmic preparations, nose drops, and other topical drugs. At one time carboxymethylcellulose (CMC) was used as an additive in the production of penicillin oral tablets. This formulation apparently increased the allergenic potential of penicillin because haptenic metabolites of penicillin G could readily bind covalently to CMC in the ratio of 0.2–0.5 haptenic groups per 100 glucose groups (6). These substituted celluloses elicited immediate-type skin responses in sensitized patients. Rarely, allergic contact dermatitis may be induced by carboxymethylcellulose (7). The drug industry subsequently recognized that polymeric cellulose and other long-chain polysaccharides could subserve a carrier function for reactive drugs or their metabolites. Methylcellulose itself lacks allergenic properties and therefore it is gradually replacing lactose as the inert ingredient in placebo tablets and capsules. Dextran, a long-chain polymer of glucose, has direct histamine-releasing properties that are more likely to occur after use of larger molecular weight homologs. However, dextrans used as additives have not caused side effects. Pectin, a purified carbohydrate product, consists chiefly of polygalacturonic acid. It is used primarily as an adsorbent and has no known allergenic characteristics. Specific instances of adverse reactions have not been reported in the literature after use of polyamides, polyesters, polyamino acids, and polycarbonates as drug additives. The polymerized form of vinyl chloride (polyvinyl chloride) is generally nonsensitizing. In the final product, however, there are frequently monomers as well as a number of other additives that include phthalate esters, phthalic acid anhydride, and epoxidized soybean oil. Workers exposed to thermal decomposition products of polyvinyl chloride have developed occupational asthma due to phthalic acid anhydride and epoxidized soybean oil (8). Objective evidence and responses to various phthalate plasticizers were not detected. Moreover, the esters of phthalic acid have very low contact dermatitis sensitizing properties, as shown by a joint patch test prospective survey conducted in 1975 by the International Contact Dermatitis Research Group (9). Occasional cases of contact dermatitis to vinyl polymer have been noted (10). Necrotizing dermatitis occurred in a patient undergoing dialysis exposed to uncoated polyvinyl chloride tubing (11). The skin lesions were reproduced by epicutaneous application of the polyvinyl chloride tubing and immunohistologic findings consisted of intravascular deposits of IgG, C3, and C9. When polyurethane-coated polyvinyl chloride tubing was substituted for uncoated tubing, there was prompt clearing of all skin lesions. There is a single case report of contact dermatitis induced by dibutylphthalate (12).

Polyvinyl polyvinylpyrrolidone is a copolymer with a mean molecular weight of 40,000 daltons. Similarly to dextran, it has potent direct histamine-releasing effects after systemic administration. However, oral administration of this substance in small amounts is not known to elicit adverse symptoms. Diffusion devices often contain ethylene–vinyl acetate copolymers that are inert insofar as allergic reactions are concerned.

Epoxy resins are rarely allergenic once they are hardened or cured. Under unusual conditions of grinding or exposure to high heat, decomposition products of resins (e.g., phthalic anhydride) have been known to cause allergic repiratory symptoms (3). Occupationally related contact dermatitis to one of the cold curing agents, triethylenetetramine, is not uncommon (13). This agent is potentially important because it cross-reacts with ethylenediamine, an important stabilizer in many drug formulations to be discussed further in this chapter (14).

Small amounts of shellac may be present in microencapsulation films and in dental impression compounds. Contact dermatitis to shellac has been observed after occupational exposure to this agent, but no recorded episodes of allergic reactivity to this material when used as an additive have been described.

Stearates, stearyl alcohol, and stearic acid are nonallergenic. Zinc dithiocarbamate was responsible for a severe adhesive tape reaction in one patient (15). Since thiocarbamates decompose to isothiocyanates, the possibility of cross-reactivity in patients previously sensitized to various diisocyanates in the workplace should be considered (16).

Buccal adhesive and transdermal delivery devices may enhance the induction of sensitivity to the active drug. The continuous and prolonged buccal or cutaneous exposure to active drug afforded by these long-term delivery systems may augment the local immune response to the drug, which ordinarily would have a low sensitization potential when administered by traditional routes (e.g., nitroglycerin) (17). There are conflicting reports concerning activation of Langerhans cells by occlusive delivery devices (18,19).

Although altered reactivity to the excipients described in this section is rare or nonexistent, it should be recognized that they are being used with increased frequency in various new formulation processes and should be monitored on a prospective basis for possible future clinical effects. Further discussion about specific biomaterials contained in medical devices will follow this chapter.

II. BUFFERS

There are no known allergic reactions to phosphate, borate, acetate, citrate, phthalate, or Tris buffers. Human serum albumin buffers may involve a small risk of anaphylaxis, as previously discussed.

III. SUSPENDING, EMULSIFYING, AND STIFFENING AGENTS

A. Anionic Agents

The substances in this category are used chiefly as emulsifying agents in topical dermatologic products. Some of the surfactant agents in this group include sodium lauryl sulfate, lauryl and myristic acid dialkanolamide, and coconut diethanolamide.

a. Type I-III immunologic reactivity

No reactions have been documented.

b. Type IV immunologic reactivity

Contact sensitivity has been reported after exposure to the most commonly used anionic surfactant agents (20-23). In the case of sodium lauryl sulfate, positive lymphocyte transformation tests were demonstrated in 10 of 12 patients suspected of having sodium lauryl sulfate contact skin allergy (22). Confirmation of allergic contact dermatitis in several other cases has been corroborated by both open and closed patch tests at concentrations between 0.5 and 1%.

c. Anatomical sites of hypersensitivity reactions: *Cutaneous*: Contact allergic dermatitis is the chief hypersensitivity manifestation. This usually appears over areas of preexisting dermatitis being treated with topical products containing one or more of these surfactants.

d. Pseudoallergic reactions

Sodium lauryl sulfate (SLS) is a known skin irritant because its surface tension properties are irritating and increase its capacity for skin penetration. At times it is used specifically to aid penetration of other substances in patch tests (the so-called SLS provocative patch test) (24). Its profound irritant effect has been observed in 52% of patients with eczema and 12% of control subjects tested with 5% aqueous solution of SLS. Because of its marked irritant effects, the diagnosis of contact allergic dermatitis induced by SLS can only be made when positive reactions occur at sites patch tested with very dilute solutions (0.05-1.0%).

B. Nonionic, Amphoteric, and Polypeptide Emulsifiers and Detergents

A wide assortment of surfactant substances are used as emulsifying and solubilizing reagents in pharmaceutical formulations. Among the most common emulsifiers are sorbitan monolaurate, various Spans (sorbitan monooleate, sorbitan monostearate), Arlacel (sorbitan sesquioleate), Tweens (polyoxyethylene sorbitan monopalmitate, poloxyethylene sorbitan monooleate), polyoxyethylene oxypropylene stearate, glycerol monostearate, and triethanolamine stearate. Cremophor EL is used as a solvent for steroids and fat-soluble vitamins as well as an emulsifying agent for topical creams and parenterally administered cyclosporine. Cocobetaine, an amphoteric detergent, may be found in therapeutic shampoos. Coconut diethanolamine is a mild surface active agent that has a synergistic detergent action in low concentration when mixed with sodium lauryl sulfate and other surface-acting agents (23). Fatty acid polypeptide conjugates complexed to triethanolamine have been used as mild surfactants in skin cleansers and eardrops (25,26).

a. Type I immunologic reactivity

Anaphylactic reactions to Cremophor EL have been reported in several patients. The immunologic mechanism of such reactions is still conjectural. Complement-mediated reactions have been suspected but not proved (27). The possibility of a type I immunologic mechanism was suggested by positive skin tests in one case and the demonstration of Cremophor-EL-specific short-term sensitizing antibody (IgG reagin) by passive transfer tests (28). A systemic reaction was induced by an oral preparation containing Cremophor El (29).

b. Type II and III immunologic reactivity

No proven cases have been reported although several authors have speculated about the possibility of complement activation and anaphylatoxin release as causes of anaphylactoid reactions.

c. Type IV immunologic reactivity

Although contact skin hypersensitivity may occur after exposure to Spans, Tweens, and various stearate surfactants, the sensitization index of these materials is low (30). The vast majority of patients with emulsifier allergy were also found to be hypersensitive to many other agents. Since emulsifiers can be expected to cause irritant reactions in epicutaneous tests, patch tests should be removed after 24 hr and read 3 times during the subsequent 4–5 days. Irritant reactions usually occur at the highest level by the first day and usually fade by 4–5 days. The reactions that occur at this time are considered to be allergic in nature. Triethanolamine stearate has the dubious distinction of having the highest irritant potential among this group of surfactants, even at the relatively low concentration of 5% (31). However, bona fide reports of contact dermatitis to triethanolamine stearate have appeared (32–34).

d. Anatomical sites of hypersensitivity reactions

Systemic: The systemic reactions to Cremophor EL are anaphylactoid in nature. If they occur during administration of an anesthetic agent containing this solvent, the only manifestation may be cyanosis and therefore the true nature of the reaction may go unrecognized for several minutes. However, the cyanosis is soon followed by diffuse erythema (28).

Cutaneous: Most of the individual cases of contact dermatitis have occurred in patients with preexisting dermatitis. These patients were treated with hydrocortisone preparations containing these emulsifiers (35,36). Contact dermatitis of the scalp has been attributed to shampoos containing the triethanolamine salt of coconut fatty acids condensed with hydrolyzed polypeptides (25). An unusual feature of this type of dermatitis is that the patient tends to be intolerant to a variety of cosmetics and soaps for some months after the acute episode of dermatitis. These persistent reactions may be due to heightened sensitivity to nonspecific irritants. Severe contact dermatitis may develop in eardrops formulated to remove cerumen (26). The active ingredient in these materials is an oleyl polypeptide that is a condensation product of oleic acid and hydrolyzed animal protein coupled to triethanolamine. Dermatitis in such cases can be severe, spreading to the neck, face, chest, and back and, in one case, periorbital edema mimicking angioneurotic edema was observed.

e. Pseudoallergic reactions

Inhalant exposure to ethanolamine compounds used in household products or in spray paints may cause nonspecific upper and lower airways symptoms (37,38). The irritant skin properties of detergents in this category are similar to those previously described for anionic detergents. To avoid confusion with such reactions, a patch test must be done with very dilute solutions and the patch test interpretation procedure should be extended 4-5 days so that irritant responses may have sufficient time to subside prior to the later development of allergic reactivity at the site of the patch.

C. Cationic Agents

Quaternary ammonium compounds are the chief offenders in this category. These compounds include benzalkonium chloride, cetrimonium bromide (cetrimide), cetalkonium chloride, and cethexonium bromide. Although quaternary ammonium compounds are most often used for their antiseptic and antibacterial properties, they are also used as cationic surface active agents in pharmaceutical preparations and medical devices. The primary preservative in most contact lens soaking solutions is benzalkonium chloride (39). Some nebulizer solutions also contain benzalkonium chloride as a preservative (40). Both benzalkonium chloride and cetrimide may be combined with bactericidal antiseptics such as chlorhexidine to enhance the effect of the primary antiseptic component. Cationic surface agents dissociate in aqueous solution into a relatively large complex cation and a small inactive anion. The large cation acts as an emulsifying bond between water and the lipid secretions of the skin surface, thereby enhancing the activity of the primary antibacterial agent (41). Benzalkonium chloride may be incorporated into plaster of Paris to improve its binding characteristics (42).

a. Types I–III immunologic reactivity

No documented instances have been reported.

b. Type IV immunologic reactivity

Isolated case reports of allergic contact dermatitis to both benzalkonium chloride and cetrimonium bromide (cetrimide) have been reported and documented by classic 48 hr closed patch tests (42-45). The proper concentration of benzalkonium chloride for patch tests is 1:750 or 1:1,000 (v/v). Cross reactions between quaternary ammonium compounds have been demonstrated (46).

c. Anatomical sites of hypersensitivity reactions

Cutaneous: Both allergic ophthalmic mucositis and contact dermatitis have been reported after sensitization to benzalkonium chloride (39-42). Sensitization is more likely to occur over areas being treated for preexisting dermatitis. There are special risk factors for contact dermatitis in medical personnel who are exposed to instruments soaked in various products containing benzalkonium chloride or related analogs. For example, allergic conjunctivitis occurred in a nurse who used an ophthalmic preparation containing benzalkonium chloride. Two years previously, he had acquired a severe hand dermatitis after using an antiseptic containing the same substance (39). Predictive maximization patch tests initially indicated that benzalkonium chloride would have minimal sensitizing potential, a prediction generally confirmed by overall clinical experience, which demonstrates that it and related compounds have a low index of contact sensitization. However, these compounds should be suspected as possible causative agents in medical and paramedical personnel. Unusual cases of contact dermatitis have been described after use of benzalkonium chloride "medicated" adhesive tape and plaster of Paris (39,42). Exacerbation of contact dermatitis may occur in previously sensitive patients by use of medical instruments or catheters disinfected with benzalkonium-containing antiseptic solutions (46). For unexplained reasons the incidence of allergic contact sensitivity to quaternary ammonium compounds is common in France (39). Moreover, generalized reactions have been observed after systemic administration of chemically related drugs such as tetraethylammonium chloride and decamethonium bromide. The immunologic significance of such reactions has not been determined.

d. Pseudoallergic reactions

Bronchodilator nebulizer solutions containing benzalkonium chloride may increase bronchial reactivity, leading to bronchoconstriction and cough in asthmatic subjects with preexisting bronchial hyperresponsiveness (40). This bronchoconstrictive effect may be inhibited by prior administration of cromolyn sodium. The concentration of benzalkonium chloride at which this effect was observed was 0.2 g/L. At lower concentrations benzalkonium chloride may release histamine in several in vitro mast cell models. The human bronchoconstrictive effect is presumably nonimmunologic.

D. Vegetable Gums

Vegetable gums are used to suspend heavy insoluble powders, as an excipient for tablets, to impart consistency to troches, and in the preparation of emulsions.

The most commonly used vegetable gums are gum arabic (derived from the tree, *Acacia senegal*), tragacanth, and karaya. Other less commonly used gums include India gum (Ghatti gum), locust gum, and gum guar. It is noteworthy that the majority of adverse reactions to vegetable gums were reported prior to 1950. These include reports of systemic (possibly anaphylactoid) reactions after intravenous injections of acacia, asthma in printers who inhaled gum arabic in the course of their occupational duties, and IgE-mediated occupational asthma after inhalation of guar gum, and respiratory and gastrointestinal symptoms after ingeastion of vegetable gums contained in foods and toothpaste (48-50). More recent and extensive studies of gum arabic in particular revealed that immune responses to the gums are comparable but not greater than those elicited by common food components such as egg ovalbumin. Furthermore, it has been determined experimentally that gum arabic acts as an immunologic tolerogen when administered by the gastrointestinal route (51). Documented occurences of adverse responses to vegetable gums contained in pharmaceuticals and topical preparations are rare.

a. Type I immunologic reactivity

A clinical history of asthma and urticaria induced by tragacanth in an antihistamine tablet was confirmed by direct intracutaneous testing followed by general urticaria within 8 min. The immunologic specificity of this acute reaction was confirmed by passive transfer testing (52). Similar hypersensitivity reactions were reported in several patients receiving prednisone tablets containing acacia and tragacanth (53). The hypersensitivity reactions in these patients were manifested by itching, rash, fever, and arthralgia. One of these patients had a positive direct skin test response to acacia, the other to tragacanth. The immunologic specificity of these reactions was not confirmed by further immunologic testing.

IgE immunologic cross-reactivity has been demonstrated between one species of acacia tree (wattle) and rye grass pollen extract (54). Thus the presence of IgE-specific antibodies in a patient with concomitant rye grass allergy may not necessarily indicate clinical sensitivity to acacia or its derivative, gum arabic.

b. Types II and III immunologic reactivity

No reactions have been documented.

c. Type IV immunologic reactivity

One case of contact dermatitis induced by tragacanth contained in electrocardiographic (ECG) electrode jelly has been reported (55). The immunologic specificity of this reaction was confirmed by a patch test with a 1% aqueous solution of gum tragacanth. Two cases of erythematous rash occurred in patients receiving transcutaneous electrical muscle stimulation with karaya-impregnated electrode pads (56). Unfortunately, the immunologic cause of these skin reactions was not confirmed. Karaya gum is also used as a skin barrier for routine care of ileostomies and colostomies. It is available in sealed rings, paste, and dry powders. A therapist developed upper and lower respiratory symptoms after exposure and sensitization to karaya gum powder. This was confirmed by a markedly positive scratch test response (57).

d. Anatomical sites of hypersensitivity reactions

Cutaneous: Generalized urticaria occurred in one patient after a challenge test with tragacanth contained in an antihistamine tablet. The reaction occurred 8 min after application of the challenge test. Several other patients developed maculopapular rashes after ingesting tablets containing acacia and tragacanth (53). Topically induced contact dermatitis has been reported after contact sensitization both to karaya gum and tragacanth (55,56).

Respiratory: A single patient developed sneezing, rhinorrhea, and asthma after sensitization and subsequent challenge with an antihistamine tablet containing tragacanth (52).

e. Pseudoallergic reactions

None have been reported.

E. Methylcellulose

Methylcellulose is inert and without adverse effects when administered as a filler or suspending product in oral medications. Because of its innocuous properties it should be considered as a more ideal filler than lactose for oral placebo tablets or capsules. However, a closely related cellulose polymer, sodium carboxymethylcellulose, may act not only as an immunologic carrier reagent but also as a contact sensitizer (6,58) (see this chapter, Section I).

F. Paraffin Products

Clinical adverse reactions to petroleum-derived paraffin products are extremely uncommon. These have been discussed in more detail previously.

G. Lubricants

Although talc induces severe granulomatous reactions in body tissues, these lesions are thought to be foreign body reactions and without allergic significance. Talc is no longer recommended for lubricating surgical gloves. However, one of the apparent benign substitutes used for this purpose (cornstarch) may induce allergic reactions. As previously discussed, the allergic potential of edible vegetable oils is extremely low. More detailed discussion of their adverse responses is found elsewhere.

H. Fatty Alcohols

Reference to topical sensitization induced by higher fatty alcohols (e.g., stearyl alcohol) may be found in Chapter 11.

IV. PRESERVATIVES

A. Antimicrobials

Many biocidal chemicals are used in the ophthalmic and dermatologic drug industries. Antimicrobials are also used to preserve parenteral preparations. Among the large number of these agents currently available, the vast majority of adverse and allergic reactions are accounted for by several main categories of chemicals.

1. Phenol, Phenol-Related Compounds, and Metabolites

Phenol may be found in topical skin preparations. Halogenated phenols such as thymol (isopropyl metacresol) and chlorocresol are found in dentifrices and mouth washes. Chlorocresols are also used as preservatives for some intravenous heparin products.

a. Type I immunologic reactivity

Documented evidence of IgE-mediated reactivity to these agents is lacking. There are several cases of anaphylactoid reactions (collapse, pallor, sweating, hypotension, and tachycardia) in patients who received chlorocresol-preserved heparin intravenously (59). In one of these cases, an intradermal skin test with preservative-free heparin was negative and future treatment with this preparation was uneventful. However, no direct skin test or in vitro evidence of an IgE response to chlorocresol was demonstrated. Late local reactions consisting of erythematous indurations have been reported in patients receiving subcutaneous injections of chlorocresol-preserved heparin. Immediate skin test responses after testing with chlorocresol-preserved heparin were obtained in a number of these patients. However, no other specific immunologic confirmation was attempted.

b. Type II and III immunologic reactivity

No clear evidence of these reactions has been recorded.

c. Type IV immunologic reactivity

Phenol itself is a rare sensitizer (60). The incidence of contact sensitivity to chlorocresol is low even though its use as a preservative in corticosteroids is extensive (61,62). In one study of 1,462 consecutive dermatitis patients who were patch tested with 2% chlorocresol and petrolatum, only 11 had positive

results (0.8%) (63). Sporadic case reports of classic contact eczematous dermatitis confirmed by patch testing have appeared in the literature over the past 20
years (61,64). The weak sensitizing potential of chlorocresol was also noted in
Draize tests of normal subjects who were tested with 5% chlorocresol as the
induction agent (65). It has been cautioned that weak contact reactions to
chlorocresol may represent cross-reactivity to chloroxylenol, a frequent contactant among users of topical medicinals in the United Kingdom (62). Contactant
allergic reactions have also been documented after exposure to phenol derivatives (2-monomethylol phenol, 2-4 dimethylol phenol and 2,6-dimethylol
phenol) and dihydroxy-diphenyl methanes present in phenol formaldehyde
resins (66–68).

d. Anatomical sites of hypersensitivity reactions

Systemic: Anaphylactoid reactions have been suspected after administration
of chlorocresol-preserved heparin. Since the immunologic specificity of such
reactions has not been demonstrated, these reactions must be currently classified as nonspecific. However, it is noteworthy that at least one of these
patients tolerated intravenous preservative-free heparin on subsequent retreat-
ment.

Cutaneous: Urticaria has been associated with the chlorocresol-associated
anaphylactoid reactions. Contact urticaria has been reported in one case after
application of an open patch test (69). Local erythematous and indurated reactions have been reported at the site of injections of chlorocresol preserved
heparin (59). Classic contact dermatitis has appeared in skin areas being treated
with topical agents containing this preservative. These reactions have been confirmed by results of 2% chlorocresol patch tests (64).

e. Pseudoallergic responses

Phenol may act as a toxicant or irritant depending on the concentration to
which patients are exposed. Significant percutaneous absorption of phenol
occurs in children being treated with local dermatologic preparations containing
4% phenol (70). In extreme cases, some of these children may become mildly
shocked and drowsy. Irritant eczematous dermatitis may occur in some patients
after use of dermatologic preparations containing less than 1% phenol (71).
There was one single case report of a patient who experienced severe burning
pain at the injection site with radiation along the veins up the forearm and into
the arm shortly after receiving 5,000 units of a chlorocresol-preserved heparin
(72). Some minutes later she felt nauseated and lightheaded and became drowsy
with pallor and sweating. The original injection site showed a bright red papule 2
days after the initial injections and later an intradermal skin test showed a positive reaction to the chlorocresol-preserved heparin. This patient tolerated
chlorocresol-free heparin on subsequent occasions. This reaction most likely

represented an irritant type of phlebitis, although an allergic component cannot be completely ruled out because of the positive intracutaneous test.

2. Parabens

Parabens are alkyl (methyl, ethyl and propyl) esters of p-hydroxybenzoic acid and have been used for about 50 years as biocidal agents in topical, oral, and parenteral drug formulations. The majority of allergic responses to these agents have been observed after topical exposure. The sensitization index of these compounds depends upon the concentrations used for incorporation into drug products. Although the chemical structure of parabens is closely related to benzoic acid, p-aminobenzoic acid, and the ester group of anesthetic agents (benzocaine and procaine), the evidence for clinical cross-sensitivity between parabens and these major drug classes is inconclusive (73,74).

a. Type I immunologic reactions

Documentation of immediate hypersensitivity reactions after parenteral administration of parabens is rare. There have been several case reports of immediate reactions occurring in dental patients receiving local anesthetics preserved with parabens (75,76). An IgE-mediated anaphylactic reaction was documented in a 10-year-old boy who was treated with intravenous hydrocortisone preserved with paraben (77). The immunologic specificity of this reaction was confirmed by passive transfer testing and there was no evidence of delayed hypersensitivity, as shown by negative patch tests to the relevant parabens. Localized contact urticaria was reported in a 31-year old man (78). Passive transfer with the patient's serum demonstrated wheal and flare reactions to methylparaben and ethylparaben in two normal volunteers. Thus this reaction was classified as contact urticaria with proven immunologic mechanism expressed as immediate hypersensitivity to the contactant.

b. Type II and III immunologic reactions

None have been recorded.

c. Type IV immunologic reactions

The contactant sensitizing potential of parabens contained in topical dermatologic products has been widely publicized, but on closer examination the role of these agents as "high-rate sensitizers" may have been overemphasized. First, there might be genetic predispositions in certain populations, such as in Denmark, where the highest numbers of contact dermatitis reactions have been reported. This factor, combined with the fact that parabens are formulated at a 5% concentration in Danish dermatologic products may account for the fact that 1% of the Danish population is hypersensitive (65). The Danish experience differs from comparable studies in the United States where parabens are most often used as 0.1–0.3% concentrations and the sensitization index in large numbers of volunteer subjects has been determined to be between 0.3 and 0.8% (65). This relatively low index potential was observed even in volunteers tested with inducing concentrations of paraben as high as 10%. The usual patch test and challenge concentration of parabens varies between 3 and 5%. The sensitization index of parabens is significantly higher in patients with preexisting dermatitis. According to a multicenter contact dermatitis study, contactant delayed hypersensitivity reactions occur in about 3% of patients with preexisting dermatitis (79). Topical contact sensitization to parabens usually occurs without concomitant evidence of immediate hypersensitivity, as demonstrated by negative scratch or intracutaneous tests in individuals with proven allergic contact dermatitis (80). Two unusual cases of generalized cutaneous reactions occurring 24–36 hr after systemic paraben exposure have been described. The first of these occurred in a young man who was proven to have allergic contact dermatitis to parabens 6 weeks before receiving local anesthesia containing 2% lidocaine and methylparaben as a preservative (74). His exacerbation was clearly eczematous and involved all previous areas that had exhibited the original contact dermatitis. This is the only documented instance of an exacerbation of allergic contact dermatitis after parenteral challenge with parabens. The second case was a hypersensitivity response manifested by an urticarial maculopapular rash appearing over the entire body of a young boy 36 hr after oral administration of a haloperidol solution containing methylparaben (81). This patient had previously received haloperidol tablets without methylparabens and had not reacted to them. The probability of a delayed hypersensitivity immunopathogenesis in this case was suggested by a positive in vitro macrophage inhibition test to methylparaben but not to the haloperidol solution.

d. Anatomical sites of hypersensitivity reactions: Systemic: Severe bronchospasm and pruritis are the chief symptoms associated with systemic reactions to paraben (77). Fortunately, these occurrences are rare, with only three cases recorded in the literature.

e. Anatomical sites of hypersensitivity reactions: Cutaneous: Localized contact urticaria has been described in one patient who originally developed the reaction after topical exposure but later also exhibited a similar reaction after parenteral administration of methylparaben (78). There were no systemic symptoms associated with this response. The most common cutaneous reaction is allergic contact dermatitis occurring after topical sensitization. As with other contactants, contact allergic sensitization to parabens is much more likely to occur after topical treatment of stasis ulcers and eczemas. Paradoxically, however, this subset of patients may continue to use paraben-containing cosmetics on normal skin with impunity (73). Thus, even patients with proven contact dermatitis may tolerate paraben-containing cosmetics as long as the cosmetic is applied to normal skin or skin that has not been dermatitic in the past. Of interest also is the fact that some patients with preexistent contact dermatitis to parabens may tolerate paraben-containing local anesthetic solutions without significant reactions. However, despite these benign observations in one or two patients, it would be prudent not to advise the use of paraben-containing local anesthetic solutions in documented paraben-sensitive patients.

It should be noted that drug manufacturers are making a conscious effort to exclude parabens from prescription topical formulations. Paradoxically, however, many of the over-the-counter topical preparations still contain paraben. This is illustrated by the large number of over-the-counter topical corticosteroids containing parabens (Table 2) (82).

f. Pseudoallergic responses

No definite pseudoallergic reactions have been reported. However, since topical methylparaben is a potent ciliotoxic agent, pulmonary mucous clearance could be significantly altered in asthmatic patients if large amounts of paraben-containing lidocaine are used for topical anesthesia of the upper airway (83).

3. Mercury Compounds

Both inorganic and organic mercury compounds have been widely used as medicinals and preservatives because of their biocidal properties. Metallic mercury is the main ingredient in mercury amalgam, which has been used for over 150 years in dental fillings. Because mercury is the common denominator in all

Table 2 OTC Topical Corticosteroids that Contain Parabens

Hydrocortisones (0.5%)
  Bactine hydrocortisone skin care cream (Miles Laboratories)
  Caldecort hydrocortisone cream (Pennwalt)
  Corticaine (Glaxo)
  Delacort (Medicon)
  Prepcort (hydrocortisone cream (Whitehall)

Hydrocortisone acetate (0.5%)
  Cortaid cream, lotion, ointment (Upjohn)
  Cortef feminine itch cream (Upjohn)
  Cortef rectal itch ointment (Upjohn)
  Gynecort antipruritic cream (Combe)
  Lanacort antipruritic cream (Combe)
  Wellcortin Cream, Lotion[a] (Burroughs Wellcome)

[a]No longer manufactured

these chemical substances, it might be assumed that sensitization profiles of inorganic and organic mercurials are similar. Clearly this is not the case. Although isolated case reports of allergic reactions to mercury amalgam have been reported, a critical assessment of this anecdotal experience must conclude that metallic mercury has an extremely low level of allergic potential (84). To allay dental patients' unwarranted fears in this regard, the American Dental Association has issued a special "questions and answers" information bulletin.*

TO THE DENTAL PATIENT:
Recent reports in the public media have raised questions as to the safety of dental amalgam. In order to provide you with accurate information on the use and safety of dental amalgam, the American Dental Association has prepared the following answers to the most commonly asked questions about dental amalgam.

What is dental amalgam?
Dental amalgam is the material most often used to fill cavities caused by tooth decay. In general, one or more metals are combined with mercury to form a pliable mass. This material is then condensed into the cavity, which the dentist has cleared of decay. There it hardens into a dental restoration or filling.

Which metals are used in dental amalgam?
Silver, copper, and tin are the metals commonly used in dental amalgam, sometimes in combination with zinc. Dental amalgam is used in about 75% of all single-tooth fillings.

Does the ADA have an acceptance program for dental amalgams?
Yes. To help dentists choose from among the various brands of dental amalgam on the market, the ADA has established an acceptance program to examine these products for safety and effectiveness. To date, more than 100 brands of dental amalgam have been accepted for dentists' use.

Why is mercury used in dental amalgam?
When combined with silver or other metals, the mercury produces a chemical reaction that causes the filling to harden after it has been placed in the cavity.

---

*Presented by permission of the American Dental Association from the *American Dental Association News*, January 2, 1984

Is this something new?
No. The basic technique has been used to restore decayed teeth for about 150 years.

Isn't mercury a poison?
When mercury is combined with the metals used in dental amalgam, its toxic properties are made harmless. Moreover, the safety of dental amalgam has been studied for nearly a century, and all documented research indicates that, for the vast majority of dental patients, mercury-containing amalgams present no health hazard. Mercury in small quantities is found naturally in the human system. And the average mercury level found in the general public is more than 100 times lower than the level at which harmful effects are usually reported.

Aren't some people allergic to mercury?
In rare cases, a patient may experience an allergic reaction to mercury, usually in the form of dermatitis or skin rash. To guard against this very remote possibility, the ADA recommends that dentists maintain a complete medical history for each patient. If the patient is known to have such an allergy, the dentist may choose some other restorative material, something other than dental amalgam.

What other filling materials are available?
Gold is often used to fill teeth, either in pure form or alloyed with some metal or element other than mercury. Some manufacturers are working to produce composite resins (plastics), which soon may be available as acceptable alternatives to dental amalgam. To date, however, these materials have not proved durable enough to withstand the great pressure generated by chewing. Dental researchers are constantly seeking safe, new methods for restoring decayed teeth. For most patients, though, dental amalgam remains a safe and effective material for filling cavities.

What is the "life span" of a dental amalgam?
On the average, amalgams serve for at least 10 years, and very often they last considerably longer. Conditions in the mouth are constantly changing, and these changes affect dental materials and their function. Your fillings will last longer if you follow proper procedures for home care and receive regular dental checkups.

In contrast, the former widespread use of an inorganic mercury formulation, ammoniated mercury, as a topical antibacterial resulted in widespread sensitization in patients with preexistent skin lesions (85). From the standpoint of drug and biological preservatives, however, organic mercurials such as thimerosal (merthiolate) and phenylmercuric salts have a relatively high potential for causing allergic reactions. Thimerosal has been used extensively as the essential antibacterial ingredient in vaccines, skin test solutions (tuberculin, histoplasmin, coccidioidin, mumps, and candida antigens) and immunoglobulin preparations. It is also used in many topical medications including creams, lotions, eye and ear drops. In recent years, one of its most common uses has been as an antibacterial preservative in saline soft lens solution used for storage and cleaning. The concentration of thimerosal varies between 0.002 and 0.01% in these various preparations. In addition, in the United States, thimerosal is used widely as a skin disinfectant (merthiolate) and is available as an over-the-counter preparation for treatment of minor skin injuries. The higher usage pattern of thimerosal in the United States may account for a somewhat increased incidence of positive patch tests in epidemiological studies conducted in the United States (86). One other organic mercurial, phenylmercuric acetate, is used widely as a spermacide and as a cosmetic preservative but less frequently as a biocidal agent for preserving biologicals, ointments, and eye drops (87). It has a high sensitization index and is also a skin irritant at 0.5% concentration (65). Of interest is the fact that phenylmercuric borate may have a much lower sensitization index (65). The chief importance of phenylmercuric compounds could be their cross-sensitization potential with other organic mercurials such as diphenylmercury and thimerosal. However, this possibility is hypothetical because equivocal cross-sensitivity was demonstrated only to diphenylmercury and not to thimerosal in a patient proven to have IgE-mediated sensitization to phenylmercuric proprionate, acetate and nitrate salts (87).

a. Type I immunologic reactivity

Life-threatening systemic reactions to mercurials have not been reported. There is one case report of acute laryngeal edema occurring after repeated daily use of an aerosol spray containing 0.033% thimerosal (88). The patient experienced marked respiratory distress 30 hr after the first use of the aerosol spray and required an emergency tracheostomy. Subsequent patch tests revealed a markedly positive test to 0.1% thimerosal but no tests were done to exclude the possibility of an IgE-mediated mechanism. The presumptive pathogenetic explanation was that the laryngeal obstruction was due to delayed hypersensitivity because there were gradual increases in severe respiratory symptoms and a strongly positive patch test reaction to thimerosal. Another immediate reaction to merthiolate was documented in a patient who had a reaction to merthiolate-preserved tetanus toxoid (89). IgE-mediated symptoms of severe asthma and urticaria were observed in a patient sensitized to phenylmercuric proprionate (87). The immunologic specificity of this reaction was corroborated by direct skin tests, passive transfer tests, and leukocyte histamine release.

b. Type II and III immunologic reactivity

None has been recorded.

c. Type IV immunologic reactivity

There are two major types of delayed hypersensitivity induced by merthiolate. Eczematous contact allergy is the most common and can be readily confirmed by patch testing with 0.1% thimerosal in petrolatum. Because of widespread exposure to thimerosal in the United States, positive patch tests are much more frequent (8–13.4%) than in Scandinavian countries (1.3–3.7%) (90). One of the epidemiologic studies in Sweden also revealed that thimerosal sensitization occurred predominantly in young age groups, compared to the expected predominance of contact allergy due to other contactants in middle-aged persons (90). Tuberculin-type delayed hypersensitivity reactions can also be induced by thimerosal. Delayed intracutaneous reactions of this type were first observed by investigators who were evaluating the possibility of immediate IgE-mediated reactions. Investigations of intracutaneous (tuberculin) reactivity have been carried out in Sweden, where it has been noted that 16% of healthy male military recruits and 26% of medical students have positive reactions. This led to the hypothesis that young adult Swedes have been accidentally sensitized in childhood either by vaccines containing thimerosal or by tuberculin skin test reagents containing this substance.

The histological features of delayed tuberculinlike reactions induced by thimerosal consist of a dense inflammatory lymphocyte infiltrate and a few eosinophils around dermal vessels and sweat glands, which are consistent with the tissue changes of an intracutaneous tuberculin reaction. These series of investigations also included cross-sensitization experiments, which demonstrated a low level of cross-reactivity to metallic mercury and various other organic mercurials including phenylmercuric acetate. These studies also demonstrated that the allergenic determinant was the ethylmercuric moiety rather thiosalicylate.

d. Anatomical sites of hypersensitivity reactions: Cutaneous: Hypersensitivity to thimerosal is more likely to occur in patients with hand eczemas, especially the variety designated as pompholyx. This was determined by a prospective study among 37 thimerosal-sensitive patients, 15 of whom were shown to have pompholyx, compared to 8 of 40 control patients with other types of skin manifestations (90). Exacerbation of atopic dermatitis was reported in a child after receiving a thimerosal-containing diptheria booster (91). Thimerosal was implicated by a positive patch test to 0.1% thimerosal. As discussed previously, upper airway manifestations of thimerosal-induced delayed hypersensitivity may result in life-threatening laryngeal obstruction. Generalized urticaria, angioedema, and erythema multiforme were described in one patient after local skin contact with phenylmercuric propionate (87). On one occasion this patient also developed dysphagia and esophageal spasm after similar exposure.

e. Anatomical sites of hypersensitivity reactions: *Ophthalmic*: A 0.01% solution of thimerosal is included in many soft lens solutions to inhibit the growth of bacteria such as *Pseudomonas aeruginosa, Acinetobacter* species, *E. coli,* and *Staphylococcus* species. A number of cases of conjunctival hyperemia and anterior stromal infiltrates of the cornea have been associated with delayed hypersensitivity reactions induced by thimerosal (92,93). Delayed hypersensitivity has been confirmed by both positive patch and intracutaneous tests using thiomerosal reagents. Slit-lamp examination revealed conjunctival injection and discrete dense, white anterior, stromal infiltrates of the cornea. A mild mixed, follicular, papillary conjunctival response was also observed. These lesions resolved completely after discontinuation of the thimerosal-containing soft lens solution.

e. Pseudoallergic reactions

There have been two case reports of elevated body temperature after topical application of thimerosal. Possible immunological mechanisms were not determined in these cases (90).

4. Formalin and Formaldehyde-Releasing Agents

Formalin was one of the earliest substances used for sterilizing kidney dialyzer membranes, especially for the reuse of these dialyzers. It is still widely used but with stringent recommendations for formaldehyde concentrations in the final rinse solution from 2 to 10 ppm. Possible reactions to formaldehyde associated with the use of these medical devices are discussed later in this chapter in the section on sterilizing agents. Formaldehyde itself currently has limited use in biologics and topical preparations. One exception is noteworthy. It is contained in a hepatitis B vaccine (HB-VAX) produced by Merck Sharp and Dohme. This vaccine contains up to 0.02 mg/ml formaldehyde (94).

Several formaldehyde-releasing agents are used as preservatives in a variety of pharmaceutical preparations, especially water-soluble creams and lotions. Among these are BNPD (2-bromo-2-nitropropane-1,3-diol), Germall (imidazolidinyl urea), and Quaternium-15. Trioxylmethylene (paraformaldehyde) is contained in root-canal-filling pastes. The use of formaldehyde in topical dermatologic preparations is not preferred because of its relatively high sensitizing potential. Among the formaldehyde-releasing agents, the majority of hypersensitivity responses have been reported after exposure to BNPD. BNPD is one of a family of halogenated nitrocompounds that effectively inhibits the growth of both gram-positive and gram-negative bacteria, particularly *P. aeruginosa* (95). The concentration of BNPD varies from 0.05 to 1% in most topical formulations. BNPD partially decomposes and releases formaldehyde at alkaline pH. Thus it is estimated that 30 ppm of formaldehyde could be generated from a 0.05% concentration of BNPD, a level attained by some currently available topical products. Quaternium 15, N-(3-chloroallyl)-hexaminium chloride, is now being used in generic brands of topical corticosteroid creams (96).

a. Type I immunologic reactivity

An apparent type I allergic response was experienced by a patient 4 hr after instillation of a root canal paste containing trioxymethylene (97). This reaction was characterized by endodontic angioedema, a generalized pruritic skin rash, and intense left periorbital and facial swelling. However, this case can only be classified as a presumptive type I reaction because neither direct skin tests nor serologic tests were performed to confirm the reaction. The immunologic potential of paraformaldehyde has been investigated in animals. Several investigators have shown that extirpated pulp tissues from the teeth of rabbits and dogs are rendered highly immunogenic after incubation with paraformaldehyde (98-100). These experiments revealed that both immediate and delayed-type hypersensitivity responses are produced by formaldehyde-treated pulp tissue. There is a documented case of anaphylactic shock occurring 26 hr after skin application of a formaldehyde patch test (101). This patient had previously experienced anaphylactic symptoms after exposure to a formaldehyde sterilized dialyzer. Prick tests performed with 0.1 and 1% formaldehyde were positive and a radioallergosorbent test to formaldehyde conjugated with human serum albumin was positive (4% binding).

b. Type II and III immunologic reactivity

The significance of IgG, IgM, IgA, and IgE antibodies directed against formaldehyde–human serum conjugates has been studied in sera from patients undergoing hemodialysis with formaldehyde-sterilized dialyzers (102). These antibodies could be detected in certain sera but no correlation of either IgG or IgE antibodies with adverse reactions was found in this series of dialysis patients. Detectable IgG antibodies to formaldehyde–human serum albumin conjugates were reported in seven of eight symptomatic persons chronically exposed to indoor formaldehyde at low concentrations (103). The clinical relevance of these antibodies has not been determined.

c. Type IV immunologic reactivity

Allergic contact dermatitis has been documented by a number of independent investigators (95,104-107). There was a marked difference of opinion about the sensitization potential of BNPD among these various investigators, some considering the overall incidence of sensitization to be infrequent and others noting a moderate to high level of sensitization. These apparent discrepancies may be explained in part by the concentration of BNPD used for patch testing and respective study populations. Early human prophetic patch testing revealed a high skin sensitization potential at a 5% inducing concentration (65). Several years later, however, a similar study was repeated using smaller concentrations of BNPD. This study demonstrated that the 5% concentration was irritative. The irritancy threshold ranged between 0.5 and 1% and it was therefore proposed that future patch skin tests to BNPD should be performed at a concentration of 0.25% (108). The low irritancy threshold of BNPD could have accounted for the high incidence of positive patch tests in 190 patients tested with 1% BNPD (97). As is the case with many other contactants, allergic contact dermatitis is much more likely to develop in patients with preexisting eczema or stasis dermatitis (95). Paradoxically, prospective "use" tests in patients with documented contact dermatitis to BNPD showed that some patients did not exhibit contact dermatitis in normal skin. This phenomenon may be comparable to the previously cited "paraben paradox." The observation of cross-sensitivity to formaldehyde has been variable. Several investigators have reported that a significant proportion of BNPD-positive patients who showed positive patch tests to formaldehyde may have had a preexisting history of sensitivity to formaldehyde (104). On the other hand, another clinical study reported that BNPD-sensitive patients do not necessarily have concomitant allergy to formaldehyde or the other formaldehyde donors such as Quaternium-15 and imidazolidinyl urea (95). Nevertheless, special caution should be observed by formalin-sensitive patients in the use of BNPD-containing products. Allergic contact dermatitis has been documented after exposure to Quaternium 15 used as a formaldehyde-releasing preservative in a generic hydrocortisone cream (96).

d. Anatomical sites of hypersensitivity reactions

Cutaneous: Diffuse maculopapular rash may be associated with sensitization to any of the formaldehyde-releasing agents. At least one case of intraoral and facial angioedema was described a few hours after exposure to one of these agents. The vast majority of cutaneous lesions are contact eczematous dermatitis. Dermatitis is much more likely to occur in areas of the skin previously involved with eczema or stasis dermatitis. Local exacerbation of contact hand eczema occurred in a patient with proven patch test reactivity to formaldehyde shortly after being vaccinated against hepatitis B vaccine. A similar reaction in the same patient was noted after a second dose of this vaccine (94).

e. Pseudoallergic responses

No clinically relevant pseudoallergic reactions have been described. However, because the irritancy threshold of these agents occurs at very low concentrations, direct erythematous and even vesicular irritant responses may be obtained at BNDP patch sites tested with concentrations of 0.25% or more.

5. Organic Acids and Their Salts

Both sorbic and benzoic acid are widely used as antimicrobial agents. Sorbic acid is 2,4-hexadienoic acid and occurs naturally in the berries of the mountain ash, cranberries, strawberries, and currants. Sorbic acid is considered to be the anti-microbial agent of choice for topically applied dermatologics containing fatty acids and polyoxyethylene esters and is incorporated in these formulations at a concentration of 0.2%. Sorbic acid is a common preservative of topical cortico-steroid creams (Table 3) (109).

Both of these organic acids are primary irritants and on rare occasions both may produce hypersensitivity reactions. Potassium sorbate is a weaker preserva-tive than sorbic acid and is used chiefly as a mold and yeast inhibitor in aqueous solutions. Two salts of benzoic acid, sodium benzoate and benzyl benzoate, are also used as preservatives in topical preparations. The esters of p-hydroxybenzoic acid have been discussed previously in the section on parabens.

a. Types I-III immunologic reactivity

No proven cases have been reported.

b. Type IV immunologic reactivity

Allergic contact dermatitis induced by sorbic acid or boric acid is rare (110-114). Moreover, prophetic patch testing in large patient populations revealed a low sensitization index of 0.8% (65). Patch test surveys in patients with preexist-ing allergic contact dermatitis also show a relatively small percentage (0.3-3%) of positive patch tests to sorbic acid (115-117). Contact dermatitis to potassium sorbate is rare but was described in a patient who became sensitized to this

Table 3 Topical Corticosteroids Containing Sorbic Acid

Aristocort Cream (Lederle)[a,b]

Florone Cream (Dermik)

Hytone Cream (Dermik)

Kenalog Cream (Squibb)

Maxiflor Cream (Herbert)

Mycolog-II Cream (Squibb)

Pramosone Cream (Ferndale)[a]

---

[a]Contains both sorbic acid and potassium sorbate
[b]Aristocort A cream is free of these preservatives.
Note: Sorbitol solution, sorbitan, and polysorbate are emulsifying agents unrelated to sorbic acid.

substance in an EKG solution (118). A prospective patch test study of 475 patients with dermatitis revealed a sensitization index of 1.9 for sodium benzoate and 1.5 for benzyl benzoate (119). Significant production of T-cell-derived leucocyte inhibitory factor in response to incubation with sodium benzoate has been demonstrated in a group of proven aspirin-intolerant patients with chronic urticaria (120).

c. Anatomical sites of hyperreactivity

Cutaneous: Contact urticaria after perioral contact with sorbic acid and benzoic acid is not uncommon and contact urticaria after airborne exposure to sodium benzoate has also been reported. Nonimmunologic mechanisms are thought to be involved in these reactions (121,122). Allergic contact dermatitis is the most common cutaneous lesion and usually occurs over skin areas that have been previously treated with a preparation containing these materials. The usual flare of contact dermatitis occurs with prominent erythema, soreness, and pruritis (112).

d. Pseudoallergic responses

It is well known that both benzoic and sorbic acids cause redness and itching when applied to human skin. These reactions may be confined to the face, especially in women who use cosmetics containing potassium sorbate (109). Sorbic acid reactors also complain of flushing after ingestion of wines, beta-blocking drugs, nitrates, and sulfite additives. Prospective studies of this phenomenon by open and closed patch test techniques demonstrated that applications of 5% benzoic acid and 2.5% of sorbic acid cause urticaria and/or erythema in more than half of volunteer subjects irrespective of their atopic status (121, 123). A recent investigation of sorbic-acid-induced erythema and edema may help to explain the nonspecific nature of this reaction (124). Sorbic acid concentrations as low as 0.1% produced transient erythema with wheal and flare after open or closed application to skin. Aspirin blocked the erythematous component of this reaction. This suggested that sorbic acid penetrates the skin and induces prostaglandin formation, which would cause further vasodilation. In this study, lidocaine and capsaicin also blocked the flare component, which suggested a similarity to histamine flares in which antidromic neural transmission is followed by release of substance P, a neuropeptide that causes vasodilation (124).

Benzoic acid was the more potent irritant than sorbic acid. Considering its background, it is not surprising that benzoic acid has been reported to cause harmful symptoms in atopic and urticarial patients when ingested orally (125–127). However, when controlled double-blind challenge tests were performed in patients suspected of having oral reactions to benzoic acid, no differences could be discerned between symptoms resulting from benzoic acid or lactose placebo (128). These recent studies suggest that the vast majority of benzoic acid reactions cannot be documented by controlled double-blind challenge tests. When they are documented objectively, in most cases they are nonimmunologic and the incidence of allergic sensitivity is minimal. Nonimmunologic contact urticaria may be induced by benzoic acid (129). Premedication with indomethacin blocked this response but this was not accompanied by concurrent changes of prostanoids sampled from urticarial blister fluid lesions. Leukotrienes were not sampled, so it is possible that the inhibitory effect of indomethacin could have affected the lipooxygenase pathway of arachidonic acid metabolism. There is a single case report of a nonimmunologic anaphylactoid reaction induced by intolerance to sodium benzoate in preoperative medications (130).

6. Alcohols (Also See Chapter 11)

Alcohols such as phenyl carbinol (benzyl alcohol) and chlorobutanol are being increasingly used as preservatives for injectable biologicals. The total number of hypersensitivity reactions after exposure to both of these agents is minimal. Although anecdotal reports have appeared in the literature, the immunologic specificity of these reactions has only been determined in a few cases. Localized and systemic reactions have been reported in several patients receiving biologicals preserved with either chlorobutanol or benzyl alcohol (131-133). Several cases of contact dermatitis to benzyl alcohol have been confirmed by positive patch tests with 1% benzyl alcohol in petrolatum (80,134). Cross-sensitization to benzyl alcohol has been reported in subjects previously sensitized to balsam of Peru (80). Fatigue, nausea, and diffuse angioedema occurred in a patient shortly after intramuscular injection of vitamin B_{12} containing benzyl alcohol as a preservative (135). A positive intradermal skin test to this preparation was obtained while a vitamin B_{12} formula without preservative was negative. Although this finding was suggestive of an IgE-mediated reaction, this could not be proved.

7. Chloramine-T

Chloramine-T, or p-toluenesulfonechloramide, is a chlorine-liberating sterilizing agent that is an occupational hazard for pharmaceutical workers, nurses, butchers, cleaners, and brewers. Insofar as medicinals are concerned, it is only used as a disinfectant for medical devices and hospital equipment (e.g., bed pans). Thus the at-risk population for hypersensitivity reactions would be almost exclusively limited to hospital personnel, although it is possible that previously sensitized individuals could develop symptoms after reexpsoure to traces of this material in the hospital. The potent sensitizing potential of chloramine-T was recognized as early as 1945 and other more recent investigations have confirmed the validity of these original observations (136-139).

a. Type I immunologic reactivity

IgE-mediated respiratory symptoms have been reported in brewery and pharmaceutical workers sensitized and subsequently reexposed to chloramine-T. These clinical reactions have been corroborated by direct scratch and prick, RAST, and leukocyte histamine release tests (132,134). Moreover, antigenic determinant investigations by a polystyrene tube radioimmunoassay revealed that the significant antigenic determinant was formed partially by the toluensulfonyl moiety of the chloramine-T molecule (138). None of these patients were found to have specific antibodies directed against IgG subclasses IgG_1, IgG_2, IgG_3, or IgG_4. Clinically sensitive individuals almost uniformly exhibit moderately high levels of total IgE, which decrease significantly after a period free from illness and further exposure to chloramine-T. Some patients also show elevated blood eosinophil counts that drop after cessation of exposure.

b. Type III immunologic reactivity

Precipitins between aqueous solutions of chloramine-T and sensitive sera have been demonstrated by agar gel diffusion tests, but the clinical relevance of these tests (i.e., immune complexes) has not been proven (136).

c. Type IV immunologic reactivity

Contact dermatitis has been reported after exposure to 0.2% aqueous solution of chloramine-T. The type IV (contact) nature of this reaction was confirmed by 48 and 96 hr patch test readings that showed erythema, induration, and papule formation (139).

d. Anatomical sites of hypersensitivity reactions: *Cutaneous*: Contact urticaria was demonstrated objectively in a patient who had developed rhinitis, shortness of breath, and edema of the eyelids after being in contact with chloramine powder that he had to dissolve in water to make 0.5 solutions for disinfection of bed pans. These symptoms appeared 15–20 min after contact with the chloramine powder and sometimes lasted several days. Closed patch tests with 0.2% solution caused erythema/wheal formation at the 48 hr patch test site. Other patch tests with stronger solutions (1.5–12.5%) had to be terminated after 8 hr because the patient developed remote urticarial lesions on the arms, trunk, and thighs (139). The contact urticaria in this patient was associated with a positive polystyrene tube radioimmunoassay (48% binding) for chloramine-T and therefore was classified as immunologically IgE-mediated contact urticaria. The eczematous contact dermatitis associated with chloramine-T sensitization may be characterized by either discrete erythematous squamous lesions or generalized eczematous contact dermatitis over areas of preexisting skin lesions.

e. Anatomical sites of hypersensitivity reactions: Respiratory: Occupational sensitization to chloramine-T may be manifested by both upper and lower respiratory symptoms. At times the nasal symptoms may precede the occurrence of cough, wheeze, and sputum production. Some patients have complained of headaches, fever, and shortness of breath after exposure to chloramine-T once the sensitization process has developed. Occupational asthma may be immediate, late, or a combination of the two: the dual response pattern.

f. Pseudoallergic responses

Chloramine-T can be toxic if ingested in excessive amounts. Formerly it was used as a sterilizing agent for canteen water used by military personnel (Halazone) and occasional episodes of oral toxicity were encountered. In high concentrations, chloramine-T is an irritant and some workers have complained of skin irritation and blistering after skin contact (236).

8. Chloracetamide

Chloracetamide is a chlorinated compound used as a preservative in many pharmaceutical and cosmetic substances. It has been reported to be a potent sensitizer in extremely low concentrations (0.015–0.1%) (64,140–142). It is now included in some standard patch test series.

V. ANTIOXIDANTS

A. Nordihydroguaiaretic Acid, Butylated Hydroxyanisole (BHA), Butylated Hydroxytoluene, Gallic Acid Esters (Propyl-,Octyl-, and Dodecyl Gallate) and Alpha-Tocopherol

These compounds are being used as antioxidants more often in the food and drug industries now that sulfite antioxidants have been barred from some fresh foods and their use greatly curtailed in packaged foods and pharmaceutical products. All of these substances are nonirritant and relatively nonsensitizing. The concentrations of these substances in drug products are low, ranging from 0.01 to 0.1%.

a. Type I immunologic reactivity

IgE-mediated allergic responses have not been well documented. There is one case report of contact urticaria 20 min after skin application of 1% ethanol solutions of butylated hydroxytoluene (BHT) and butylated hydroxyanisole (BHA). This reaction was not obtained with dilutions of 0.1 and 0.01% (143). Some patients with chronic urticaria demonstrate recurrence of urticarial lesions after oral challenge with BHT and BHA, but these occurrences are most likely nonimmunologic and should properly be classified as pseudoallergic reactions (127).

b. Type II immunologic reactivity

This has not been demonstrated.

c. Type III immunologic reactivity

There is an isolated case report of a systemic urticarial rash occurring after exposure to oral BHT. The urticarial rash gradually developed into an erythematous macular eruption, which finally evolved into violet–brown lesions over a 3-week course. A skin biopsy revealed significant vascular deposits of IgM, $C1_q$, C3, and C9 complement components as well as fibrinogen (144). Cutaneous lesions were reproduced by a controlled, single-blind challenge experiment. Although specific antibodies were not demonstrated in this case, an immune-complex-mediated lesion was suggested by the immunofluorescent deposition of immunoglobulins and complement components.

d. Type IV immunologic reactivity

There are only scattered case reports of patch-test-positive contact dermatitis after exposure and sensitization to nordihydroguaiaretic acid (NDGA), BHA, BHT, and the gallic acid esters (145–147). The contact sensitization index of this group of antioxidants is extremely low. Modified Draize experiments in 60 human volunteers did not reveal sensitivity to BHT after daily applications of this agent in volunteers for 60 consecutive days (148). Similarly, large-scale patch test surveys with BHT and BHA allergens revealed only 1 positive reaction to 5% BHA in petrolatum and no reactions to BHT in petrolatum in 360 consecutive patients (149). It is of interest that propylgallate has a high propensity for contact sensitization in guinea pigs, but this is easily abolished by prior oral ingestion of 10% propylgallate (150). Several human volunteers were also readily sensitized by daily maximization applications of propylgallate. The apparent paradox between the ease of experimental contact sensitization and the relative lack of spontaneously occurring contact sensitization in the general public was explained by the relative ease in inducing tolerance by oral administration of propylgallate in guinea pigs. Presumably, the same phenomenon could occur in humans constantly exposed to gallate esters in food products.

Positive patch tests to alpha-tocopherol (natural or synthetic vitamin E) are extremely rare, probably because it is no longer used as an antioxidant in dermatologic preparations. Topical use of vitamin E caused generalized erythema multiforme reactions in two patients (151). A patch test with vitamin E oil revealed positive local reactions in both cases.

e. Anatomical sites of hypersensitivity reactions: *Cutaneous*: One case of contact urticaria has been documented (143). The presentation involved an ulcer of the left arm occurring shortly after the patient used an antibiotic ointment containing 0.1% propylgallate. The histologic characteristic of the lesion was that of a hyperkeratotic eczema (152). Antioxidant-induced contact dermatitis commonly presents on the face and hands (137,138). Cheilitis has also been described after oral contact with BHA-containing foods or creams. Two patients with hand eczema due to BHT and BHA experienced marked exacerbation of vesicular lesions after oral challenge with the respective antioxidants (145).

f. Pseudoallergic reactions

As discussed above, anecdotal reports of urticarial responses after challenge with BHA or BHT in patients with chronic urticaria were not associated with immunologic reactions and therefore represent pseudoallergic reactions (127). Moreover, the high prevalence of these references appearing after these initial uncontrolled observations has not been confirmed by controlled investigations in a number of other medical centers. In attempting to replicate these studies, it is absolutely essential that tests be conducted according to a controlled, double-blind protocol.

Both nasal and bronchial symptoms were reported to be exacerbated in seven patients in a double-blind challenge protocol with 125–250 mg doses of BHA and BHT (153). Controlled groups of aspirin-intolerant patients and patients with other pulmonary diseases did not exhibit similar reactions. Patients exhibiting the positive challenge responses also demonstrated an increase in bleeding times. The exacerbation of symptoms in the rhinitis group of patients occurred within 5–75 min. The asthmatic patients developed asthmatic symptoms between 5 and 60 min after the challenge. Other symptoms recorded were diaphoresis, somnolence, flushing, and headache. The results of this study were not confirmed by a similar controlled investigation of seven patients with nonallergic asthma and rhinitis (154). In the latter study there were no objective changes of respiratory function nor were bleeding times increased. Some of the patients in this study did complain of somnolence. Thus, the presumption of respiratory pseudoallergic reactions after ingestion of BHA and BHT must be considered equivocal at the present time.

B. Sulfites

There are five sulfite salts (potassium metabisulfite, sodium metabisulfite, potassium bisulfite, sodium bisulfite, and sodium sulfite) that may be used as preservatives in nebulizer solutions, parenteral solutions, and peritoneal dialysis solutions. The amount of sulfite ion available for absorption into body tissues varies widely from product to product for several reasons (155). Added sulfites are subject to inactivation because of autooxidation or chemical interactions with other materials in the preparations. Thus it has been determined that sulfites disappear quickly from infusion solutions in plastic bottles whereas a similar loss does not occur in glass bottles. It is presumed that loss from plastic bottles occurs because of increased permeability to air, which causes auto-oxidation of sulfite. Autooxidation of sulfites in peritoneal dialysis solutions also occurs during the autoclaving process, which may destroy as much as 90% of sulfites in the solution. In addition, sulfites may combine with glucose in peritoneal dialysis solutions to form a hydroxysulfonate adduct. High-dose exposures of sulfites (500 mg) may occur in patients receiving parenteral infusion solutions in a matter of a few hours or in patients undergoing peritoneal dialysis receiving 10 L of solution over a relatively short period of time. Sulfite exposure in patients receiving unit dose injectables or nebulizer solutions is generally much lower but, on the other hand, a number of these preparations are used in asthmatic patients who may be particularly susceptible to sulfite reactions. Table 4 contains a partial list of pharmaceuticals containing sulfites.

Adverse responses to sulfites encompass a broad spectrum of immunologic and nonimmunologic mechanisms, which are often difficult to differentiate. It is therefore not surprising that the terminology of these responses has included a wide variety of descriptive terms, the most common of which are sulfite sensitivity and sulfite hypersensitivity. Since only a small percentage of affected cases are mediated by hypersensitivity reactions (i.e., types I–IV), neither of these terms appear to be entirely appropriate. There is no consensus on an all-inclusive term, but for the purpose of this discussion all adverse clinical responses induced will be termed "sulfite reactivity."

The majority of adverse reactions to sulfite occur after ingestion of foods containing this antioxidant. In recent years the number of reported severe adverse reactions including death had increased to the point where the FDA banned the use of sulfites in fresh fruits and vegetables and required packaged foods containing sulfites to be labeled if sulfites were present in concentrations of 10 ppm or greater. Sulfites were not banned in drug products because of the lack of suitable sulfite substitutes for maintaining potency in certain medications. Instead, the FDA recommended that prescription drugs contain a warning about possible sulfite-induced allergic type reactions, including anaphylaxis. This warning is required in the physician package insert for prescription drugs. Many forms of aqueous epinephrine contain sulfites as essential antioxidants for preserving the potency of this life-saving drug. A special labeling accommodation has been made in the case of injectable epinephrine, which states that the "presence of sulfite(s) in this product should not deter the administration of the drug for treatment of serious allergic or other emergency situations" (156). The rationale for this recommendation is based on the fact that subcutaneous doses of small amounts of sulfites (10 mg or less) ordinarily present in parenteral medications are usually well-tolerated by known sulfite-reactive asthmatic patients (157). However, it is possible that anaphylaxis could occur after injections of small amounts in those rare patients with exquisite IgE-mediated anaphylactic sensitivity.

Table 4   Partial List of Pharmaceuticals Containing Sulfites

Bronchodilator inhalant solutions[a]
  Alupent (metaproterenol sulfate)[b]
  Bronkephrine (ethylnorepinephrine HCl)
  Bronkosol (isoetharine HCl)
  Isuprel hydrochloride solution (isoproterenol HCl)
  Metaprel (metaproterenol sulfate)
  Micronefrin (racemic epinephrine)
Tablets
  Isuprel HCl Glossets (isoproterenol HCl)
  Bactrim, Septra
  Aldomet
Injectables
  Miscellaneous
    Adrenalin 1/1,100 (epinephrine)
    Aldomet ester HCl injection (methyldopa HCl, MSD)
    Aramine (metaraminol bitartrate)
    Celestone phosphate (brand of metamethasone sodium)
    Compazine (prochlorperazine)
    Decadron-LA suspension (dexamethasone acetate)
    Decadron phosphate injection (dexamethasone sodium phosphate)
    Decadron phosphate with Xylocaine (dexamethasone sodium phosphate and lidocaine HCl)
    Dopastat (dopamine HCl)
    Intropin (dopamine HCl)
    Isuprel HCL sterile injection 1:5,000 (isoproterenol HCl)
    Largon (propiomazine HCl)
    Levophen bitartrate (norepinephrine bitartrate)
    Levoprome (methotrimeprazine)
    Lidocaine HCl with epinephrine
    Marcaine HCl with epinephrine (bipivacaine HCL and epinephrine)
    Mepergan (meperidine and promethazine HCl)

  Nesacaine (chloroprocaine HCl)
  Nesacaine-CE (chloroprocaine HCl)
  Novocaine (procaine HCl injection [USP])
  Nubain (nalbuphine HCl)
  Phenergan (promethazine HCl)
  Prednisolone sodium phosphate
  Pronestyl (procainamide HCl)
  Reglan (metoclopramide HCl)
  Serpasil (reserpine USP)
  Solu-pred
  Thorazine (chlorpromazine HCl)
  Tofranil (imipramine HCL [USP])
  Torecan (brand of thiethylperazine [USP])
  10% Travasol (amino acid) injection without electrolytes
  Trilafon (perphenazine [USP])
  Tubocurarine chloride injection (USP)
  Yutopar (ritodrine (HCl)
Antibiotics
  Amikin (amikacin sulfate)
  Bactrim IV infusion (trimethoprim and sulfamethoxazole)
  Bristagen (gentamicin sulfate)
  Gantrisin (sulfisoxazole)
  Garamycin injectable (gentamicin sulfate)
  Kantrex injection (kanamycin sulfate injection)
  Nebcin (tobramycin sulfate)
  Septra IV infusion

Skin topicals
  Corticosporin
  Neo-cort-dome
  Neodecadron

Eye and ear products
  Cortisporin otic solution (polymyxin B-neomycin-hydrocortisone)
  Decadron in ocumeter (dexamethasone sodium phosphate)

Decadron phosphate 0.1% sterile
ophthalmic solution (neomycin
sulfate–dexamethasone sodium phosphate)
Neodecadron sterile ophthalmic
solution (neomycin sulfate–dexamethasone sodium phosphate)

Otocort ear drops
Pred-forte ophthalmic suspension
Pred-mild ophthalmic suspension
Propine ophthalmic solution
(dipivefrin HCl)

---

[a]Only solutions, not metered dose dispensers. The unit-dose Alupent formulation does not
contain sulfites.
[b]Except unit dose, which does not contain sulfites.

a. Type I immunologic reactivity

Documentation of an IgE-mediated mechanism for inducing acute sulfite reactions is sparse. The first serious adverse clinical reaction to sulfites was a case of
anaphylaxis that was corroborated by positive skin tests and passively transferable antibody (158). However, systemic symptoms were induced in this patient
only after ingestion of sulfite additives in food. Immediate anaphylactoid
symptoms have been reported in patients exposed to sulfites in nebulizer solutions and several forms of parenterally administered drugs (159–162). Positive
skin tests were elicited only in those patients whose leukocytes also demonstrated positive sulfite-specific histamine release (159). Positive prick tests
passively transferred with unheated serum were also demonstrated in a sulfite-
reactive asthmatic (163). Although the involvement of type I immunologic
mechanisms is unequivocal in these few cases, it is generally recognized that the
vast majority of sulfite reactions cannot be ascribed to immediate hypersensitivity.

b. Type II and III immunologic reactivity

No reactions have been reported.

c. Type IV immunologic reactivity

In general, the contactant sensitizing potential of sulfites in concentrations used
either in food or drugs is low. Several cases of contact dermatitis to sulfites have
been reported. The immunologic specificity of these reactions was confirmed by
patch tests with the appropriate sulfite salts at concentrations of 2, 5, and 10%
in aqueous solution (164).

d. Anatomical sites of hypersensitivity reactions: Systemic: Anaphylactic reac-
tions due to sulfite additives in drugs are characterized by diffuse pruritus,
flushing, urticaria, fullness in the head, nasal congestion, and severe wheezing.
The combination of these symptoms is often life-threatening. At least 12 fatal

cases allegedly involving sulfites in foods have been reported to the FDA (155). Some of these reports point out that death occurred within seconds or minutes of the subject ingesting sulfite additives.

e. Anatomical sites of hypersensitivity reactions: Respiratory: The occurrence of bronchoconstriction is the chief clinical manifestation associated with sulfite ingestion, injection, or inhalation. In the majority of instances, bronchospasm occurs without systemic manifestations. Inhalation of sulfites (e.g., in nebulizer solutions) is likely to induce bronchoconstriction in sulfite-reactive asthmatics at one-tenth to one-hundredth the dose required by oral sulfite ingestion or challenge (155). Asthmatics may become symptomatic after sulfite challenge because of the sulfur dioxide (SO_2) generated from inhalation, the act of swallowing oral solutions, the acidity produced after the dissolving of SO_2 in body fluids, or a combination of these effects. It should be emphasized that high concentrations of inhaled SO_2 can cause bronchoconstriction in all individuals but asthmatics respond to this gas at much lower concentrations. Inhalation of either acidic sulfites or SO_2 accounts for the vast majority of asthmatic reactions experienced by sulfite-reactive patients. On the other hand, in a small number of patients sulfite ions themselves will elicit immunologic release of allergic mediators that account for bronchoconstriction and/or generalized symptoms of anaphylaxis.

The prevalence of sulfite reactivity in known asthmatic populations with no prior history of sulfite reactivity has been investigated by use of spirometric changes after controlled oral provocation tests. The incidence of positive reactions in several studies ranged between 3.9 and 37% (155). Steroid-dependent asthmatics were more likely to exhibit positive oral challenge reactions. Asthmatic patients may develop paradoxical bronchospasm after inhalation of nebulizer solutions containing sulfite additives. Since significant quantities of SO_2 are generated by sulfite aerosols, it is postulated that bronchoconstriction induced by nebulized bisulfite saline solutions is due chiefly to the generation of SO_2 (165). Respiratory distress and decline of respiratory function were reported to occur in one patient after use of a glaucoma eye solution containing a small amount (0.075%) of potassium metabisulfite (166). Asthmatic reactions can be induced in susceptible individuals by dose–response challenges with either sulfite aqueous solutions or sulfite capsules. Challenge with oral sulfite solutions will identify SO_2-reactive asthmatic patients more readily while oral challenge with sulfite capsules will detect patients with susceptibility to the sulfite ion itself. A suggested protocol for oral challenge with sulfite capsules is shown in Table 5.

f. Anatomical sites of hypersensitivity reactions: Cutaneous: Urticarial and erythematous cutaneous reactions are expressed by the relatively few individuals who show anaphylactoid symptoms. Several cases of contact dermatitis have

Table 5 Suggested Double-Blind Dose Response Challenge Protocol (mg) for
Sodium/Potassium Metabisulfite Oral Challene on Two Separate Days

Time (hr)	0	½	1	1½	2
Dose (mg)	Placebo or 10	Placebo or 25	Placebo or 50	Placebo or 100	Placebo or 200

[a]The order of place bo or sulfite administration is determined by random selection.

been observed. Overall, skin reactions to sulfite exposure or challenge are in-frequent.

Gastrointestinal: Isolated symptoms of retching and vomiting occurred in a 7-year-old child after an oral challenge dose of a sulfite agent. These symptoms occurred within minutes. A positive scratch test was later demonstrated in this child (167).

g. Pseudoallergic reactions

The vast majority of sulfite reactions are nonimmunologic in nature. If exposure is by the inhaled route with drugs containing sulfite additives, the most likely mechanism is sulfur dioxide-induced bronchoconstriction. This phenomenon has been extensively studied by many investigators (155). The mechanism of bronchoconstriction induced by inhaled SO_2 is a reflex effect mediated through parasympathetic nerve pathways. Sulfur-dioxide-induced bronchoconstriction in humans can be abolished by prior inhalation of atropine, an effect easier to demonstrate in nonasthmatic subjects. Prior administration of cromolyn sodium also attenuates the effects of sulfite exposure in susceptible patients. While cromolyn sodium is thought to exert its chief effect by stabilizing mast cell membranes, recent evidence indicates that it also may be effective in abro-gating various reflex-induced stimuli that induce asthma. Oral administration of 1-5 mg vitamin B_{12} may fully or partially block bronchoconstriction in sulfite reactive asthmatic patients. The effectiveness of vitamin B_{12} is postulated to be due to its ability to catalyze sulfite oxidation (155).

Predisposing susceptibility to sulfite reactivity is of special interest because a relatively small number of asthmatic patients develop this life-threatening problem. It has been suggested that sulfite oxidase deficiency in chronic asthmatics may play a key role in the sulfite reactivity syndrome (155). It is postulated that chronic asthmatics with sulfite oxidase deficiency are unable to catabolize sulfite additives present in foods and drugs. This permits increased absorption and persistence of the sulfite ion within the systemic circulation and the tissues of vital organs. In support of this theory are some preliminary experimental data showing that sulfite-reactive asthmatics have decreased tissue sulfite oxidase levels compared to normal individuals. Once the syndrome has become manifest, patients must be cautioned to avoid further contact with sulfite additives contained in parenteral drugs, ophthalmic preparations, and infusion fluids. The only situation in which sulfite antioxidant might be permitted is the injection of epinephrine containing sulfites for treatment of life-threatening anaphylactic reaction due to some other substance.

VI. STABILIZERS: ETHYLENEDIAMINE

Ethylenediamine is a versatile chemical reagent. It is widely used in industry as a solvent for shellac, a corrosion inhibitor, a lubricant, a stabilizer for dyes, emulsifiers, and resin adhesives, and for making ethylenediamine derivatives (e.g., antihistamines and aminophylline). It has been widely used in topical pharmaceutical creams, especially a widely used commercial brand, Mycolog cream, a mixture of triamcinolone acetonide, neomycin, gramicidin, and nystatin, because its dibasic chemical characteristics impart an excellent stabilizing property to the cream. Similar product formulations in other parts of the world also contain this additive. Other important medical sources of ethylenediamine are aminophylline, which is an ethylenediamine salt of theophylline, and many types of thimerosal topical products (168,169). Occupational exposure to ethylenediamine may occur in many industries (preparation of dyes, rubber accelerators, fungicides, synthetic waxes, resins, insecticides, asphalt wetting agents, handling of photographic chemicals). Prior exposure by these routes may serve as the initial sensitizing dose for full-blown clinical sensitization that appears after the use of pharmaceuticals containing ethylenediamine. Of particular importance in this regard are pharmacists and nurses who handle aminophylline suppositories. It is also noteworthy that ethylenediamine cross-reacts with a large number of polyamines, structurally similar drugs, and drugs derived from ethylenediamine (170). Prior exposure to these substances could be the sensitizing stimulus for subsequent clinical sensitivity reactions.

a. Type I immunologic reactivity

Although industrial exposure and sensitization to ethylenediamine have been purported to induce rhinitis, coughing, and delayed-type asthma, the immunologic significance of such clinical responses is unknown (171). Positive direct skin test reactions to ethylenediamine were demonstrated in workers exposed to this chemical in the rubber, lacquer, and shellac industries (172). Sera from two of these patients passively transferred allergic antibody to the skin of normal persons, suggesting that specific IgE antibodies were responsible for the skin test reactions and respiratory symptoms in these patients. Type I sensitization to ethylenediamine contained in pharmaceutical preparations has not yet been proven.

b. Type II and III immunologic reactivity

No reactions have been reported.

c. Type IV immunologic reactivity

Several large-scale patch test surveys in patients with a clinical diagnosis of contact dermatitis revealed a high prevalence of sensitization to ethylenediamine ranging from 2 to 12.5% (173,174). This human experience combined with guinea pig sensitization experiments suggest that ethylenediamine has a high sensitization index (175). Confirmatory patch tests for ethylenediamine hydrochloride sensitivity should be performed with 1% ethylenediamine in petrolatum. This recommended concentration of ethylenediamine for routine patch testing is 10 times higher than the concentration found in one of the most common ethylenediamine-containing products on the market, Mycolog. However, this 10-fold increment is essential for patch test purposes because false-negative patch tests have been obtained when the Mycolog cream itself is used as the patch test reagent. These false-negative tests are attributed to the fact that the corticosteroid (triamcinolone) component in the Mycolog cream may retard the clinical expression of contact delayed hypersensitivity and the concentration of ethylenediamine may be too low in the cream to elicit a positive reaction on normal skin. A new formulation of Mycolog, Mycolog II cream, no longer contains neomycin and therefore ethylenediamine has also been eliminated. Patch tests with this proprietary preparation would therefore be negative in ethylenediamine patients. However, generic nystatin creams still contain ethylenediamine (176).

As noted above, many drugs and polyamines cross-react with ethylenediamine. Most of the data concerning cross-reactions have been gleaned by studies in small numbers of ethylenediamine-sensitive patients who also demonstrated positive patch tests to chemicals and drugs such as aminophylline, piperazine, triethylenetetramine, triethanolamine, aminoethylethanolamine, and hydroxyzine (170,177). A prospective patch test study of 50 cases of ethylenediamine-proven contact sensitization confirmed the presence of cross-reactivity to all of the above chemicals (178). This prospective study also established the fact that ethylenediamine tetraacetic acid (EDTA) did not cross-react with ethylenediamine. A subsequent patch test survey in 32 ethylenediamine-sensitive patients confirmed the high incidence of skin test cross-reactions to aliphatic polyamines and piperazine (diethylenediamine), but not to other ethylenediamine-related antihistamines (179). Oral challenges with hydroxyzine hydrochloride and the piperazine antihistamine derivative, cinnarizine, in five of these patients did not cause systemic reactions or exacerbation of contact dermatitis. However, there are at least two case reports of systemic contact dermatitis induced by oral ingestion of hydroxyzine in ethylenediamine-sensitive persons (180).

d. Anatomical sites of hypersensitivity reactions: *Cutaneous*: The first two case reports of contact dermatitis induced by ethylenediamine occurred in pharmacists who developed generalized papular eczematous eruptions after preparing aminophylline suppositories (168). Later, many more instances of ethylenediamine-induced contact dermatitis were observed in patients sensitized by topical creams containing this agent. Systemic exacerbation of contact dermatitis is apparently common after intravenous infusion of aminophylline in patients with preexisting sensitivity reactions to ethylenediamine (177,181). Two case reports of generalized severe exfoliative erythroderma occurred in ethylenediamine-sensitive patients (177,182). A patch test in one of these individuals reproduced the prior exfoliative erythroderma. The histologic lesion of this patch test showed dermal and epidermal edema and a lymphocyte infiltrate. Contact cutaneous reactivity to ethylenediamine has also been observed in patients receiving oral aminophylline treatment (168). Urticarial reactions have been recorded in one patient after intravenous infusion of aminophylline (183). This reaction was not thought to be due to the theophylline portion of the aminophylline because this patient was later able to tolerate oral theophylline without any reaction. However, objective tests to identify immediate or contact sensitivity to ethylenediamine were negative. An erythema-multiforme-like eruption occurred at a site distant from the original ethylenediamine-induced dermatitis (184).

Photocontact dermatitis appearing over exposed surfaces of the body has been observed in several patients (185,186). The diagnosis was confirmed by negative 48 hr covered patch tests, positive exposed patch tests, and controlled ultraviolet irradiation.

Respiratory: Upper and lower respiratory symptoms have occurred after occupational exposure and sensitization to ethylenediamine (172,187). These symptoms were verified by controlled laboratory bronchoprovocation with ethylenediamine that elicited a late response asthmatic reaction in several patients.

Because of extensive cross-reactions between ethylenediamine, many drugs, and industrial agents, patients with known ethylenediamine cutaneous sensitivity should avoid the use of topical creams containing ethylenediamine, antihistamines that are ethylenediamine-derivatives (tripelennamine, hydroxyzine), piperazine, aminophylline, thimerosal preparations, and various aliphatic polyamines.

e. Pseudoallergic reactions

A single case of urticaria appearing during intravenous aminophylline appears to be nonimmunologic (177). One patch with ethylenediamine-induced asthma under occupational conditions also did not demonstrate specific immune reactions but did exhibit histamine release from his blood when it was incubated with ethylenediamine (187). This suggested that ethylenediamine caused nonspecific release of mediators in this particular case.

VII. CHELATING AGENTS

Ethylenediaminetetracetic acid (EDTA) is the prototype agent in this category. EDTA in solution has a strong affinity for metals such as lead, calcium, and magnesium. EDTA is utilized as a preservative to prevent discoloration by binding trace metals that are essential reagents for catalytic or enzymatic processes in the preparation of antibiotic, antihistamine, and local anesthetic preparations. It is present in ear, eye, and nosedrops, local anesthetics (e.g., Monocaine), antibiotics, antihistamines and dermatologic creams and lotions. In ophthalmic solutions it enhances the antibacterial activity of benzalkonium chloride, chlorobutanol, and thimerosal by disrupting the lipid–protein complexes of cell walls. EDTA is also incorporated into a number of dental preparations including chemical disinfectants and local anesthetic solutions. It may also be added to medical appliances such as tampons.

a. Type I–III immunologic reactivity

No documented cases have been observed. There is one anecdotal report of vasculitis and hemolytic anemia occurring in two patients being treated by "chelation therapy" for coronary artery disease (188).

b. Type IV immunologic reactivity

Contact dermatitis has been documented by patch tests with 1% EDTA in petrolatum in several patients exposed and sensitized to this substance contained in local dermatologic creams (189). Several other reactions were described in patients using eyedrops or eye ointments containing EDTA. Contrary to popular belief, patients with known EDTA sensitization do not exhibit cross-reactions with ethylenediamine and the converse also applies (190).

c. Anatomical sites of hypersensitivity reactions: *Cutaneous*: Only a few cases of contact dermatitis have been described (189,190). The sensitization index is extremely small: routine patch testing with EDTA elicits only an occasional reaction.

d. Pseudoallergic reactions

Such reactions have not been reported.

VIII. STERILIZING AGENTS

1. Ethylene Oxide

Ethylene oxide gas is widely used as a sterilizing agent for plastics that cannot be subjected to gas or steam sterilization. It is a very potent alkylator of sulfhydryl, amino, carboxyl, and hydroxyl components of membrane proteins, thereby rendering microorganisms nonviable (191). Following sterilization, trace amounts of breakdown products or new products derived from interaction with plastic materials may be demonstrated (192). These include ethylene oxide itself, ethylene glycol, polyethylene glycol, ethylene chlorohydrin, and epichlorohydrin. Furthermore, trace amounts of ethylene oxide may persist for long periods of time in porous plastics, so gas desorption by aeration is not an effective means of ridding plastics of ethylene oxide contamination following sterilization (193). Adverse reactions to ethylene oxide gas were first discovered as a result of many investigations into the causes of the first-use syndrome (FUS), which was a descriptive term coined to describe an assortment of adverse symptoms occurring during hemodialysis on exposure to a fresh (previously unused) dialyzer (191,194). Hemodialyzer reactions are classifed into two main categories, type A and type B. Type A reactions begin immediately or up to 30 min. Symptoms include dyspnea, angioedema, flushing, urticaria, pruritis, rhinorrea, lacrimation, and abdominal cramping. Type B reactions occur during the first hour, with the most prominent symptoms being chest and back pains. Type A reactions are severe and often have to be treated with epinephrine. Type B reactions are mild and do not require discontinuation of the dialysis procedure. Adverse ethylene oxide gas reactions have been associated primarily with type A hemodialysis reactions. Similar adverse occurrences induced by ethylene oxide gas have been described in patients on peritoneal dialysis, plasmapheresis donors, and plateletpheresis donors (193,195,196).

a. Type I immunologic reactivity

The initial report of ethylene-oxide-specific IgE anaphylactic senstivity in patients with type A hemodialysis reactions has been corroborated by many centers throughout the world (191,193,195,197,198). In these studies, the allergenic reagent is prepared by incubating human serum albumin or other protein carriers with ethylene oxide gas as ordinarily generated during a routine sterilization process. Type I specificity in many type A hemodialysis reactions has been confirmed by direct skin tests with ethylene oxide–human serum albumin (EO–HSA) conjugates, RAST, enzyme-linked immunosorbent assay

(ELISA), polystyrene tube radioimmunoassay, passive cutaneous anaphylaxis in subhuman primates, and human leukocyte histamine release (191,193,195,197–201). One of the earlier reports suggested that IgE-specific antibodies were directed primarily against the haptenic moiety (ethylene oxide) (199). However, subsequent inhibition experiments with dialyzer rinsing fluid residues and ethylene oxide linked to simple amino acids (glycine and lysine) suggested that IgE antibody specificity is directed primarily to new antigenic determinants that occur after the interaction of ethylene oxide and carrier protein (200,202). In contrast to the vast majority of natural and chemical-allergen specific IgE-mediated reactions, direct skin tests with EO–HSA conjugates are less sensitive than RAST in the identification of sensitized patients (202). This paradox was explained by a marked decrease of cutaneous responsiveness in renal failure patients receiving chronic hemodialysis. However, not all patients experiencing immediate-type hypersensitivity reactions to ethylene oxide are RAST-positive (193). Several patients who demonstrated significant specific leukocyte histamine release induced by EO–HSA had negative skin and RAST tests. The estimated specificity and sensitivity of RAST are 0.89 and 0.63, respectively (203). The estimated false-positive and false-negative rates of RAST are 0.11 and 0.007, respectively.

b. Type II and III immunologic reactivity

IgG antibody specific for ethylene oxide has been demonstrated by radioimmunoprecipitation, ELISA, and total antibody techniques (199,195,200). These antibodies are significantly elevated in patients with dialysis tubing reactions compared to normal, unexposed controls. However, the precise role of these IgG antibody responses in the pathogenesis of the reaction is unknown.

c. Type IV immunologic reactivity

Type IV reactions are all of the contact dermatitis type. The conditions for performing and interpreting valid patch tests must be carefully differentiated from the known irritant effects of ethylene oxide gas on human skin. Different patch materials will rapidly lose ethylene oxide gas after varying periods of aeration. For example, ethylene oxide in petrolatum will produce irritative skin reactions in normal volunteers 4–8 hr after contact (204). Thus, the concentration of ethylene oxide should be less than 1,000 ppm in petrolatum in order to avoid such nonspecific skin irritation. Very sensitive patients will show markedly positive patch tests with gauze sterilized by ethylene oxide and aerated for as long as 48–96 hr.

d. Anatomical sites of hypersensitivity reactions: Systemic: The majority of type

A hemodialysis reactions are thought to be anaphylactic and mediated by IgE antibody. In addition to the usual symptoms and signs of anaphylaxis, these patients often describe a sensation of burning or heat throughout the body or at the vascular access site before systemic symptoms are manifest. These reactions are severe, occur within 30 min, and require immediate therapy with epinephrine and other supportive measures. The reported incidence of type A reactions is 3–5:100,000 dialyzers sold (194). The prevalence rate of immediate hypersensitivity reactions among patients undergoing long-term chronic hemodialysis ranges from 12 to 42%. Reactions to dialysis are much less frequent among peritoneal dialysis populations, repeat plasmapheresis donors (0.002%), and plateletpheresis donors (188,196,193).

e. Anatomical sites of hypersensitivity reactions: *Respiratory*: In one clinical study of symptomatic dialysis patients, 5 of 19 patients with increased RAST values were found to have asthma. Four of these patients had developed asthma only after the start of dialysis treatment, and in one case it was markedly aggravated during continuation of dialysis using ethylene-oxide-sterilized equipment (198).

f. Anatomical sites of hypersensitivity reactions: *Cutaneous*: A pruritic macular papular and erythematous rash of face, trunk, and extremities occurred in a 6-month-old infant, 5½ months after peritoneal dialysis had been started (195). This case was associated with IgE antibodies against ETO–HSA, peripheral eosinophilia, and marked peritoneal eosinophilia. The most common cutaneous lesion is contact dermatitis, which has been reported after exposure to face masks, gauze, and prepacked nitrofurazone dressings sterilized by ethylene oxide gas (205).

g. Pseudoallergic reactions

Ethylene oxide gas can be extremely irritating and irritant reactions must be clearly differentiated from allergic contact dermatitis. In the industrial setting, solutions of ethylene oxide act as vesicants and also may cause conjunctivitis if splashed in the eye. One hospital outbreak of ethylene oxide-induced burns in 19 hospitalized women was especially noteworthy (205). These women developed severe burns of the buttocks and back from contact with reusable surgical gowns and drapes that had been sterilized with ethylene oxide and had not been aerated. Tests of the reusable gowns revealed ethylene oxide gas residuals of 3,600–10,800 ppm ethylene oxide, compared to the safe level of retained ethylene oxide gas of 200 ppm. This outbreak illustrates that high levels of ethylene oxide gas in sterilized equipment and lack of proper degassing techniques could cause irritant rather than contact dermatitis.

2. Gluteraldehyde

Gluteraldehyde is an excellent cold sterilizing agent because it has a potent in vitro bactericidal, tuberculocidal, fungicidal, sporicidal, and viricidal activity.

It is used widely for cold sterilization of medical and dental equipment and is particularly useful for sterilizing fiberoptic endoscopes.

a. Type I immunologic reactivity

Several nurses developed upper and/or lower respiratory symptoms within weeks after being exposed to alkaline gluteraldehyde sterilizing solutions. Open and uncontrolled respiratory provocation studies (nasal and bronchial) revealed late nasal reactions in one instance and a late bronchial reaction in another case. Delayed challenge responses in both of these patients suggested the possibility of an IgE-mediated reaction but this was not confirmed by skin or in vitro serologic tests (206).

b. Type II and III immunologic reactivity

No reactions have been reported.

c. Type IV immunologic reactivity

Although a number of contact dermatitis cases induced by gluteraldehyde have been documented, this substance is a relatively infrequent sensitizer (208). Suspected cutaneous reactivity should be confirmed with a 1% aqueous solution of gluteraldehyde. Repeat insult patch tests in 706 normal unsensitized and 16 previously sensitized volunteers with 0.5% aqueous gluteraldehyde did not sensitize any of the subjects (207). Sensitized individuals may differ markedly in their responses to patch tests applied at different sites (208). Application of 25% gluderaldehyde to the soles of the feet failed to elicit positive skin responses in previously sensitive volunteers. In contrast, when the same patients were tested with 2.5% gluteraldehyde on the antecubital fossae, all developed severe dermatitis within 48 hr.

d. Anatomical sites of hypersensitivity reactions: Cutaneous: Allergic contact dermatitis is the only cutaneous manifestation that has been reported. In medical workers, this is most likely to appear on the hands of those who handle medical instruments that require cold sterilization.

e. Anatomical sites of hypersensitivity reactions: Respiratory: A general survey of medical staffs exposed to gluteraldehyde revealed conjunctival, nasal, and asthmatic symptoms. One case of pseudomembranous laryngotracheitis was reported from an anesthetic unit where gluteraldehyde had been used to sterilize endotracheal tubes (206). Direct proof that gluteraldehyde was the causal agent has only been determined in two patients by means of direct provocation tests.

3. Formaldehyde

Adverse reactions to formaldehyde as it is used for its antimicrobial properties in pharmaceutical preparations has been described. Formaldehyde is also used extensively as a sterilizing method for disposable hollow-fiber dialyzers. It has been suggested that some adverse responses in patients receiving chronic hemodialysis could be due to immunologically induced formaldehyde antibodies (209). One study suggested that these antibodies could be specifically directed to the N blood group antigen of formaldehyde-treated red blood cells. The search for significant formaldehyde antibodies in chronic hemodialysis patients has not been productive and the evidence to date that such antibodies are clinically significant is nil (102,210). Erythema multiforme with liver involvement has been described in two patients after occupational exposure to formaldehyde (211). One documented instance of an IgE-mediated anaphylactic reaction has been reported in a young woman exposed to a formaldehyde-sterilized dialyzer appparatus (101).

4. Chloramine-T

Adverse responses to this agent may occur in pharmaceutical workers and nurses who are exposed to this material as a sterilizing agent. This has been discussed previously.

IX. PROPELLANTS

The chief concerns about adverse reactions to propellants have been their possible cardiotoxic properties. Based on animal experiments, there has been a long-standing suspicion that fluorocarbon propellants, in particular, are capable of sensitizing the heart to epinephrine and beta-adrenergic agonists, effects that could lead to serious cardiac arrhythmias in humans. Although this controversy is not completely resolved, data on the cardiotoxic potential of the most commonly used propellants are equivocal in humans. The worst case scenario involves patients who deliberately inhale fluorocarbons and sympathomimetic drugs, as they do in the treatment of asthma. Although fluorocarbon concentrations of up to 5 μg/ml are found in arterial blood after 1-2 puffs of an inhaler, the concentrations of these propellants required to sensitize conscious dogs challenged with epinephrine were at least four to seven times higher (212). Only with extreme abuse of metered dose inhalers could equivalent conditions of cardiac sensitization occur in humans. Therefore, the FDA has concluded that the use of fluorocarbon aerosol propellants in metered dose dispensers is safe and should be permitted. A recent report of ventricular tachycardia associated with nonfreon aerosol propellants (isobutane, n-butane, and propane) requires further confirmation (213). Hypersensitivity reactions have not been documented after use of freon or nonfreon dispensed medical appliances. One possible exception to this is the possibility that patients with halothane-induced hepatitis could experience recrudescence of symptoms after exposure to structurally related fluorocarbons. The chief adverse responses to fluorocarbon propellants are related to their nonspecific effects in the lungs.

a. Pseudoallergic reactions

Several independent investigators have demonstrated that aerosol propellants, particularly fluorohydrocarbons, cause measurable increases in airway resistance after inhalation of 2 puffs from metered dose dispensers (214-216). Normal subjects also show slight decrease in specific airway conductance after inhalation of propellant sprays (214). The bronchoconstrictive effects of propellants are readily reversed by addition of $beta_2$-adrenergic agonists to the aerosol or by prior treatment with atropine. More detailed studies in dogs revealed that many freon and nonfreon propellants increased pulmonary resistance and decreased pulmonary compliance, with the single exception of fluorocarbon 11 (217). In humans, the bronchoconstrictive effects of these agents are not associated with significant changes in arterial oxygen tension (215). The mechanisms of propellant-induced bronchoconstriction appear to be reflex mediated through irritant receptors in the tracheobronchial tree. The refrigerant properties of propellants raise the question of possible supercooling of bronchial mucous membranes to achieve the bronchospastic effect, but it is highly unlikely that sufficient quantities of cooled gas would be delivered to the lower air space after 2 inhalations from a metered dose dispenser.

REFERENCES

1. Moscato, G., Naldi, L. and Candura, F. Bronchial asthma due to spiramycin and adipic acid. Clin. Allergy 14:355-361 (1984).
2. deWeck, A.L. Immunological effects of aspirin anhydride, a contaminant of commercial acetylsalicylic acid preparations. Int. Arch. Allergy Appl. Immunol. 41:393-418 (1971).
3. Bernstein, I.L. and Bernstein, D.I. Respiratory allergy to synthetic resins. In Clinics In Immunology and Allergy, 4. W.B. Saunders, London, pp 83-101 (1984).
4. Chung, C.W. and Giles, A.L. Jr. Sensitization potentials of methyl, ethyl, and n-butyl methacrylates and mutual cross-sensitivity in guinea pigs. J. Invest. Dermatol. 68:187-190 (1977).
5. Rietschel, R.L., Huggins, R., Levy, N. et al. In vivo and in vitro testing of gloves for protection against UV-curable acrylate resin systems. Contact Derm. 11:279-282 (1984).
6. Schneider, C.H., deWeck, A.L. and Stauble, E. Carboxylmethylcellulose additives in penicillins and the elicitation of anaphylactic reactions. Experimentia 27:167-168 (1971).
7. Hamada, T. and Horiguchi, S. Allergic contact dermatitis due to sodium carboxymethylcellulose. Contact Derm. 4(4):244 (1978).
8. Pauli, G., Bessot, J.C., Kopferschmitt, M.C. et al. Meat wrapper's asthma: Identification of the causal agent. Clin. Allergy 10:263-269 (1980).
9. Vidovic, R. and Kansky, A. Contact dermatitis in workers processing polyvinyl chloride plastics. Derm.-Beruf.-Umwelt 33(3):104-105 (1985).

10. Fisher, A.A. Allergic contact dermatitis in early infancy. Cutis 35:315–316 (1985).
11. Bommer, J., Ritz, E. and Andrassy, K. Necrotizing dermatitis resulting from hemodialysis with polyvinylchloride tubing. Ann. Intern. Med. 91: 869–870 (1979).
12. Calnan, C.D. Dibutyl phthalate. Contact Derm. 1:388 (1975).
13. Krajewska, D. and Rudzki, E. Sensitivity to epoxy resins and triethylenetetramine. Contact Derm. 2:135–138 (1976).
14. Fisher, A.A. Cross reactions between ethylenediamine base in merthiolate tincture with ethylenediamine HCI. Contact Derm. 14(3):181 (1986).
15. Calnan, C.D. Diethyldithiocarbamate in adhesive tape. Contact Derm. 4(1): 61 (1978).
16. Fregert, S., Trulson, L. and Ximerson, E. Contact allergic reactions to diphenylthiourea and phenylisothiocyanate in PVC adhesive tape. Contact Derm. 8:38–42 (1982).
17. Fisher, A.A. Dermatitis due to transdermal therapeutic systems. Cutis 34: 526–531 (1984).
18. Lindberg, M. and Forslind, B. The effects of occlusion of the skin on the Langerhans' cells. Acta Derm. Venereol. 61:201–205 (1981).
19. Nieboer, C., Bruynzeel, D.P., and Boorsma, D.M. The effect of occlusion of skin with transdermal therapeutic system on Langerhans' cells and the induction of skin irritation. Arch. Dermatol. 123:1499–1502 (1987).
20. Hannuksela, M., Kousa, M. and Pirila, V. Allergy to ingredients of vehicles. Contact Derm. 2:105–110 (1976).
21. Prater, E., Goring, H.D. and Schubert, H. Sodium lauryl sulphate—a contact allergen. Contact Derm. 4(4):242–243 (1978).
22. Eubanks, S. and Patterson, J.W. Dermatitis from sodium lauryl sulfate in hydrocortisone cream. Contact Derm. 11(4):250–251 (1984).
23. Nurse, D.S. Sensitivity to coconut diethanolamine. Contact Derm. 6(7):502 (1980).
24. Kligman, A.M. The SLS provocative patch test in allergic contact sensitization. J. Invest. Dermatol. 46:573–583 (1966).
25. Emmett, E.A. and Wright, R.C. Allergic contact dermatitis from TEA-Coco hydrolyzed protein. Arch. Dermatol. 112:1008–1009 (1976).
26. Kroon, S. Contact dermatitis from oleyl polypeptide in Xeruminex ear drops. Contact Derm. 7(5):271–272 (1981).
27. Howrie, D.L., Ptachcinski, R.J., Griffith, B.P. et al. Anaphylactoid reactions associated with parenteral cyclosporine use: Possible role of cremophor EL. Drug Intell. Clin. Pharm. 19:425–427 (1985).
28. Moneret-Vautrin, D.A., Laxenaire, M.C. and Viry-Babel, F. Anaphylaxis caused by anti-cremophor EL IgG STS antibodies in a case of reaction to althesin. Br. J. Anaesth. 55:469–471 (1983).
29. van Hooff, J.P., Bessems, P., Beuman, G.H. et al. Absence of allergic reaction to cyclosporin capsules in patient allergic to standard oral and intravenous solution of cyclosporin. Lancet 1456 (1987).

30. Hannuksela, M., Kousa, M. and Pirila, V. Contact sensitivity to emulsifiers. Contact Derm. 2:201–204 (1976).

31. Warning for Prescriptive Drugs Containing Sulfites. FDA Drug Bull. April: 1–10, 1987.

32. Samsoen, M. and Jelin, G. Allergy to daktarin gel. Contact Derm. 6:351–342 (1977).

33. Edwards, E.K. Jr. and Edwards, E.K. Allergic reaction to triethanolamine stearate in a sunscreen. Cutis 31:195–196 (1983).

34. Suurmond, D. Patch test reactions to Phenergan cream, promethazine and triethanolamine. Dermatologica 133:503–506 (1966).

35. Finn, O.A. and Forsyth, A. Contact dermatitis due to sorbitan monolaurate. Contact Derm. 1(5):318 (1975).

36. Austad, J. Allergic contact dermatitis to sorbitan monooleate (Span 80). Contact Derm. 8(6):426–427 (1982).

37. Herman, J.J. Intractable sneezing due to IgE-mediated triethanolamine sensitivity. J. Allergy Clin. Immunol. 71:339–344 (1983).

38. Vallieres, M., Cockcroft, D.W., Taylor, D.M. et al. Dimethylethanolamine-induced asthma. Am. Rev. Respir. Dis. 115:867–871 (1977).

39. Fisher, A.A. Allergic contact dermatitis and conjunctivitis from benzalkonium chloride. 39:381–383 (1987).

40. Beasley, C.R.W., Rafferty, P. and Holgate, S.T. The role of preservatives in atrovent-induced bronchoconstriction. Thorax 42:702 (1987).

41. Haidar, Z. An adverse reaction to a topical antiseptic (Cetrimide). Br. J. Oral Surg. 15:86–91 (1977–78).

42. Staniforth, P. Allergy to benzalkonium chloride in plaster of paris after sensitization to cetrimide. J. Bone Joint Surg. 62:500–501 (1980).

43. Cruickshank, C.N.D. and Squire, J.R. Skin sensitivity to cetrimide (CTAB). Br. J. Ind. Med. 6:164–167 (1949).

44. Morgan, J.K. Iatrogenic epidermal sensitivity. Br. J. Clin. Pract. 22:261–264 (1968).

45. Haider, Z. An adverse reaction to a topical antiseptic (cetrimide). Br. J. Oral Surg. 15:86–91 (1977–78).

46. Shmunes, E. and Levy E.J. Quaternary ammonium compound contact dermatitis from a deodorant. Arch. Dermatol. 105:91–93 (1972).

47. Padnos, E., Horwitz, I.D. and Wunder, G. Contact dermatitis complicating tracheostomy. Am. J. Dis. Child. 109:90–91 (1965).

48. Bayliss, W.M. Acacia for transfusion. J.A.M.A. 78(24):1885–1887 (1922).

49a. Lagier, F., Cartier, A., Dolovich, J., and Malo, J. L.: Occupational asthma due to guar gum. J. Allergy Clin. Immunol. 83: 172 (1989).

50. Gelfand, H.H. The vegetable gums by ingestion in the etiology of allergic disorders. J. Allergy 20:311–321 (1949).

51. Anderson, D.M.W. Evidence for the safety of gum arabic (Acacia senegal (L) Willd.) as a food additive—a brief review. Food Additives Contamin. 3(3):225–230 (1986).

52. Brown, E.B. and Crepea, S.B. Allergy (asthma) to ingested gum tragacanth. J. Allergy 18:214–215 (1947).
53. Rubinger, D., Friedlander, M. and Superstine, E. Hypersensitivity to tablet additives in transplant recipients on prednisone. Lancet 689 (1978).
54. Howlett, B.J., Hill, D.J. and Knox, R.B. Cross-reactivity between Acacia (wattle) and rye grass pollen allergens. Clin. Allergy 12:259–268 (1982).
55. Coskey, R.J. Contact dermatitis caused by ECG electrode jelly. Arch. Dermatol. 113:839–840 (1977).
56. Ronnen, M., Suster, S., Kahana, M. et al. Contact dermatitis due to Karaya gum induced by the application of electrodes. Int. J. Dermatol. 25:24–25 (1986).
57. Wagner, W. Karaya gum hypersensitivity in an enterstomal therapist. Letters to the Editor. J.A.M.A. 243(5):432 (1980).
58. Hamada, T. and Horiguchi, S. Allergic contact dermatitis due to sodium carboxymethylcellulose. Contact Derm. 4(4):244 (1978).
59. Hancock, B.W. and Naysmith, A. Hypersensitivity to chlorocresol-preserved heparin. Br. Med. J. 3(5986):746–747 (1975).
60. Baer, R.L., Serri, F. and Weissenbach-Vial, C. Studies on allergic sensitization to certain topical therapeutic agents. Arch. Dermatol. 71:19 (1955).
61. Archer, C.B. and MacDonald, D.M. Chlorocresol sensitivity induced by treatment of allergic contact dermatitis with steroid creams. Contact Derm. 11:144–145 (1984).
62. Burry, J.N., Kirk, J., Reid, J.G. et al. Chlorocresol sensitivity. Contact Derm. 1:41–42 (1975).
63. Anderson, K.E. Contact allergy to chlorocresol, formaldehyde and other biocides. Acta Derm. Venereol. 125:1–21 (1986).
64. Dooms-Goossens, A., Degreef, H., Vanhee, L. et al. Chlorocresol and chloracetamide: Allergens in medications, glues and cosmetics. Contact Derm. 7(1):51–52 (1981).
65. Marzulli, F.N. and Maibach, H.I. Antimicrobials: Experimental contact sensitization in man. J. Soc. Cosmet. Chem. 24:399–421 (1973).
66. Rycroft, R.J.G. Contact sensitization to 2-monomethylol phenol in phenol formaldehyde resin as an example of the recognition and prevention of industrial dermatoses. Clin. Exp. Dermatol. 7:285–290 (1982).
67. Bruze, M. and Zimerson, E. Contact allergy to 3-methylol phenol, 2,4-dimethylol phenol and 2,6-dimethylol phenol. Acta Derm. Venereol. (Stockh.) 65:548–551 (1985).
68. Bruze, M., Fregert, S., Persson, L. et al. Contact allergy to 4,4'-dihydroxy-(hydroxymethyl)-diphenyl methanes: Sensitizers in a phenol-formaldehyde resin. J. Invest. Dermatol. 87(5):617–623 (1986).
69. Freitas, J.P. and Brandao, F.M. Contact urticaria to chlorocresol. Contact Derm. 15:252 (1986).
70. Rogers, S.C.F., Burrows, D. Neill D. Percutaneous absorption of ophenol and methyl alcohol in Magenta patient BPC. Br. J. Dermatol. 98:559 (1978).

71. Fisher, A.A. Irritant and toxic reactions to phenol in topical medications. Cutis 26:363–392 (1980).
72. Kopelman, P. and Morgan, P.G.M. Adverse reaction to chlorocresol-preserved heparin. Lancet 1:705 (1977).
73. Fisher, A.A. Paraben dermatitis due to a new medicated bandage: The "paraben paradox." Contact Derm. 5(4):273–274 (1979).
74. Aeling, J.L. and Nuss, D.D. Systemic eczematous "contact type" dermatitis medicamentosa caused by parabens. Letters to the editor. Arch. Dermatol. 110:640 (1974).
75. Aldrete, A.J. and Johnson, D.A. Allergy to local anesthetics. J.A.M.A. 207: 356–357 (1969).
76. Latronica, R.J., Goldberg,A.F. and Wrightman, J.R. Local anesthetic sensitivity: Report of a case. Oral Surg. 28:439–441 (1969).
77. Nagel, J.E., Fuscaldo, J.T. and Fireman, P. Paraben allergy. J.A.M.A. 237 (15):1594–1595 (1977).
78. Henry, J.C., Tschen, E.H. and Becker, L.E. Contact urticaria to parabens. Arch. Dermatol. 115:1231–1232 (1979).
79. North American Contact Dermatitis Group. Epidemiology of contact dermatitis in North America 1972. Arch. Dermatol. 108:437–540 (1973).
80. Fisher, A.A. Allergic paraben and benzyl alcohol hypersensitivity relationship of the "delayed" and "immediate" varieties. Contact Derm. 1:281–284, 1975.
81. Kaminer, Y., Apter, A., Tyano, S. et al. Delayed hypersensitivity reaction to orally administered methylparaben. Clin. Pharm. 1:469–470 (1982).
82. Fisher, A.A. Allergic reactions to the preservatives in over-the-counter hydrocortisone topical creams and lotions. Cutis 32:222–230 (1983).
83. Mostow, S.R., Dreisin, R.B., Manawadu, B.R. et al. Adverse effects of lidocaine and methylparaben on tracheal ciliary activity. Laryngoscope 89: 1697–1701 (1979).
84. Fisher, A.A. The misuse of the patch test to determine "hypersensitivity" to mercury amalgam dental fillings. Cutis 35:110–117 (1985).
85. Calnan, C.D. Contact dermatitis from drugs; symposium on drug sensitization. Proc. R. Soc. Med. 55:39 (1962).
86. Rudner, E.J., Clendenning, W.E., Epstein, E. et al. Epidemiology of contact dermatitis in North America: 1972. Arch. Dermatol. 108:537 (1973).
87. Mathews, K.P. Immediate type hypersensitivity to phenylmercuric compounds. Am. J. Med. 44:310–318 (1968).
88. Maibach, H. Acute laryngeal obstruction presumed secondary to thiomersal (merthiolate) delayed hypersensitivity. Contact Derm. 1:221–222 (1975).
89. White, W.G., Barnes, G.M., Barker, E. et al. Reactions to tetanus toxoid. J J. Hyg. (Camb.) 71:283 (1973).
90. Moller, H. Merthiolate allergy: A nationwide iatrogenic sensitization. Acta. Derm. Venereol. (Stockh.) 57:509–517 (1977).
91. Cox, N.H. and Morley, W.N. Vaccination reactions and thiomersal. Br. Med. J. 294:250 (1987).

92. Mondino, H.J., Salamon, S.M. and Zaidman, G.W. Allergic and toxic reactions in soft contact lens wearers. Surv. Ophthalmol. 26(6):337–343 (1982).

93. Zadnik, K. Severe allergic reaction to saline preserved with thimerosal. J. Am. Opthom. Assoc. 55(7):507–509 (1984).

94. Heyderman, E. and Brown, B.M.E. Exacerbation of eczema of formalin-containing hepatitis B vaccine in formaldehyde-allergic patient. Lancet: 522–523 (1986).

95. Storrs, F.J. and Bell, D.E. Allergic contact dermatitis to 2-bromo-2-nitropane-1,3-diol in a hydrophilic ointment. J. Am. Acad. Dermatol. 8:157–170 (1983).

96. Fisher, A.A. Preservative (Quaternium 15) dermatitis from the "generic equivalent" of a "brand name" hydrocortisone cream (Hytone® cream, Dermik). Cutis 41:153–154 (1988).

97. Forman, G.H. and Ord, R.A. Allergic endodontic angioedema in response to periapical endomethasone. Br. Dent. J. 160:348–350 (1986).

98. Block, R.M., Lewis, R.D., Sheats, J.B. et al. Antibody formation to dog pulp tissue altered by N2 type paste within the root canal. J. Endodont. 3:309–315 (1977).

99. Block, R.M., Lewis, R.D., Sheats, J.B. et al. Cell-mediated immune responses to dog pulp tissue altered by Formocresol within the root canal. J. Endodont. 3:424–430 (1977).

100. Dilley, G.J. and Courts, E.J. Immunological response to four pulpal medicaments. Pediatr. Dent. 3:179–183 (1981).

101. Maurice, F., Rivory, J.-P., Larsson, P.H. et al. Anaphylactic shock caused by formaldehyde in a patient undergoing long-term hemodialysis. J. Allergy Clin. Immunol. 77:594–597 (1986).

102. Patterson, R., Pateras, V., Grammer, L.C. et al. Human antibodies against formaldehyde-human serum albumin conjgates or human serum albumin in individuals exposed to formaldehyde. Int. Arch. Allergy Appl. Immunol. 79:53–59 (1986).

103. Thrasher, J.D., Wojdaani, A., Cheung, G. et al. Evidence for formaldehyde antibodies and altered cellular immunity in subjects exposed to formaldehyde in mobile homes. Arch. Environ. Health 42:347–350 (1987).

104. Peters, M.S., Connolly, S.M. and Schroeter, A.L. Bronopol allergic contact dermatitis. Contact Derm. 9:397–401 (1983).

105. Camarasa, J.G. Contact dermatitis due to Bronopol. Contact Derm. 14(3): 191–192 (1986).

106. Bryce, D.M., Croshaw, B., Hall, J.E. et al. The activity and safety of the anti-microbial agent bronopol (2-bromo-2-nitropropane-1, 3-diol). J. Soc. Cosmet. Chem. 29:3–24 (1978).

107. Rudner, E.J. North American Group results. Contact Derm. 3:208–209 (1981).

108. Maibach, H.I. Dermal sensitization potential of 2-bromo-2-nitropropane-1,3-diol (Bronopol). Contact Derm. 3:99–108 (1977).

109. Fisher, A.A. Erythema limited to the face due to sorbic acid. Cutis 40: 395–397 (1987).
110. Goransson, K. and Liden, S. Contact allergy to sorbic acid and unguentum Merck.
111. Fisher, A.A. The contact dermatitis syndrome—a commentary on the Tokyo report. Cutis 31:28–34 (1983).
112. Saihan, E.M. and Harman, R.M. Contact sensitivity to sorbic acid in "unguentum Merck." Br. J. Dermatol. 99:583–584 (1978).
113. Brown, R. Another case of sorbic acid sensitivity. Contact Derm. 5:268 (1979).
114. Simpson, J.R. Sorbic acid sensitivity from cortacream bandages. Contact Derm. Newsletter 10:232 (1971).
115. Hjorth, N. and Trolle-Larsen, C. Skin reactions to preservatives in cream with special regard to paraben esters and sorbic acid. Am. Perfum. 77:43 (1962).
116. Klaschka, F. and Biersdorff, H. Allergic eczematous reaction for sorbic acid used as a preservative in external medicaments. Munch. Med. Wochenschr. 107:185 (1965).
117. Rudzki, E. and Kleniewska, D. The epidemiology of contact dermatitis in Poland. Br. J. Dermatol. 83:543 (1970).
118. Kerstin, G. and Liden, S. Contact allergy to sorbic acid and unguentum Merck. Contact Derm. 7(5):277 (1981).
119. Meynadier, J.M., Meynadier, J., Colmas, A. et al. Allergie aux conservateurs. Ann. Dermatol. Venereol. (Paris) 109:1017–1023 (1982).
120. Warrington, R.J., Sauder, P.J. and McPhillilps, S. Cell-mediated immune responses to artificial food additives in chronic urticaria. Clin. Allergy 16: 527–533 (1986).
121. Lahti, A. Non-immunologic contact urticaria. Acta Derm. Venereol. (Stockh.) 60:23 (1980).
122. Nethercott, J.R., Lawrence, M.J., Roy, A.M. et al. Airborne contact urticaria due to sodium benzoate in a pharmaceutical manufacturing plant. J. Occup. Med. 26:734–736 (1978).
123. Lahti, A. Skin reactions to some antimicrobial agents. Contact Derm. 4(5):302–303 (1978).
124. Soschin, D. and Leyden, J.J. Sorbic acid-induced erythema and edema. J. Am. Acad. Dermatol. 14:234–241 (1986).
125. Michaelsson, G. and Juhlin, L. Urticaria induced by preservatives and dye additives in food and drugs. Br. J. Dermatol. 88:525–532 (1983).
126. Warin, R.P. and Smith, R.J. Challenge test battery in chronic urticaria. Br. J. Dermatol. 94:401–406 (1976).
127. Juhlin, L. Recurrent urticaria: Clinical investigation of 330 patients. Br. J. Dermatol. 104:369–381 (1981).
128. Lahti, A. and Hannuksela, M. Is benzoic acid really harmful in cases of atopy and urticaria? Lancet 2:1055, (1981).
129. Lahti, A., Oikarinen, A., Viinikka, L. et al. Prostaglandins in contact urti-

caria induced by benzoic acid. Acta Derm. Venereol. (Stockh.) 63:425–427 (1983).

130. Moneret-Vautrin, D.A., Moeller, R., Malingrey, L. et al. Anaphylactoid reaction to general anaesthesia: A case of intolerance to sodium benzoate. Anaesth. Intens. Care 10:156–157 (1982).

131. Dux, S., Pitlik, S., Perry, G. et al. Hypersensitivity reaction to chlorbutanol-preserved heparin. Lancet 1:149 (1981).

132. Itabashi, A., Katayama, S. and Yamaji, T. Hypersensitivity to chlorobutanol in DDAVP solution. Lancet 1:108, (1982).

133. Hoffman, H., Goerz, G. and Plewig, G. Anaphylactic shock from chlorobutanol-preserved oxytocin. Contact Derm. 15:241–260 (1986).

134. Shmunes, E. Allergic dermatitis to benzyl alcohol in an injectable solution. Arch. Dermatol. 120:1200–1201 (1984).

135. Grant, J.A., Bilodeau, P.A., Guernsey, B. et al. Unsuspected benzyl alcohol hypersensitivity. N. Engl. J. Med. 306:108 (1982).

136. Bourne, M.S., Flindt, M.L.H. and Walker, J.M. Asthma due to industrial use of chloramine. Br. Med. J. 2:10–12 (1979).

137. Dijkman, J.H., Vooren, P.H. and Kramps, J.A. Occupational asthma due to inhalation of chloramine-T. I. Clinical observations and inhalation-provocation studies. Int. Arch. Allergy Appl. Immunol. 64:422–427 (1981).

138. Kramps, J., van Toorenenbergen, A.Q., Vooren, P.H. et al. Occupational asthma due to inhalation of chloramine-T. II. Demonstration of specific IgE antibodies. Int. Arch. Allergy Appl. Immunol. 64:428–438 (1981).

139. Dooms-Goossens, A., Gevers, D., Mertens, A. et al. Allergic contact urticaria due to chloramine. Contact Derm. 9(4):319–320 (1983).

140. Prins, F.J. and Smeenk, G. Contacteczeem door Hirudoidsalf. Ned. Tijdschr. Geneeskd. 46:115 (1934–1938).

141. Nater, J.P. Allergic reactions due to chloracetamide. Dermatologica 142:191–192 (1971).

142. Marzulli, F.N. and Maibach, H.I. Antimicrobials: Experimental contact sensitization in man. J. Soc. Cosmet. Chem. 24:399 (1973).

143. Osmundsen, P.E. Contact urticaria from nickel and plastic additives (Butylhydroxytoluene, oleylamide). Contact Derm. 6:452–454 (1980).

144. Moneret-Vautrin, D.A., Faure, G. and Bene, M.C. Chewing gum preservative induced toxidermic vasculitis. Allergy 41:546–548 (1986).

145. Roed-Peterson, J. and Hjorth, N. Contact dermatitis from antioxidants. Hidden sensitizers in topical medications and foods. Br. J. Dermatol. 94:233–241 (1976).

146. White, I.R., Lovell, C.R. and Cronin, E. Antioxidants in cosmetics. Contact Derm. 11:265–267 (1984).

147. Liden, S. Alphosyl® sensitivity and propyl gallate. Contact Derm. 1(4):257–258 (1975).

148. Maibach, H., Gellin, G. and Ring, M. Is the antioxidant butylated hydroxytoluene a depigmenting agent in man? Contact Derm. 1:295–296 (1975).

149. Meneghini, C.L., Rantuccio, F. and Lomuto, M. Additives, vehicles and

active drugs of topical medicaments as causes of delayed-type allergic dermatitis. Dermatologica 143:137 (1971).

150. Kahn, G., Phanuphak, P. and Claman, H.N. Propyl gallate-contact sensitization and orally-induced tolerance. Arch. Dermatol. 109:506–509 (1974).

151. Saperstein, H., Rapaport, M. and Rietschel, R.L. Topical vitamin E as a cause of erytheme multiforme-like eruptions. Arch. Dermatol. 120:906 (1984).

152. Pigatto, P.D., Boneschi, V., Riva, F. et al. Allergy to propylgallate, with unusual clinical and histological features. Contact Derm. 11(1):43 (1984).

153. Fisherman, E.W. and Cohen, G. Chemical intolerance to butylated-hydroxyanisole (BHA) and butylated-hydroxytoluene (BHT) and vascular response as an indicator and monitor of drug intolerance. Ann. Allergy 31:126–133 (1973).

154. Cloninger, P. and Novey, H.S. The acute effects of butylated hydroxyanisole ingestion in asthma and rhinitis of unknown etiology. Ann. Allergy 32:131–133 (1974).

155. Gunnison, A.F. and Jaconsen, D.W. Sulfite sensitivity. A critical review. Crit. Rev. Toxicol. 17(3):185–214 (1987).

156. Warning for Prescriptive Drugs Containing Sulfites. FDA Drug Bull. April, 1987, pp. 1–10.

157. Goldfarb, G. and Simon, R. Provocation of sulfite sensitive asthma. J. Allergy Clin. Immunol. 73(Abst):135 (1984).

158. Prenner, M. and Stevens, J.J. Anaphylaxis after ingestion of sodium bisulfite. Ann. Allergy 37:180 (1976).

159. Twarog, F.J. and Leung, D.Y.M. Anaphylaxis to a component of isoetharine (sodium bisulfite). J.A.M.A. 248(16):2030–2031 (1982).

160. Koepke, J.W., Christopher, K.L., Chai, H. et al. Dose-dependent bronchospasm from sulfites in isoetharine. J.A.M.A. 251(22):2982–2983 (1984).

161. Baker, G.J., Collett, P. and Allen, D.H. Bronchospasm induced by metabisulphite-containing foods and drugs. Med. J. Aust. Nov. 28: 614–617 (1981).

162. Schwartz, H.J. and Sher, T.H. Bisulfite sensitivity manifesting as allergy to local dental anesthesia. J. Allergy Clin. Immunol. 75:525–527 (1985).

163. Simon, R.A. Sulfite sensitivity. Ann. Allergy 56:281–291 (1986).

164. Apetato, M. and Marques, M.S.J. Contact dermatitis caused by sodium metabisulphite. Contact Derm. 14(3):194 (1986).

165. Koepke, J.W., Selner, J.C. and Dunhill, A.L. Presence of sulfur dioxide in commonly used bronchodilator solutions. J. Allergy Clin. Immunol. 72: 504 (1983).

166. Schwartz, H.J. and Sher, T.H. Bisulfite intolerance manifest as bronchospasm following topical dipiverfrin hydrochloride therapy for glaucoma. Arch. Ophthalmol. 103:14 (1985).

167. Wolf, S.I. and Nicklas, R.A. Sulfite sensitivity in a seven-year-old child. Ann. Allergy 54:420–423 (1985).

168. Provost, T.T. and Jillson, O.F. Ethylenediamine contact dermatitis. Arch. Dermatol. 96:231–234 (1967).
169. Fisher, A.A. Cross reactions between ethylenediamine base in merthiolate® tincture with ethylenediamine HCI. Contact Derm. 14(3):181 (1986).
170. Fisher, A.A. Cross-reactions between epoxy resin "amine" hardeners and ethylenediamine. Curr. Contact News 17:839–841 (1976).
171. Aldrich, F.D., Stange, A.W. and Geesaman, R.E. Smoking and ethylenediamine sensitization in an industrial population. J. Occup. Med. 29(4): 311–314 (1987).
172. Gelfand, H.H. Respiratory allergy due to chemical compounds encountered in the rubber lacquer, shellac and beauty culture industries. J. Allergy 34:374–381 (1963).
173. Eriksen, K.E. Allergy to ethylenediamine. Arch. Dermatol. 111:791 (1975).
174. White, M.I., Douglas, W.S. and Main, R.A. Contact dermatitis attributed to ethylenediamine. Br. Med. J. 415–416 (1978).
175. Eriksen, K. Sensitization capacity of ethylene diamine in the guinea pig and induction of unresponsiveness. Contact Derm. 5:193–296 (1979).
176. Fisher, A.A. Problems associated with "generic" topical medications. Cutis 41:313–314 (1988).
177. Elias, J.A. and Levinson, A.I. Hypersensitivity reactions to ethylenediamine in aminophylline. Am. Rev. Repsir. Dis. 123:550–552 (1981).
178. Balato, N., Cusano, F., Lembo, G. et al. Ethylenediamine contact dermatitis. Contact Derm. 11:112–114 (1984).
179. Balato, N., Cusano, F., Lembo, G. et al. Ethylenediamine dermatitis. Contact Derm. 15:263–265 (1986).
180. Fisher, A.A. Conact dermatitis: Highlights from the 1987 meeting of the American Academy of Dermatology, San Antonio, Texas. Cutis 41:87–88 (1988).
181. DeShazo, R.D. Ethylenediamine-aminophylline hypersensitivity. Arch. Intern. Med. 141:1267 (1981).
182. Petrozzi, J.W. and Shore, R.N. Generalized exfoliative dermatitis from ethylenediamine. Arch. Dermatol. 112:525–526 (1976).
183. Booth, B.H., Coleman, W.P. and Mitchell, D.Q. Urticaria following intravenous aminophylline. Ann. Allergy 43:289–290 (1979).
184. Fisher, A.A. Erythema multiforme-like eruptions due to topical medications: Part II. Cutis 37:158–161 (1986).
185. Burry, J.N. Photocontact dermatitis from ethylenediamine. Contact Derm. 16(5):305–306 (1986).
186. Romaguera, C., Grimalt, F. and Lecha, M. Photoallergic dermatitis from ethylenediamine. Contact Derm. 14(2):130 (1986).
187. Lam, S. and Chan-Yeung, M. Ethylenediamine-induced asthma. Am. Rev. Respir. Dis. 121:151–155 (1980).
188. Peterson, G.R. Adverse effects of chelation therapy. J.A.M.A. 250:2926 (1983).

189. DeGroot, A.C. Contact allergy to EDTA in a topical corticosteroid preparation. Contact Derm. 15(4):250-252 (1986).
190. Fisher, A.A. (ed). Contact Dermatitis, 3rd edition. Lea & Febiger, Philadelphia, (1986).
191. Poothullil, J., Shimizu, A., Day, R.P. et al. Anaphylaxis from the product(s) of ethylene oxide gas. Ann. Intern. Med. 82:58-60 (1975).
192. Limitation of ethylene oxide sterilization. J. Hosp. Res. 7:39-54 (1969).
193. Leitman, S.F., Boltansky, H., Alter, H.J. et al. Allergic reactions in healthy plateletpheresis donors caused by sensitization to ethylene oxide gas. N. Engl. J. Med. 315(19):1192-1196 (1986).
194. Ing, T.S., Ivanovich, P.T. and Daugirdas, J.T. First-use syndrome and hypersensitivity during hemodialysis: Some pieces of the puzzle are falling into place. Artif. Organs 11:(2):79-81 (1987).
195. Patterson, R., Lerner, C., Roberts, M. et al. Ethylene oxide (ETO) as a possible cause of an allergic reaction during peritoneal dialysis and immunologic detection of ETO from dialysis tubing. Am. J. Kidney Dis. VIII:64-66 (1986).
196. Dolovich, J., Sagona, M., Pearson, F. et al. Sensitization of repeat plasmapheresis donors to ethylene oxide gas. Transfusion 27(1):90-93 (1987).
197. Bommer, J., Barth, H.P., Wilhelms, O.H. et al. Anaphylactoid reactions in dialysis patients: Role of ethylene-oxide. Lancet 2: 1382-1384, (1985).
198. Rumpf, K.W., Seubert, A., Valentin, R. et al. Association of ethylene-oxide-induced IgE antibodies with symptoms in dialysis patients. Lancet 2:1385-1387 (1985).
199. Dolovich, J. and Bell, B. Allergy to a product(s) of ethylene oxide gas. J. Allergy Clin. Immunol. 62(1):30-32 (1978).
200. Grammer, L.C., Shaugnessy, M.A., Paterson, B.F. et al. Characterization of an antigen in acute anaphylactic dialysis reactions: Ethylene oxide-altered human serum albumin. J. Allergy Clin. Immunol. 76:670-675 (1985).
201. Grammer, L.C. and Patterson, R. IgE against ethylene oxide-altered human serum albumin (ETO-HSA) as an etiologic agent in allergic reactions of hemodialysis patients. Artif. Organs 11(2):97-99 (1987).
202. Marshall, C., Shimizu, A., Smith, E.K.M. et al. Ethylene oxide allergy in a dialysis center: Prevalence in hemodialysis and peritoneal dialysis populations. Clin. Nephrol. 21(6):346-349 (1984).
203. Pearson, F., Bruszer, G., Lee, W. et al. Ethylene oxide sensitivity in hemodialysis patients. Artif. Organs 11(2):100-103 (1987).
204. Shupack, J.L., Andersen, S.R. and Romano, J.S. Human skin reactions to ethylene oxide. J. Lab. Clin. Med. 98:723 (1981).
205. Fisher, A.A. Ethylene oxide dermatitis. Cutis 34:20-24 (1984).
206. Corrado, O.J., Osman, J. and Davies, R.J. Asthma and rhinitis after exposure to glutaraldehyde in endoscopy units. Hum. Toxicol. 5:325-327 (1986).
207. Weaver, J.E. and Maibach, H.I. Dose response relationships in allergic

contact dermatitis: Glutaraldehyde-containing liquid fabric softener. Contact Derm. 3:65–68 (1977).

208. Maibach, H.I. and Prystowsky, D.S. Glutaraldehyde (Pentanedial) allergic contact dermatitis. Arch. Dermatol. 113:170–171 (1977).

209. Lynen, R., Rothe, M. and Gallasch, E. Characterization of formaldehyde-related antibodies encountered in hemodialysis patients at different stages of immunization. Vox Sang. 44:81–89 (1983).

210. Dolovich, J., Evans, S., Baurmeister, U. et al. Antibody responses to hemodialysis-related antigens in chronic hemodialysis patients. Artif. Organs 11(2):93–96 (1987).

211. Nethercott, J.R., Alberts, J., Gurguis, S. et al. Erythema multiforme exudativum linked to the manufacture of printed circuit boards. Contact Derm. 8:314 (1982).

212. Dollery, C.T., Williams, F.M., Draffan, G.H. et al. Arterial blood levels of fluorocarbons in asthmatic patients following use of pressurized aerosols. Clin. Pharm. Ther. 15:59 (1974).

213. Wason, S., Gibler, B. and Hassan, M. Ventricular tachycardia associated with non-freon aerosol propellants. J.A.M.A. 256(1):78–80 (1986).

214. Sterling, G.M. and Batten, J.C. Effect of aerosol propellants and surfactants on airway resistance. Thorax 24:228 (1969).

215. Brooks, S.M., Mintz, S. and Weiss, E. Changes occurring after freon inhalation. Am. Rev. Respir. Dis. 105:640–642 (1972).

216. Graff-Lonnevig, V. Diurnal expiratory flow after inhalation of freons and fenoterol in childhood asthma. J. Allergy Clin. Immunol. 64(1):534–538 (1979).

217. Belej, M.A. and Aviado, D.M. Cardiopulmonary toxicity of propellants for aerosols. J. Clin. Pharmacol. 105–115 (1975).

Part IV
Device Materials

Chapter 16 Reactions to Materials Used in the Construction
of Devices 343

16
Reactions to Materials Used in the Construction of Devices

I. Background 343
II. Medical plastic appliances 346
III. Rubber appliances 346
IV. Dialyzer devices 347
V. Needles and sutures 348
VI. Hearing devices 349
VII. Pacemaker devices 349
VIII. Skin adhesive devices 349
IX. Transdermal delivery systems 349
X. Intradermal implants 350
XI. Vaginal and intrauterine devices 350
XII. Skeleton system appliances 351
XIII. Eye appliances 352
References 353

I. BACKGROUND

The development of new medical devices and appliances has expanded greatly in the past three decades. A recent government survey revealed that there are more than 1,700 different types of medical devices and 50,000 separate products. To regulate shortcomings and/or adverse reactions of these devices, a set of new amendments was enacted by Congress to determine that new devices satisfied conditions of safety and efficacy before being widely marketed (the Medical Device Amendments of 1976 to the Federal Food, Drug and Cosmetic Act). The 1976 Amendments established seven categories of medical devices, one of which was termed "transitional." This category included devices that were regulated as drugs before enactment of the new statute but were redefined as medical devices. These included such biomaterials as bone heterografts, injectable silicone, intraocular lenses, surgical sutures, and soft contact lenses (1). The new trends in biomaterials research are focused on implantable materials that may actually interact with and/or form chemical bonds with body tissues.

As research into and technology of biomaterial development became more sophisticated, the number of transitional medical devices has expanded. One of the most important prerequisites of any biomaterial for use within or on the body is that it be totally inert. However, the possibility exists that these "inert" substances could cause adverse reactions similar to "inert" excipients of drugs.

Transitional appliances contain many of the same materials commonly used as traditional excipients in drug formulations. The concept of excipient as applied to transitional medical devices has not been clearly defined nor can "active" principles in these devices by clearly differentiated from "excipients" in every case. Because of these unique interrelationships it must be recognized that medical appliances must be looked upon as containing excipients. Their innate "inertness" also qualifies them in the general category of excipients.

A multitude of chemical polymers form the chief inert backbones of most of these products. For example, polyurethane-based polymers are used in cardiovascular appliances. Another important polymer is bone cement (polymethyl methacrylate) used to cement metallic implants (2). Polycarbonates, polyethylene, and polyvinyl chloride are used in a wide variety of microporous devices and plastics. Plasticizers such as diethylhexylphthalate impart pliability to the final product. These materials are important because they may be leached from plastic blood containers.

Microscopic implantable spheres are not only used for obtaining long-term drug effects but also for encapsulating normal functioning tissue such as pancreatic beta cells. In the latter system, pancreatic cell clusters are encapsulated by a composite material of an amino acid polymer and sodium alginate. The amino acid polymer provides strength and the sodium alginate provides structure. Together they form a membrane that is porous enough to allow insulin to leave and glucose to enter the capsule (2). Other encapsulation materials for implants include gelatin, gluteraldehyde, serum albumin, and phospholipid dispersions.

Ophthalmic medical devices include hard and soft plastic lenses and ocular inserts. The latter treatment devices are fashioned with polypeptides and are preserved with trace amounts of formaldehyde. Bioerodible ocular devices consist of polyanhydride polymers and several organic acids (adipic, pimelic, and azelaic acids). Implantable lenses are manufactured from polymethyl methacrylate because this material is relatively inert in the eye. More recently foldable lenses have been made of silicone rubber or of hydrogel, a viscous jellylike polymer.

Drug delivery systems for the skin may involve many microporous materials including polycarbonates, polyvinyl chlorides, polyamides, polysulfones, halogenated polymers, acrylic resins, and silicone rubbers. Injectable bovine collagen is widely used for the correction of contour defects of the skin due to scarring and age-induced wrinkles. A polymer derived from bovine collagen fibers is also used as a biodegradable skin substitute.

Dispensers for the digestive tract are usually composed of humidified mixtures of cellulose derivatives. There are inflatable devices for the stomach that work on the principle of osmotic dispensing. They consist of cellulose acetate, polyethylene terephthalate, and polyurethane. There are also devices that become buoyant in gastric juices. Some of these devices contain cellulose acetate phthalate and/or acrylic/methacrylic acids.

Gynecologic appliances used for dispensing medications and for contraceptive purposes contain a variety of primary and secondary amines, monoethanolamines, siloxanes, and EDTA. Intrauterine shields consist of some of the following metals: copper, zinc, silver, platinum, and cadmium. Erodible drug dispensers can also be placed within the uterus. Such dispensers may contain collagen, animal muscle protein, vegetable gums, or traces of formaldehyde.

Colorants in medical devices are subject to similar regulations as are applied to drug products. Table 1 is a partial list of colorants permitted in medical devices. As is the case with drugs, the requirement for Food and Drug Administration (FDA) certification is based upon the safety profile of individual colors.

It is beyond the scope of this book to discuss every possible ingredient of each device. Not only would this be a formidable task but it would yield low dividends because there are few documented reports about clinical adverse reactions to medical devices and their respective components. In part, this may be due to a failure to recognize some reactions and in part to limited surveillance of these devices. To focus attention on possible adverse reactions of "inert" components of medical devices and appliances, some representative appliances will be considered in this section.

Table 1 Colorants Permitted in Medical Devices

FDA official name	Limitations	Current status
Subject to certification		
D&C Green No. 6	Contact lenses only; 0.03% (w/w) max	Listed
[Phthalocyaninato (2-1)] Copper	Polypropylene sutures for use general and ophthlamic surgery; 0.5% (w/w) max. Contact lenses; 0.01% (w/w) max.	Listed
Exempt from certification		
2-[[2,5-Diethoxy-4-[(4-Methylphenyl) Thio] Phenyl] Azo]-1,3,5-Benzenetriol	To mark soft (hydrophilic) contact lenses with the letters R and L only; 1.1×10^{-7} μg/lens maximum	Listed

II. MEDICAL PLASTIC APPLIANCES

The chief concern about medical plastic products is focused on the extensive use of polyvinyl chloride in these products. Polyvinyl chloride itself is inert but it may contain leachable and potentially toxic monomeric vinyl chloride as well as the plasticizer, di (2-ehtylhexyl)phthalate (DEHP), at concentrations as high as 40%. Unusual efforts are made to prevent the trapping of vinyl chloride monomer in the walls of plastic products in order to prevent the vinyl chloride syndrome previously described in workers exposed to this substance. Possible implications of immunologic mechanisms in the pathogenesis of this unusual syndrome were reported by Ward et al. in 1987. These investigators demonstrated the presence of circulating immune complexes in 19 of 28 patients with the disease and in 2 other patients of a group of 30 exposed to vinyl chloride. These results were interpreted as suggesting that vinyl chloride disease may be an immune complex disorder and that the immune response may be triggered by conjugation of vinyl chloride or one of its metabolites to one or more tissue or plasma proteins (3). The plasticizing agent, di-2 ethylhexylphthalate, is not firmly bound but in loose attachment with the polymer, thereby forming a gel-like structure. Thus DEHP is readily extracted from plastic products by a variety of organic solvents and is also leached into blood from plastic blood containers. After leaching into plasma, DEHP is converted to mono (2-ethylhexyl) phthalate (MEHP) by a plasma enzyme. The toxicity of DEHP and MEHP has been studied in various animal species. Hepatocellular carcinoma and testicular atrophy are known long-term toxic effects of large doses of DEHP and MEHP in rats and mice, while acute side effects of MEHP are decreases in heart rate and blood pressure (4). While these animal toxic effects of DEHP are undisputed, there is at yet no direct evidence that phthalates induce significant human toxicity despite the fact that DEHP is known to accumulate in human tissues (5). Far less is known about the allergenicity of plasticizers leached from polyvinyl chloride storage products. Allergic antibodies to DEHP and other plasticizers have not been demonstrated by direct skin tests or serologic methods in either dialysis patients or workers exposed to polyvinyl chloride film thermal decomposition products (5,6). However, there is evidence obtained by radioallergosorbent (RAST) inhibition experiments that DEHP exhibits modest cross-sensitivity to phthalic anhydride, the precursor chemical used to manufacture DEHP (5). Although these studies suggest that DEHP is potentially allergenic, direct proof of this assumption must await the demonstration of positive skin and/or serologic tests. Similarly, the allergenic potential of other plasticizers (polyethylene terephthalate, cellulose acetate phthalate) has yet to be determined.

III. RUBBER APPLIANCES

Rubber glove intolerance is a common medical problem. Both immediate and delayed types of hypersensitivity reactions have been reported. Allergic contact dermatitis due to rubber is usually caused by sensitivity to one or more rubber antioxidants or accelerators. To detect specific causes, patch tests should be performed with the most common rubber chemicals, which include mercapto-benzothiazole, tetramethylthiuram, and zinc dithiocarbamate. Patients who demonstrate allergy to tetramethylthiuram may develop a severe systemic reaction and generalized dermatitis after ingestion of Antabuse for the treatment of alcoholism. Rubber-glove-induced contact dermatitis may also be induced by contactant allergens that penetrate and contaminate the gloves. This has been well documented in the case of nickel salts, which pass through rubber but not polyvinyl chloride glove material (7). Localized contact urticaria with or without systemic anaphylactoid reactions may be provoked by rubber latex gloves (8). Some of these immediate reactions are immunologically mediated, as indexed by positive scratch and RAST tests to extracts of the rubber tree (*Hevea brasiliensis*). Contact urticaria to one of the common components of rubber gloves, zinc diethyldithiocarbonate, has also been reported and verified by positive scratch tests (9). Immediate hypersensitivity reactions due to rubber ingredients should be differentiated from contact urticaria due to cornstarch surgical glove powder (10). Even though soluble protein is almost totally removed from cornstarch, positive prick tests to cornstarch glove powder have been demonstrated in a few cases. Whether positive reactions are due to cornstarch, which is a derivative of the polysaccharides amylose and amylopectin, or to traces of corn or rubber latex protein has not been determined. Cornstarch in rubber gloves may also be responsible for granulomatous starch peritonitis (11). Intradermal skin tests of these patients with starch glove powder suspended in 0.1 ml sterile water reveal erythematous reactions at least 5 mm wide between 3 and 8 days after the inoculation. The histologic morphology of these lesions suggested immunologically mediated delayed hypersensitivity with epithelioid cell granulomas being present in the majority of patients. A special form of rubber appliance dermatitis is that due to condoms (12). Contact dermatitis may occur in rubber-sensitive men or women. Some rubber-sensitive patients may react only to certain brands of rubber condoms and tolerate others. Contact dermatitis may be induced by condom lubricants, (including guar gum), perfumes, and parabens.

IV. DIALYZER DEVICES

Although the majority of hemodialysis reactions have been attributable to ethylene-oxide-gas-mediated type I antibody mechanisms, these devices are also associated with a number of adverse clinical responses that cannot be attributed to ethylene oxide gas contamination. All commonly used dialyzers use membranes composed of either cellulose or polyacrylonitrile. Most adverse first-use responses have been observed with the use of capillary and plate dialyzers made of cuprammonium cellulose. Symptoms occurring after first use have also been associated with the use of regenerated cellulose membranes, while no reactions have been reported after the use of polyacrylonitrile dialzyers (13). Besides anaphylaxis there are three other major types of dialyzer-associated adverse events that may have immunologic significance: hypereosinophilia, asthmatic attacks, and pulmonary leukostasis with abnormal pulmonary function (14). Cuprophan dialyzers are often associated with chronic reactions (including eosinophilia) in some patients. Activation of complement components is more likely to occur after use of new cuprophan dialyzers compared to reused cuprophan dialyzers and polyacrylonitrile-based devices (15). Various contaminants within hollow-fiber dialyzers have been suspected as causes of these atypical, non-IgE responses. At various times formaldehyde, isocyanates, phthalates, or cotton linter derived from cellulose have been suggested as sources of antigenic stimulation. Despite these widely published speculations about possible antigens, the source of antigenic materials in dialysis fluids has not been discovered. There is one reported case of presumptive cutaneous hypersensitivity to nickel administered intravenously during hemolysis in a patient with preexisting nickel hypersensitivity (16). The source of the nickel was a stainless steel fitting that came in contact with solutions of the dialysis system. The amount of copper contained in cuprammonium cellulose hemodialyzers is insignificant as a possible cause of adverse responses.

V. NEEDLES AND SUTURES

Both anaphylactoid reactions and generalized exanthemata have been observed in nickel-sensitive persons receiving intravenous infusions. Presumably these reactions were caused by leaching of nickel from the needles used in the infusions (17). Allergic contact dermatitis from acupuncture needles also occurs in nickel-sensitive patients exposed to nickel-plated needles (18). However, nickel does not necessarily leach from some stainless steel sutures containing as much as 10% nickel (19). This can be confirmed by a negative results of a dimethylglyoxime test. Modern biomaterial research has led to the development of many new types of nonabsorbable sutures. One new development of special interest cosists of multifilament sutures incorporated with antimicrobial agents and coated with a polyurethane polymer (methylene diphenyldiisocyanate, MDI). To what extent the latter substance, a well-known occupational sensitizer, could cause adverse reactions in the body is unknown. Catgut and plain collagen sutures occasionally cause adverse local reactions but the immunologic significance of these is unknown. It is possible that both chromic catgut and chromic collagen could exacerbate eczematous skin reactions in patients with preexisting contact hypersensitivity reactions to chromium.

VI. HEARING DEVICES

Contact dermatitis may develop after various periods of exposure to plastics used in hearing aids (20). In such cases, positive patch test reactions were demonstrated against methylmethacrylate, polyvinyl chloride, and vulcanite. Contact dermatitis to the methylmethacrylate in acrylic plastic hearing aids presumably occurs because the cold-curing polymerization process leaves enough residual monomer to sensitize the skin soon after the plastic appliances are applied to the skin of the ear. Heat-cured methylmethacrylae devices usually are inert.

VII. PACEMAKER DEVICES

Several cases of severe redness, swelling, and itching at the site of implantable pacemaker generators have been reported. One of these patients developed necrotic lesions over each of the implant sites. Extensive patch tests with various plastic and metals revealed a markedly positive patch test to a titanium-encased pacemaker in one of these cases (21). Other cases of pacemaker hypersensitivity reactions were discovered to be sensitive to epoxy-coated pacemakers and several of the transition metallic salts (22,23).

VIII. SKIN ADHESIVE DEVICES

Contact dermatitis to various brands of adhesive tape is very common and is due to a variety of adhesive materials. Both contact urticaria and contact dermatitis have been observed in patients using self-adhesive pads (24). Positive patch tests to Cu (II)-acetyl acetonate and acetyl acetone were demonstrated in one case. Eczematous eruptions caused by adhesives in and around colostomy devices have been induced by water-soluble coated polymers (N-butylmonoesters of poly-methyl vinyl ether maleic acid), epoxy resins, rubber, polyacrylate, and a mixture of pectin, gelatin, and sodium carboxymethylcellulose (25,26). Karaya seal rings induce unusual lesions of denuded mucosa around ileostomy stomata (27). Contact dermatitis was induced by an ostomy bag deodorant, citronella oil (28). There is an isolated case report of chronic urticaria to tantalum contained in metal staples. This symptom disappeared after removal of the skin staples (29).

IX. TRANSDERMAL DELIVERY SYSTEMS

Severe contact dermatitis has been reported after use of nitroglycerin patches (30). Thirty percent of patients who used clonidine patches eventually become sensitized to the drug. Irritant reactions at the site of transdermal skin patches must be clearly differentiated from contact dermatitis. In these cases of drug-induced dermatitis, the transdermal delivery system is clearly an adjuvant when it enhances drug absorption and the opportunity for sensitization. Acrylate adhesives in some of the transdermal skin patches may cause contact dermatitis but these are relatively infrequent sensitizers. Irritant reactions to transdermal patches tend to occur in hot humid weather as a result of sweat retention. When dimethylsulfoxide (DMSO) is used as a patch test vehicle it may cause erythema and contact urticaria, both of which are thought to be nonimmunologic. A few cases of generalized dermatitis have been reported after local application of DMSO (31).

X. INTRADERMAL IMPLANTS

Bovine collagen implants may induce adverse reactions of erythema, induration, and urticaria at implantation sites. Prior to treatment patients are skin tested with 0.1 ml of the material to detect potential sensitivity. It is estimated that 5% of the general population will show evidence of sensitization to bovine collagen detected by this test. A negative test reaction predicts that the patient will tolerate the bovine implant without any adverse reactions (32). Bovine specific enzyme-linked immunosorbent assay (ELISA) antibodies have been demonstrated in 10 patients who had adverse treatment reactions while 29 of 30 control patients without adverse reactions did not show high levels of antibody (33). Investigation of possible association of major histocompatibility complex antigens and immune responses to bovine collagen implants revealed that all patients with adverse clinical reactions to bovine collagen implants were lacking the HLA–DR4 class II antigen (34). Bovine collagen implants may be contraindicated in patients with thromboangiitis obliterans because almost 80% of these patients exhibit cellular sensitivity to human type I or type III collagens (35). Whether these antibodies cross-react with bovine collagens is speculative but it is known that other bovine–human protein cross-reactions occur.

XI. VAGINAL AND INTRAUTERINE DEVICES

Apart from the well-known sensitizers contained in douches, feminine hygiene deodorants, and vaginal spermicides, the excipient constituents of intravaginal appliances may, on occasion, act as local sensitizing agents. Vaginitis and vulvitis may be produced by rubber support pessaries and contraceptive diaphragms in rubber-sensitive women. Rubber condoms may also induce allergic dermatitis of the vulva and the inner aspect of the thighs. Various vaginal dispensers contain primary and secondary amines as well as ethanolamine excipient components. Some U-shaped devices contain soluble fibrous materials and siloxanes. Tampons contain trace amounts of edetic acid (EDTA) but no adverse effects from this have been thus far reported.

A few allergic reactions to copper-containing intrauterine devices have been reported (36,37). One of these patients developed a papulovesicular eruption with excoriations over the trunk, thighs, and groin areas. This reaction was corroborated by a positive patch test to copper, which was unusual because copper is an extremely rare contact sensitizer. One interesting case report of cholinergic urticaria appeared to be associated with the presence of a copper-containing intrauterine device (37). In this instance, histologic examination of urticarial lesions developing after exercise revealed a significant increase in acetylcholine receptors. It was postulated that copper and acetylcholine acted in a collaborative manner to stimulate the release of histamine and other mediators from mast cells. Erodible intrauterine drug dispensers contain structural animal protein such as bovine collagen as well as vegetable gums and formaldehyde. Other intrauterine devices serving as drug reservoirs contain methylmethacrylate. Thus far, there have not been any specific instances of allergic adverse responses to the latter type of device.

XII. SKELETAL SYSTEM APPLIANCES

Polymethyl methacrylate (PMMA) is used extensively for artificial hips, knees, shoulders, elbows, wrists, and tooth replacement implants. If the appliance is heat cured, there is no evidence that patients are likely to become sensitized to the polymeric form of methylethacrylate. However, incompletely cured acrylics contain methacrylate monomers that are fully capable of inducing hypersensitivity reactions (38,39). This is more likely to occur after exposure to acrylic bone cement used in orthopedic surgery and dentistry. Residual monomers in these preparations can penetrate rubber and polyvinyl gloves, resulting in classic allergic contact dermatitis in orthopedic surgeons documented by positive patch test reactions to methylmethacrylate. Chronic handling of the methacrylate monomer may also cause paresthesia of the fingers because of a direct inflammatory effect of the monomer on peripheral nerve endings. Dizziness, hypotension, and bradycardia have been described both in operators and patients exposed to the mixing of acrylic cement (40–42). Nausea and vomiting have also been described, presumably as a result of an inhibitory effect on gastric motor function (40). Severe foreign body reactions to polymeric debris following cemented total hip arthroplasty have been described (43). The debris consisted of polyethylene and polymethyl methacrylate microfragments. These microfragments were thought to cause extensive lytic reactions manifested by inflammatory responses, which presumably led to loosening of the cemented hip implants. Various metals are used for bone plates, screws, wires, intramedullary nails, rods, and for vertebral spacers and extensors. Anecdotal reports of delayed hypersensitivity reactions to cobalt and nickel have appeared in the literature, but the causal role of metallic substances in the loosening process of metal-to-metal prosthesis is extremely controversial (44). No definitive studies have proved that this occurs. Although titanium has been implicated as a contact sensitizer in the case of implantable pacemakers, there are no documented reports that titanium implants used in orthopedic surgery or oral surgey have caused hypersensitivity reactions (45). Aluminum oxide (Al_2O_3) is used for vertical spacers and for coating bioglass used in alveolar bone and tooth replacement prostheses. Although granulomatous formation may occur after subcutaneous injections of vaccines containing aluminum hydroxide, reactions to aluminum oxide implants have not been noted (46). There is considerable controversy about whether rejection of an artificial hip joint could be caused by allergic reactions to the methylmethacrylate monomer. A prospective study revealed that allergy to prosthetic components could not be implicated in cases of hip loosening (47). In this study, however, there were isolated instances of patch test skin reactivity to metal components (cobalt, nickel, chromium) and methacrylate.

XIII. EYE APPLIANCES

Polymethyl methacrylate and hydrogels are used for corneal prostheses. Intraocular lenses may contain PMMA or polypropylene. Silicone teflon sponge material or polyglycerylmethacrylate are used as artificial vitrous humors (48). Adverse reactions to these materials have not been reported. Ocular inserts may have small concentrations of formaldehyde or preservatives and although sensitization to this potent sensitizer can always occur, no reports have appeared thus far. Other bioerodible ocular devices contain polyanhydride polymers, adipic acid, pimelic acid, azelaic acid, and metallic salts including nickel and chromium. Allergic reactions to any of these substances are possible but have not yet been documented. "Daily wear" soft contact lenses have low water content and must be removed from the eye at night whereas "constant" or "permanent" wear soft contact lenses have higher water contact, greater oxygen permeability, and can be worn by the patient for weeks or months without being taken out (49). The most serious allergic reactions to soft contact lenses is the contact-lens-associated giant papillary conjunctivitis syndrome (50). In patients who develop this problem, lenses have been satisfactorily worn for 3 to 30 months before the onset of symptoms. These patients develop a very severe form of vernal conjunctivitis of the upper tarsal conjunctivae. Although this is most often caused by soft lenses, it has also been described after hard lens use. This problem is not associated with preexisting atopy and can be clearly differentiated from classic vernal conjunctivitis. It is postulated that denatured proteins and lens coatings that accumulate on the inner surfaces of these lenses may act as antigens and initiate an allergic reaction, causing the final manifestations of the contact lens giant papillary conjunctivitis syndrome (51). Whether excipient chemicals could interact with lens coatings to form hapten–protein conjugates is highly speculative but, as previously discussed, various preservatives (thimerosal, benzalkonium chloride, parabens, sorbic acid, chlorobutanol, chlorhexidine, and phenylmercuric nitrate) in contact lens cleaning solutions may cause conjunctival mucositis and contact dermatitis in sensitized patients (52). In addition, papain, an enzyme used to remove protein deposits from soft contact lenses, may also cause IgE-mediated sensitization in the eye itself and periorbital tissues. The IgE nature of this reaction has been amply documented by direct skin tests and positive RAST results. Discontinuation of the papain cleanser results in complete cure (52,53).

REFERENCES

1. Kessler, D.A., Pape, S.M. and Sundwall, D.N. The federal regulation of medical devices. N. Engl. J. Med. 317(6):357–366 (1987).
2. Fuller, R.A. and Rosen, J.J. New polymers, ceramics, glasses and composites are among the many materials now enabling medical engineers to design innovative, and increasingly biocompatible, replacements for damaged human tissues. Sci. Am. 255:118–125 (1986).
3. Ward, A.M., Udnoon, S., Watkins, J. et al. Immunological mechanisms in the pathogenesis of vinyl chloride disease. Br. Med. J. 17:936–938 (1976).
4. Boruchoff, S.A. Hypotension and cardiac arrest in rats after infusion of mono (2-ethylhexyl)phthalate (MEHP), a contaminant of stored blood. N. Engl. J. Med. 316(19):1218–1219 (1987).
5. Gallagher, J.S., Ataman, G., Maccia, C.A. and Bernstein, I.L. *In vitro* cross sensitivity between phthalic anhydride and diethyl-hexyl-phthalate. J. Allergy Clin. Immunol. 57:205 (1976).
6. Dolovich, J., Evans, S., Baurmeister, U. et al. Antibody responses to hemodialysis-related antigens in chronic hemodialysis patients. Artif. Organs 11 (2):93–96 (1987).
7. Wall, L.M. Nickel penetration through rubber gloves. Contact Derm. 6: 461–463 (1980).
8. Wrangsjo, J., Mellstrom, G. and Axelsson, G. Discomfort from rubber gloves indicating contact urticaria. Contact Derm. 15:79–84 (1986).
9. Helander, I. and Makela, A. Contact urticaria to zinc diethyldithiocarbamate (ZDC). Contact Derm. 9(4):327 (1983).
10. Fisher, A.A. Contact urticaria due to cornstarch surgical glove powder. Cutis 38(5):307–308 (1986).
11. Grant, J.B.F., Davies, J.D., Espiner, H.J. et al. Diagnosis of granulomatous starch peritonitis by delayed hypersensitivity skin reactions. Br. J. Surg. 69:197–199 (1982).
12. Fisher, A.A. Condom dermatitis in either partner. Cutis 39:281–285 (1987).

13. Ing, T.S., Daugirdas, J.T., Popli, S. et al. First-use syndrome with cuprammonium cellulose dilayzers. Int. J. Artif. Organs 6(5):235–239 (1983).
14. Michelson, E.A., Cohen, L. Dankner, R.E. et al. Eosinophilia and pulmonary dysfunction during Cuprophan hemodialysis. Kidney Int. 24:246–249 (1983).
15. Chenoweth, D.E. Complement activation during hemodialysis: Clinical observations, proposed mechanisms and theoretical implications. Artif. Organs 9(3):281–287 (1984).
16. Olerud, J.E., Lee, M.Y., Uvelli, D.A. et al. Presumptive nickel dermatitis from hemodialysis. Arch. Dermatol. 12:1066-1068 (1984).
17. Fisher, A.A. Nickel dermatitis in men. Cutis 35(5):424–426 (1985).
18. Fisher, A.A. Allergic dermatitis from acupuncture needles. Cutis 38(4): 226 (1986).
19. Fisher, A.A. Medico-legal aspects of the use of stainless steel sutures in nickel-sensitive persons. Cutis 41:25–26 (1988).
20. Cockerill, D. Allergies to ear moulds. Br. J. Audiol. 21:143-145 (1987).
21. Peters, M.S., Schroeter, A.L., van Hale, H.M. et al. Pacemaker contact sensitivity. Contact Derm. 11:214-218 (1984).
22. Anderson, K.E. Cutaneous reaction to an epoxy-coated pacemaker. Arch. Dermatol. 115:97–98 (1979).
23. Tilsley, D.A. and Rotstein, H. Sensitivity caused by internal exposure to nickel, chrome and cobalt. Contact Derm. 6:175-178 (1980).
24. Sterry, W. and Schmoll, M. Contact urticaria and dermatitis from self-adhesive pads. Contact Derm. 13(4):284–285 (1985).
25. Heskel, N.S. Allergic contact dermatitis from stomadhesive paste. Contact Derm. 16:119-121 (1987).
26. Bergman, B., Lowhagen, G.B. and Mobacken, H. Irritant skin reactions to urostomal adhesives. Urol. Res. 10:153-155 (1982).
27. Colwell, J.C. Karaya sensitivity. J. Enterostom. Ther. 11(4):159-160 (1984).
28. Davies, M.G., Hodgson, G.A. and Evans, E. Contact dermatitis from an ostomy deodorant. Contact Derm. 4:11-13 (1978).
29. Werman, B.S. and Rietschel, R.L. Chronic urticaria from tantalum staples. Arch. Dermatol. 117:438–439 (1981).
30. Lasagna, L. and Greenblatt, D.J. More than skin deep: Transdermal drug-delivery systems. N. Engl. J. Med. 314(25):1638–1639 (1986).
31. Fisher, A.A. Dimethyl sulfoxide as a vehicle for food allergy patch tests. Cutis 36(2):109-110 (1985).
32. Trentham, D.E. Adverse reactions to bovine collagen implants. Arch. Dermatol. 122:643-644 (1986).
33. Siegle, R.J., McCoy, J.P. Jr., Schade, W. et al. Intradermal implantation of bovine collagen. Arch. Dermatol. 120:183-187 (1984).
34. Vanderveen, E.E., McCoy, J.P. Jr., Schade, W. et al. The association of HLA and immune responses to bovine collagen implants. Arch. Dermatol. 122:65–654 (1986).

35. Adar, R., Papa, M.Z., Halpern, Z. et al. Cellular sensitivity to collagen in thromboangiitis obliterans. N. Engl. J. Med. 308(19):1113–1116 (1983).
36. Rongioletti, F., Rivara, G. and Rebora, A. Contact dermatitis to a copper-containing intra-uterine device. Dermatologica 175(1):41–44 (1987).
37. Shelley, W.B., Shelley, E.D. and Ho A.K.S. Cholinergic urticaria: Acetyl-choline-receptor-dependent immediate-type hypersensitivity reaction to copper. Lancet 1:843 (1983).
38. Fisher, A.A. Reactions to acrylic bone cement in orthopedic surgeons and patients. Cutis 37(6):425 (1986).
39. Rajaniemi, R. Clinical evaluation of occupational toxicity of methyl-methacrylate monomer to dental technicians. Occup. Med. 36(2):56–59 (1986).
40. Burchman, S. and Wheater, R.H. Hazard of methyl methacrylate to operating room personnel. J.A.M.A. 235:2652 (1976).
41. Brittain, G.J.C. and Ryan, D.J. Hypotension and methylmethacrylate cement. Br. Med. J. 4:667–668 (1972).
42. Wong, K.C., Martin, W.E., Kennedy, W.F. et al. Cardiovascular effects of total hip placement in man with observation on the effect of methyl-methacrylate on the isolated rabbit heart. Clin. Pharmacol. Ther. 21:709 (1977).
43. Maguire, J.K. Jr., Coscia, M.F. and Lynch, M.H. Foreign body reaction to polymeric debris following total hip arthroplasty. Clin. Orthop. Rel. Res. 216:213–223 (1987).
44. Fisher, A.A. The safety of artificial hip replacement in nickel-sensitive patients. Cutis 37(5):333 (1986).
45. Williams, D.F. Titanium as a metal for implantation. Part 2: Biological properties and clinical applications. J. Med. Eng. Tech. 266–270 (1977).
46. Fawcett, H.A. and Smith N.P. Injection-site granuloma due to aluminum. Arch. Dermatol. 120:1318–1322 (1984).
47. Waterman, A.H. and Schrik, J.J. Allergy in hip arthroplasty. Contact. Derm. 13:294 (1985).
48. Hench, L.L. Biomaterials. Science 208:826–831 (1980).
49. Ruben, M. Soft contact lenses. Br. Med. J. 1:138 (1976).
50. Allansmith, M.R., Korb, D.R., Greiner, J.V. et al. Giant papillary conjunctivitis in contact lens wearers. Am. J. Ophthalmol. 83:697–708 (1977).
51. Mondino, B.J., Salamon, S.M. and Zaidman, G.W. Allergic and toxic reactions in soft contact lens wearers. Sur. Ophthalmol. 26:337–344 (1982).
52. Fisher, A.A. Allergic reactions to contact lens solutions. Cutis 36:209–211 (1985).
53. Bernstein, D.I., Gallagher, J.S., Grad, M. et al. Local ocular anaphylaxis to papain enzyme contained in a contact lens cleansing solution. J. Allergy Clin. Immunol. 74(3):258–260 (1984).

Part V

Tabulation of Inactive Ingredients   359

Tabulation of Inactive Ingredients

This section reproduces information from the latest available version (January 1988) of the *Inactive Ingredient Guide* prepared by the Food and Drug Administration. The tables of ingredients are preceded by three brief sections:

I. A list of current liaison representatives from the various FDA divisions to their Division of Drug Information Resources (DDIR), which compiles and periodically updates the *Guide*.

II. An outline describing the *Inactive Ingredients Guide* including purpose, design, warnings, and a description of the column headings in the *Guide* tables. If an agent can be identified by a Chemical Abstract Service number, that number appears under the column headed "CAS" in the major table. The "Approval Date" column gives the date of the most recently approved NDA with that ingredient in its formulation. The "NDA count" gives the number of currently marketed products that contain this excipient. Columns headed "colors" and "new" are described under "listed colors," but are not included in the tabulation here because this information was not made available.

III. Routes of administration tabulated alphabetically, giving the page numbers in which inactive ingredients used in formulations intended for each of these routes are listed. Routes that involve injectable formulations are identified by an asterisk.

I. LIAISON REPRESENTATIVES

Division of Cardio-Renal Drug Products, HFN-110: Kevin Dermanoski, R.Ph.

Division of Neuropharmacological Drug Products, HFN-120: James Cobb, R.Ph.

Division of Oncology and Radiopharmaceutical Drug Products, HFN-150: William Hess, R.Ph.

Division of Surgical-Dental Drug Products, HFN-160: Herbert Thornton, R.Ph.

Division of Generic Drugs, HFN-230: Richard Lipov, R.Ph.

Division of Metabolism and Endocrine Drug Products, HFN-810: Janet Anderson, R.Ph.

Division of Anti-Infective Drug Products, HFN-815: Stephen Wickizer, R.Ph.

All DDIR Liaison Representatives can be contacted at (202) 443-0500.

II. INACTIVE INGREDIENT GUIDE

A. Purpose

The *Inactive Ingredient Guide* contains all inactive ingredients present in approved drug products or conditionally approved drug products currently marketed for human use. The *Guide* is compiled by the Division of Drug Information Resources (DDIR) and is updated semiannually. It provides reviewers from the FDA Center for Drug Evaluation and Research and the Center for Biologies Evaulation and Research CDER/CBER with information on inactive ingredients in products that have been approved by the Agency. Once an inactive ingredient appears in a currently approved drug product for a particular route of administration, the inactive ingredient would not usually be considered new and may require a less extensive review.

B. Design

The *Inactive Ingredient Guide* has been sorted alphabetically by route of administration. Routes of administration are derived from current approved labeling. The index that precedes the list will allow users to locate particular routes of administration without having to go through the entire document.

C. Warnings

The *Inactive Ingredient Guide* lists inactive ingredients specifically designated as such by the manufacturer. Some of these inactive ingredients could also be considered as active ingredients under different circumstances. Furthermore, reactants in radiopharmaceutical kits, or inactive ingredients that physically or chemically combine with active ingredients to facilitate drug transport are considered as inactive ingredients for the purposes of this *Guide*.

D. CAS Number

Many inactive ingredients have Chemical Abstract Service (CAS) numbers associated with them. These can be found in the column to the right of the inactive ingredients. CAS numbers may be helpful to CDER/CBER Reviewers when initiating computer-assisted searches with the National Library of Medicine's online data bases.

E. Qualitative NDA Data

The next four columns to the right of the CAS number serve to qualify the data presented. The 'NDA COUNT' reflects the total number of NDA's in which a particular inactive ingredient currently appears. The 'Last NDA' specifies which NDA was the most recent one to be approved by the Agency with this inactive ingredient. The 'APPROVAL DATE' and 'DIV' specify the approval date and Review Division responsible for evaluating this most recent NDA.

F. Procedure for Obtaining Further Assistance

The Division of Drug Information Resources can also provide you with specialized searches on the automated data base from which the *Inactive Ingredient Guide* is generated. For assistance in using the *Guide*, to schedule a presentation on the *Guide*, or for a more detailed search, contact your DDIR Liaison Representative or Mr. William A. Hess at (202) 443-0500.

lll. INDEX FOR ROUTES OF ADMINISTRATION

Anesthesia, caudal nerve block	364*	Intrathecal	384*
intrathecal		Intratacheal	384
Anesthesia, infiltration	364*	Intratumor	384*
Anesthesia, sympathetic nerve block	365*	Intrauterine	384
Buccal	365	Intravascular	385*
Buccal/sublingual	366	Intravenous	385
Caudal block	366*	Irrigation	388*
Dental	367	IV-SC	388*
Epidural	368*	IV (infusion)	388*
Extracorporeal	368	Nasal	390
IM-IV	369*	Nerve block	391*
IM-IV-SC	371*	Ophthalmic	392
IM-SC	372*	Oral	395
Implantation	373	Oral birth control	423
Inhalation	373	Otic	425
Inhalation/nasal	374	Percutaneous	426
Interstitial	375*	Perfusion, biliary	427*
Intra-amniotic	375*	Perfusion, cardiac	427*
Intra-arterial	375*	Periarticular	427*
Intra-articular	376*	Peridural	427*
Intrabursal	377*	Rectal	427
Intracardiac	377*	Retrobulbar	429
Intradermal	378*	Soft tissue	430
Intradiscal	378*	Subarachnoid	430*
Intralesional	378*	Subcutaneous	430*
Intralymphatic	379*	Sublingual	431
Intramuscular	379*	Topical	433
Intraocular	382*	Transmucosal	445
Intraperitoneal	382*	Ureteral	445
Intrapleural	382*	Urethral	445
Intraspinal	383*	Vaginal	445
Intrasynovial	383*		

---

*Denotes injectables.

INACTIVE INGREDIENTS FOR CURRENTLY MARKETED DRUG PRODUCTSa

Route Ingredient	CAS #	NDA Count	Approval Date
Anesthesia, caudal nerve block, intrathecal			
Acetone sodium bisulfite	000540921	1	07/10/79
Benzyl alcohol	000100516	1	11/01/71
Citric acid	000077929	1	09/02/83
Hydrochloric acid	007647010	5	05/21/86
Sodium bicarbonate	000144558	1	02/18/82
Sodium chloride	007647145	5	05/21/86
Sodium hydroxide	001310732	5	05/21/86
Sodium metabisulfite	007757746	1	09/02/83
Anesthesia, infiltration			
Acetic acid, glacial	000064197	1	07/21/77
Acetone sodium bisulfite	000540921	4	11/15/79
Ascorbic acid	000050817	1	10/03/72
Benzyl alcohol	000100516	1	12/08/72
Calcium chloride	010035048	3	12/01/86
Chlorobutanol	000057158	3	11/15/79
Citric acid	000077929	5	10/13/87
Citric acid monohydrate	005949291	1	02/04/80
Edetate calcium disodium	023411349	2	10/03/72
Edetate disodium	006381926	15	01/22/85
Hydrochloric acid	007647010	57	10/13/87
Isotonic sodium chloride solution	008028771	1	02/04/80
Lactic acid	008012213	1	07/29/76
Methylparaben	000099763	43	10/13/87
Potassium chloride	007447407	4	12/01/86
Potassium metabisulfite	004429429	2	01/22/85
Potassium phosphate, monobasic	007778770	2	07/29/76

Anesthesia, infiltration (cont)

Propylparaben	000094133	4	07/29/76
Sodium Bisulfate acetone	007546125	1	04/04/68
Sodium bisulfite	007631905	11	09/09/80
Sodium carbonate	000497198	1	12/08/72
Sodium chlorate	007775099	1	09/15/72
Sodium chloride	007647145	89	10/13/87
Sodium citrate	006132043	1	03/13/72
Sodium hydroxide	001310732	79	10/13/87
Sodium L-lactate	000867561	1	10/03/72
Sodium metabisulfite	007757746	25	10/13/87
Sodium phosphate, dibasic	007782856	2	12/03/73
Thioglycerol	000096275	1	10/03/72

Anesthesia, sympathetic nerve block

Hydrochloric acid	007647010	2	08/21/84
Sodium chloride	007647145	2	08/21/84
Sodium hydroxide	001310732	2	08/21/84

Buccal

Alcohol, diluted	008000166	1	02/15/73
Anise oil	008007703	1	10/19/64
Aromatics		1	03/02/44
Benzoic acid	000065850	1	02/15/73
Carboxymethyl starch sodium salt	009063381	1	02/09/81
Cassia, synthetic		1	10/19/64
Citric acid	000077929	1	07/05/55
Clove oil	008000348	1	10/19/64
Dye FDC blue #1	002650182	1	02/15/73
Dye FDC blue #2	000860220	1	08/03/79
Dye FDC blue #40		1	08/03/79
Flavor mint		1	03/02/44
Flavor peppermint		11	04/21/86
Flavor spearmint		11	04/21/86
Glycerin	000056815	1	02/15/73
Lactose	000063423	13	04/21/86
Magnesium stearate	000557040	2	02/09/81
Menthol	000089781	1	10/19/64
Methyl salicylate	000119368	1	10/19/64
Methylcellulose	009004675	1	04/02/79
Peppermint		1	11/20/81

Buccal (cont)

Peppermint oil	008006904	1	10/19/64
Polyethylene glycols		1	08/03/79
Polysorbate 80	009005656	1	02/15/73
Saccharin sodium	006155573	1	02/15/73
Silica gel	007699414	11	04/21/86
Sodium hexametaphosphate	010124568	1	07/05/55
Sodium phosphate, dibasic	007782856	1	02/15/73
Sodium phosphate, monobasic	007558807	1	02/15/73
Sodium pyrophosphate	007722885	1	07/05/55
Spearmint oil	008008795	1	11/20/81
Starch	009005258	1	02/09/81
Stearic acid	000057114	13	04/21/86
Sucrose	000057501	1	02/09/81
Synchron oral carrier		11	04/21/86
Tartrazine	001934210	2	10/19/64
Thymol	000089838	1	10/19/64

Buccal/sublingual

Acacia	009000015	3	02/02/77
Cellulose		1	07/16/74
Dye FDC yellow #6-aluminum lake	012227600	1	06/24/76
Flavor apricot		1	06/24/76
Guar gum	009000300	1	07/16/74
Lactose	000063423	5	02/02/77
Magnesium stearate	000557040	3	09/07/76
Mannitol	000069658	1	12/20/40
Methylcellulose	009004675	1	02/02/77
Polyethylene	009002884	1	06/24/76
Saccharin sodium	006155573	1	07/16/74
Sodium lauryl sulfate	000151213	1	07/16/64
Starch	009005258	3	09/07/76
Stearic acid	000057114	2	02/02/77
Sucrose	000057501	3	02/02/77
Talc	014807966	2	06/24/76
Tartrazine	001934210	3	02/02/77
Tragacanth	009000651	1	12/20/40

Caudal block

Ascorbic acid	000050817	1	10/03/72
Calcium chloride	010035048	1	10/05/82

Caudal block (cont)

Edetate calcium disodium	023411349	1	10/03/72
Edetate disodium	006381926	1	12/11/73
Hydrochloric acid	007647010	13	03/03/87
Methylparaben	000099763	5	03/03/87
Potassium chloride	007447407	1	10/05/82
Sodium bisulfite	007631905	1	10/03/72
Sodium chloride	007647145	17	03/03/87
Sodium hydroxide	001310732	17	03/03/87
Sodium l-lactate	000867561	1	10/03/72
Sodium metabisulfate	007757746	3	04/16/82
Thioglycerol	000096275	1	10/03/72

Dental

Acetone sodium bisulfite	000540921	1	10/10/84
Alcohol		1	08/13/86
Alcohol, denatured	008024451	1	06/03/87
Anethole	012002403	1	08/13/86
Calcium phosphate, dibasic	007757939	1	08/03/70
Calcium pyrophosphate	007790763	1	12/19/58
Carboxymethylcellulose sodium	009004324	5	07/06/87
Cellulose		1	08/03/70
Dye DC yellow #10	008004920	1	06/03/87
Dye FDC blue #1	002650182	3	06/03/87
Dye FDC green #3	002353459	1	08/06/86
Eucalyptol	000470826	1	08/13/86
Flavor		2	08/13/86
Flavor DF-119		1	06/03/87
Flavor DF-1530		1	08/06/86
Flavor enhancer		1	06/03/87
Flavor natural and artificial herb alpine		1	08/13/86
Flavor peppermint		1	08/13/86
Gelatin	009000708	3	07/06/87
Glycerin	000056815	3	08/13/86
Hydrocarbon gel, plasticized	008049658	1	03/04/60
Magnesium aluminum silicate	001327431	1	12/19/58
Menthol	000089781	1	08/13/86
Mineral oil	008012951	2	10/01/86
Pectin	009000695	3	07/06/87
Polyethylene	009002884	2	10/01/86
Polyethylene glycol 1500		1	05/12/55

Dental (cont)

Polyethylene glycol 1540		1	06/03/87
Polyethylene glycol 4000		1	05/12/55
Polyols		1	06/03/87
Polyoxyl 40 stearate	009004993	1	08/13/86
Propylene glycol	000057556	1	05/12/55
Saccharin sodium	006155573	4	06/03/87
Silica gel	007699414	1	06/03/87
Sodium alkyl sulfate	008036542	1	12/19/58
Sodium benzoate	000532321	2	06/03/87
Sodium bisulfate acetone	007546125	1	04/04/68
Sodium chloride	007647145	2	10/10/84
Sodium coconut monoglyceride sulfonate		1	12/19/58
Sodium hydroxide	001310732	1	10/10/84
Sodium lauryl sulfate	000151213	2	06/03/87
Sodium pyrophosphate	007722885	1	08/03/70
Sorbitol	000050704	1	12/19/58
Stannous pyrophosphate	015578264	1	12/19/58

Epidural

Ascorbic acid	000050817	1	10/03/72
Benzyl alcohol	000100516	1	04/09/86
Calcium chloride	010035048	2	12/01/86
Citric acid	000077929	2	08/30/76
Edetate calcium disodium	023411349	2	10/03/72
Edetate disodium	006381926	1	12/11/73
Hydrochloric acid	007647010	30	03/03/87
Methylparaben	000099763	10	03/03/87
Potassium chloride	007447407	3	12/01/86
Sodium bisulfite	007631905	2	10/03/72
Sodium chloride	007647145	35	03/03/87
Sodium citrate	006132043	1	04/09/86
Sodium hydroxide	001310732	36	03/03/87
Sodium l-lactate	000867561	1	10/03/72
Sodium metabisulfite	007757746	5	04/16/82
Sodium sulfite	007757837	1	04/09/86
Thioglycerol	000096275	1	10/03/72

Extracorporeal

Benzyl alcohol	000100516	1	04/20/83
Cellulose paper		1	07/08/75

Extracorporeal (cont)

Hydrochloric acid	007647010	1	04/20/83
Methyl alcohol	000067561	1	07/08/75
Poloxamer		1	02/10/77
Sodium chloride	007647145	2	04/20/83
Sodium hydroxide	001310732	1	04/20/83
Sodium oxalate	000062760	1	12/06/41

IM–IV

Acetic acid, glacial	000064197	13	11/10/83
Alcohol		17	10/13/87
Alcohol, dehydrated	000064175	14	10/22/87
Alcohol, diluted	008000166	1	09/19/73
Ammonium sulfate	007783202	1	03/11/81
Ascorbic acid	000050817	5	12/08/77
Benzethonium chloride	000121540	7	07/16/81
Benzoic acid	000065850	13	10/22/87
Benzyl alcohol	000100516	110	12/21/87
Calcium chloride	010035048	5	01/29/74
Chlorobutanol	000057158	11	10/01/82
Citric acid	000077929	24	03/18/87
Creatinine	000060275	4	07/01/82
Dextrose	005996101	4	07/23/86
Dicyclohexyl-carbodiimide		1	03/11/81
Diethylamine		1	03/11/81
Edetate calcium disodium	023411349	1	01/21/74
Edetate disodium	006381926	50	12/21/87
Edetate sodium	000064028	2	09/28/77
Glutamic acid hydrochloride	000138158	1	08/30/63
Glycerin	000056815	3	06/30/76
Hydrochloric acid	007647010	136	12/21/87
Isotonic sodium chloride solution	008028771	4	02/28/83
Lactic acid	008012213	3	11/17/86
Lactic acid, DL-	000598823	1	06/11/70
Lactose	000063423	7	06/08/84
Lactose monohydrate	010039266	1	07/22/82
Lysine	000056871	2	11/26/84
Magnesium stearate	000557040	1	03/20/74
Mannitol	000069658	6	07/07/86
Methanesulfonic acid	000075752	1	04/12/46
Methylparaben	000099763	43	11/17/86
N,N-dimethylacetamide	000127195	1	03/11/81

IM-IV (cont)

Phenol	000108952	21	04/29/87
Phosphoric acid	007664382	2	05/29/81
Polyethylene glycol 300	025322683	2	07/03/80
Polyethylene glycol 400	009004960	1	07/25/80
Polyethylene glycols		1	05/02/75
Polysorbate 40	009005667	1	03/29/65
Potassium metabisulfite	004429429	1	03/28/49
Potassium phosphate, monobasic	007778770	1	10/19/84
Povidone	009003398	1	07/22/82
Propylene glycol	000057556	39	10/22/87
Propylparaben	000094133	37	11/17/86
Saccharin sodium	006155573	2	07/08/87
Saccharin sodium anhydrous	000128449	1	12/23/57
Sodium acetate	006131904	14	11/10/83
Sodium acetate, anhydrous	000127093	1	09/19/73
Sodium benzoate	000532321	14	10/22/87
Sodium bicarbonate	000144558	10	10/13/87
Sodium bisulfate	007681381	5	03/28/83
Sodium bisulfite	007631905	57	07/08/87
Sodium carbonate	000497198	9	03/06/86
Sodium chloride	007647145	68	11/30/87
Sodium citrate	006132043	42	05/07/87
Sodium citrate anhydrous	000068042	8	02/03/86
Sodium formaldehyde sulfoxylate	000149440	10	10/01/82
Sodium hydroxide	001310732	183	12/21/87
Sodium L-lactate	000867561	1	04/20/61
Sodium metabisulfite	007757746	25	03/18/87
Sodium phosphate	007632055	20	07/22/82
Sodium phosphate, dibasic	007782856	32	08/18/87
Sodium phosphate, dibasic, anhydrous		2	06/08/84
Sodium phosphate, dibasic, dihydrate	010028247	1	07/08/87
Sodium phosphate, dried		1	05/28/81
Sodium phosphate, monobasic	007558807	37	08/18/87
Sodium phosphate, monobasic, monohydrate	010049215	8	07/08/87
Sodium sulfate	007727733	2	02/28/83
Sodium sulfite	007757837	16	07/08/87

IM-IV (cont)

Sodium tartrate	000868188	3	07/08/87
Sodium thiomalate	030245513	1	12/24/81
Starch	009005258	1	03/20/74
Succinic acid	000110156	1	06/25/82
Sulfuric acid	007664939	14	11/30/87
Tartaric acid, DL-	000133379	1	03/23/73
Thiazoximic acid		1	03/11/81
Thimerosal	000054648	1	03/28/60
Thioglycerol	000096275	3	04/30/87
Trithiazoximic acid		1	03/11/81
2-ethyl-mexanoic acid		1	03/11/81
7-amino-cephalosporic acid		1	03/11/81

IM-IV-SC

Acetic acid		2	06/15/84
Acetic acid, glacial	000064197	5	11/21/84
Benzyl alcohol	000100516	14	05/28/87
Buffer, acetic acid–sodium acetate		1	02/13/74
Chlorobutanol	000057158	3	07/15/77
Citric acid	000077929	5	05/28/87
Citric acid monohydrate	005949291	2	07/02/86
Creatinine	000060275	1	06/08/60
Dextrose	005996101	1	07/14/61
Edetate sodium	000064028	1	12/26/74
Gelatin	009000708	2	11/21/84
Glycerin	000056815	2	03/04/87
Glycine	000056406	1	08/16/57
Hydrochloric acid	007647010	52	11/18/87
Lactic acid	008012213	5	01/06/76
Lactose	000063423	3	03/04/87
Methylparaben	000099763	27	12/22/87
Phenol	000108952	3	01/22/75
Phenol, liquified		2	03/04/87
Phosphoric acid	007664382	1	06/13/45
Polyoxyethylene fatty acid		1	07/14/61
Propylparaben	000094133	27	12/22/87
Sodium acetate	006131904	5	06/15/84
Sodium bisulfite	007631905	6	12/22/87
Sodium chloride	007647145	50	12/22/87
Sodium citrate	006132043	7	05/28/87

IM-IV-SC (cont)

Sodium dithionite	007775146	1	02/05/62
Sodium hydroxide	001310732	36	05/28/87
Sodium l-lactate	000867561	3	01/06/76
Sodium lactate	000072173	1	05/23/56
Sodium metabisulfite	007757746	15	05/28/87
Sodium phosphate, dibasic	007782856	1	01/22/75
Thimerosal	000054648	1	11/29/73
Thioglycerol	000096275	1	12/06/72

IM-SC

Acetic acid		1	07/03/86
Acetic acid, glacial	000064197	8	10/31/86
Benzyl alcohol	000100516	26	07/14/87
Chlorobutanol	000057158	3	06/24/75
Citric acid	000077929	1	01/11/84
Cresol, M-	000108394	1	01/23/85
Cysteine		1	02/06/56
Dextrose	005996101	3	07/25/83
Edetate disodium	006381926	1	07/28/72
Gelatin	009000708	5	02/21/78
Glycerin	000056815	1	12/05/79
Glycine	000056406	1	06/23/87
Hydrochloric acid	007647010	19	01/23/85
Isotonic sodium chloride solution	008028771	1	09/12/79
Mannitol	000069658	3	06/23/87
Methylparaben	000099763	3	06/10/87
PEG vegetable oil	003051352	1	07/25/83
Phenol	000108952	8	01/23/85
Phosphoric acid	007664382	1	06/23/87
Polyoxyethylene fatty acid		2	07/25/83
Propylparaben	000094133	2	07/05/77
Protamine sulfate	009009658	1	01/23/85
Sesame oil	008008740	4	07/14/87
Sodium acetate	006131904	5	06/10/87
Sodium acetate, anhydrous	000127093	1	10/02/77
Sodium chloride	007647145	21	06/10/87
Sodium citrate	006132043	1	01/11/84
Sodium formaldehyde sulfoxylate	000149440	1	06/24/75
Sodium hydroxide	001310732	21	06/23/87

IM-SC (cont)

Sodium phosphate dihydrate		1	01/23/85
Sodium phosphate, dibasic	007782856	1	06/23/87
Thimerosal	000054648	1	01/23/79
Zinc chloride	007646857	1	01/23/85
Zinc oxide	001314132	1	06/10/87

Implantation

Butylated hydroxytoluene	000128370	1	08/29/73
Calcium carbonate, precipitated	000471341	1	08/29/73
Calcium stearate	001592230	1	08/29/73
Crospovidone	009003398	1	07/13/72
Dye DC blue #6	000482893	1	08/29/73
Dye DC green #6	000128803	2	10/29/76
Hydroquinone	000123319	2	10/07/71
Paraffin	008002742	1	12/20/76
Polybutilate	024936978	2	10/29/76
Resin		2	10/29/76
Stearic acid	000057114	1	07/13/72

Inhalation

Acetone sodium bisulfite	000540921	2	01/30/81
Acetylcysteine	000616911	1	09/15/86
Air		3	10/01/82
Alcohol		6	12/28/84
Alcohol, dehydrated	000064175	5	04/23/83
Alcohol, denatured	008024451	1	06/12/79
Ammonia	007664417	1	03/12/58
Ascorbic acid	000050817	24	09/15/86
Benzalkonium chloride	008001545	3	01/16/87
Butylated hydroxytoluene	000128370	1	05/25/78
Carbon dioxide	000124389	1	10/10/74
Cetylpyridinium chloride	000123035	2	07/10/62
Chlorobutanol	000057158	2	08/10/71
Citric acid	000077929	5	06/30/81
Cryofluorane	000076142	14	12/29/86
Dichlorodifluoromethane	000075718	20	12/30/86
Dye DC yellow #10	008004920	1	01/05/79
Dye FDC yellow #6	002783940	1	01/05/79
Edetate disodium	006381926	17	08/17/87
Edetate disodium, anhydrous	000139333	1	08/11/87
Edetate sodium	000064028	1	08/17/87

Inhalation (cont)

Flavor		1	03/09/56
Fluorochlorohydrocarbons		1	09/17/62
Gelatin	009000708	1	12/03/82
Glycerin	000056815	31	09/15/86
Hydrochloric acid	007647010	22	08/17/87
Hydrochloric acid, diluted		1	08/17/87
Lactose	000063423	1	06/20/73
Lecithin, soy bean	008030760	1	12/29/86
Menthol	000089781	3	12/28/84
Methylparaben	000099763	9	09/15/86
Nitric acid	007697372	3	05/23/84
Nutmeg oil	008008435	1	06/27/63
Oleic acid	000112801	4	05/01/81
Poloxamer		1	06/27/63
Propylene glycol	000057556	1	01/05/79
Propylparaben	000094133	9	09/15/86
Saccharin	000081072	2	12/28/84
Saccharin sodium	006155573	2	12/16/61
Sodium bisulfate	007681381	1	09/16/83
Sodium bisulfite	007631905	16	03/26/84
Sodium chloride	007647145	38	08/17/87
Sodium citrate	006132043	21	09/15/86
Sodium hydroxide	001310732	12	08/17/87
Sodium metabisulfite	007757746	13	03/14/84
Sodium sulfite	007757837	9	03/26/84
Sorbitan trioleate	005960065	11	12/30/86
Sulfuric acid	007664939	2	01/16/87
Thymol	000089838	4	07/14/76
Trichloromonofluoromethane		13	12/30/86
Trichlorotrifluroethane	000076131	1	01/13/60
Turpentine oil	008006642	1	06/27/63
Xenon	007440633	1	10/10/74

Inhalation/nasal

Benzalkonium chloride	008001545	3	12/23/87
Butylated hydroxyanisole	008003245	1	09/24/81
Carboxymethylcellulose sodium	008004324	2	12/23/87
Cellulose microcrystalline/ carboxymethylcellulose sodium		1	12/23/87
Cellulose, microcrystalline	009004346	1	07/27/87

Inhalation/nasal (cont)

Citric acid	000077929	1	09/24/81
Dextrose	005996101	2	12/23/87
Dichlorodifluoromethane	000075718	2	09/30/81
Edetate disodium	006381926	1	09/24/81
Hydrochloric acid	007647010	3	12/23/87
Oleic acid	000112801	2	09/30/81
Phenylethyl alcohol	000060128	2	12/23/87
Polyethylene glycol 3350		1	09/24/81
Polysorbate 80	009005656	2	12/23/87
Propylene glycol	000057556	1	09/24/81
Sodium citrate	006132043	1	09/24/81
Sodium hydroxide	001310732	1	09/24/81
Trichloromonofluoromethane		2	09/30/81

Interstitial

Benzyl alcohol	000100516	1	09/23/74
Dextrose	005996101	1	09/23/74
Hydrochloric acid	007647010	1	09/23/74
Sodium acetate	006131904	1	09/23/74
Sodium hydroxide	001310732	1	09/23/74

Intra-amniotic

Citric acid	000077929	1	12/22/76
Edetate disodium	006381926	1	10/08/71
Hydrochloric acid	007647010	2	10/08/71
Sodium hydroxide	001310732	2	12/22/76

Intra-arterial

Benzyl alcohol	000100516	1	07/10/86
Diatrizoic acid	000117964	2	08/29/74
Edetate calcium disodium	023411349	2	10/21/86
Edetate disodium	006381926	2	10/19/76
Hydrochloric acid	007647010	11	07/17/87
Meglumine	006284408	2	08/17/72
Methylparaben	000099763	1	10/19/76
Propylparaben	000094133	1	10/19/76
Sodium bisulfite	007631905	1	10/19/76
Sodium chloride	007647145	8	03/10/87
Sodium citrate	006132043	1	08/29/74
Sodium citrate anhydrous	000068042	1	10/19/76
Sodium hydroxide	001310732	14	07/17/87
Tromethamine	000077861	1	10/21/86

Intra-articular

Acetic acid, glacial	000064197	6	03/14/79
Benzalkonium chloride	008001545	1	03/03/65
Benzyl alcohol	000100516	39	03/18/87
Buffer, acetic acid-sodium acetate		1	11/15/77
Carboxymethylcellulose	009000117	2	03/06/78
Carboxymethylcellulose sodium	009004324	23	05/24/82
Citric acid	000077929	12	03/18/87
Creatine	000057001	1	11/08/78
Creatinine	000060275	4	06/19/80
Diatrizoic acid	000117964	1	08/29/74
Edetate disodium	006381926	11	05/24/82
Hydrochloric acid	007647010	13	11/05/81
Isotonic sodium chloride solution	008028771	2	12/06/79
Methylcellulose	009004675	5	01/13/81
Methylparaben	000099763	10	01/13/81
Phenol	000108952	3	01/30/79
Phosphoric acid	007664382	2	05/29/81
Polyethylene glycol 3350		3	09/09/75
Polyethylene glycol 4000		9	10/20/82
Polysorbate 80	009005656	34	02/17/84
Potassium phosphate, dibasic	007758114	1	03/29/74
Potassium phosphate, monobasic	007778770	2	03/29/74
Propylparaben	000094133	10	01/13/81
Sodium acetate	006131904	5	03/14/79
Sodium bisulfite	007631905	9	05/24/82
Sodium chloride	007647145	35	10/20/82
Sodium citrate	006132043	15	03/18/87
Sodium citrate anhydrous	000068042	2	08/08/75
Sodium hydroxide	001310732	32	03/18/87
Sodium metabisulfite	007757746	5	03/18/87
Sodium phosphate	007632055	4	02/27/79
Sodium phosphate, dibasic	007782856	5	12/31/74
Sodium phosphate, monobasic	007558807	1	03/03/65
Sodium sulfite	007757837	4	04/09/86
Sorbitol	000050704	1	02/17/84
Sorbitol solution	003959533	2	07/29/69
1-tetradecyl-4-picolinium chloride	002748881	5	10/20/82

Intrabursal

Benzalkonium chloride	008001545	1	03/03/65
Benzyl alcohol	000100516	7	03/07/78
Carboxymethylcellulose	009000117	1	03/07/78
Carboxymethylcellulose sodium	009004324	6	02/11/77
Citric acid	000077929	5	02/11/77
Creatinine	000060275	1	07/11/62
Edetate disodium	006381926	3	08/08/75
Hydrochloride acid	007647010	1	01/04/60
Methylparaben	000099763	2	08/08/75
Polysorbate 80	009005656	7	03/07/78
Propylparaben	000094133	2	08/08/75
Sodium bisulfite	007631905	1	07/11/62
Sodium chloride	007647145	8	03/07/78
Sodium citrate anhydrous	000068042	1	08/08/75
Sodium hydroxide	001310732	5	03/07/78
Sodium metabisulfite	007757746	1	08/08/75
Sodium phosphate	007632055	1	02/11/77
Sodium phosphate, dibasic	007782856	4	02/13/74
Sodium phosphate, monobasic	007558807	1	03/03/65

Intracardiac

Citric acid	000077929	1	11/15/74
Diatrizoic acid	000117964	1	10/27/72
Edetate disodium	006381926	1	10/27/72
Hydrochloric acid	007647010	3	01/06/76
Lactic acid	008012213	4	01/06/76
Sodium bisulfite	007631905	2	01/06/76
Sodium chloride	007647145	5	01/06/76
Sodium citrate	006132043	2	11/15/74
Sodium hydroxide	001510732	1	10/27/72
Sodium L-lactate	000867561	3	01/06/76
Sodium lactate	000072173	1	05/25/56
Sodium metabisulfite	007757746	3	02/25/75

Intracavitary

Benzyl alcohol	000100516	2	09/23/74
Dextrose	005996101	1	09/23/74
Hydrochloric acid	007647010	2	09/23/74
Sodium acetate	006131904	1	09/23/74
Sodium chloride	007647145	1	03/15/49
Sodium hydroxide	001310732	2	09/23/74

Intradermal

Benzalkonium chloride	008001545	1	03/03/65
Benzyl alcohol	000100516	2	09/06/73
Carboxymethylcellulose sodium	009004324	2	09/06/73
Creatinine	000060275	1	09/06/73
Cresol, M-	000108394	1	02/08/77
Edetate disodium	006381926	2	09/06/73
Glycerin	000056815	3	02/08/77
Hydrochloric acid	007647010	7	02/08/77
Methylparaben	000099763	3	02/08/77
Phenol	000108952	3	02/08/77
Polysorbate 80	009005656	2	09/06/73
Protamine sulfate	009009658	2	02/08/77
Sodium acetate	006131904	3	02/08/77
Sodium bisulfite	007631905	1	09/06/73
Sodium chloride	007647145	6	02/08/77
Sodium hydroxide	001310732	8	02/08/77
Sodium phosphate	007632055	3	02/08/77
Sodium phosphate, dibasic	007782856	1	03/05/65
Sodium phosphate, monobasic	007558807	1	03/03/65
Zinc chloride	007646857	5	02/08/77

Intradiscal

Cysteine hydrochloride mono-hydrate	007048046	1	01/18/84
Diatrizoic acid	000117964	1	08/21/69
Edetate calcium disodium	023411349	1	08/21/69
Edetate disodium	006381926	1	01/18/84
Meglumine	006284408	1	08/21/69
Sodium bisulfite	007631905	1	01/18/84
Sodium hydroxide	001310732	1	01/18/84
Sodium l-cysteinate hydro-chloride		1	08/21/84

Intralesional

Acetic acid, glacial	000064197	1	03/14/79
Benzalkonium chloride	008001545	1	03/03/65
Benzyl alcohol	000100516	16	10/16/87
Carboxymethylcellulose sodium	009004324	5	10/16/87
Citric acid	000077929	5	03/18/87
Creatine	000057001	1	11/08/78

Intralesional (cont)

Creatinine	000060275	4	06/19/80
Edetate disodium	006381926	8	06/19/80
Hydrochloric acid	007647010	9	10/16/87
Isotonic sodium chloride solution	008028771	2	12/06/79
Methylcellulose	009004675	1	12/06/79
Methylparaben	000099763	4	06/19/80
Phenol	000108952	3	01/30/79
Phosphoric acid	007664382	2	05/29/81
Polyethylene glycol 3350		2	09/09/75
Polyethylene glycol 4000		7	10/20/82
Polysorbate 80	009005656	11	10/16/87
Propylparaben	000094133	4	06/19/80
Sodium acetate	006131904	1	03/14/79
Sodium bisulfite	007631905	8	06/19/80
Sodium chloride	007647145	12	10/16/87
Sodium citrate	006132043	11	03/18/87
Sodium hydroxide	001310732	21	10/16/87
Sodium metabisulfite	007757746	4	03/18/87
Sodium phosphate	007632055	1	01/30/79
Sodium phosphate, dibasic	007782856	2	12/31/74
Sodium phosphate, monobasic	007558807	1	03/03/65
Sodium sulfite	007757837	2	01/25/84
Sorbitol	000050704	1	02/17/84
Sorbitol solution	003959533	2	07/29/69
1-tetradecyl-4-picolinium chloride	002748881	5	10/20/82

Intralymphatic

Poppy seed oil	008002117	1	03/31/54

Intramuscular

Acetic acid		2	07/09/80
Acetic acid, glacial	000064197	19	11/26/82
Alcohol		2	04/17/80
Alcohol, denatured	008024451	1	01/30/78
Ammonium acetate	000631618	1	02/28/83
Ascorbic acid	000050817	7	02/13/74
Benzalkonium chloride	008001545	1	03/03/65
Benzethonium chloride	000121340	2	06/12/79
Benzyl alcohol	000100516	129	01/02/87

Intramuscular (cont)

Benzyl benzoate	000120514	14	01/02/87
Buffer, acetic acid–sodium acetate		2	11/26/82
Butylated hydroxyanisole	008003245	1	05/18/49
Butylated hydroxytoluene	000128370	1	05/18/49
Butylparaben	000094268	2	11/01/50
Calcium chloride	010035048	1	07/26/72
Carboxymethylcellulose	00900117	1	02/23/35
Carboxymethylcellulose sodium	009004324	35	08/23/83
Castor oil	008001794	6	01/02/87
Chlorobutanol	000057158	30	02/09/87
Chlorobutanol hemihydrate	006001645	1	02/11/86
Citric acid	000077929	25	04/03/87
Corn oil	008001307	1	09/12/41
Cottonseed oil	008001294	8	02/09/87
Creatine	000057001	1	11/08/78
Creatinine	000060275	1	09/06/73
Croscarmellose sodium		2	07/01/77
Dextrose	005996101	3	05/24/79
Diatrizoic acid	000117964	4	09/23/82
Docusate sodium	000577117	3	08/23/83
Edetate calcium disodium	023411349	4	09/23/82
Edetate disodium	006381926	16	04/03/87
Edetate sodium	000064028	1	08/06/74
Gelatin	009000708	2	09/12/79
Glutathione	000070188	1	02/20/59
Glycerin	000056815	3	01/30/87
Glycine	000056406	3	03/08/87
Hydrochloric acid	007647010	58	12/22/87
Isotonic sodium chloride solution	008028771	4	12/06/79
Lactic acid	008012213	7	12/14/87
Lactose	000063423	3	09/18/86
Lecithin	008002435	7	05/24/79
Magnesium chloride	007791186	3	11/30/54
Maleic acid	000110167	1	07/21/61
Mannitol	000069658	11	03/08/87
Meglumine	006284408	1	09/23/82
Methylcellulose	009004675	10	08/23/83
Methylparaben	000099763	42	12/14/87

Intramuscular (cont)

Peanut oil	008002037	3	06/16/54
Phenol	000108952	26	04/03/87
Phenylmercuric nitrate	000055685	1	04/17/57
Phosphoric acid	007664382	1	10/01/76
Polyethylene glycol 200		1	09/28/55
Polyethylene glycol 3350		2	09/09/75
Polyethylene glycol 4000		12	10/20/82
Polyoxyethylene sorbitan monoisostearate		1	12/23/75
Polysorbate 40	009005667	1	06/27/52
Polysorbate 80	009005656	39	05/24/82
Potassium phosphate, dibasic	007758114	1	03/29/74
Potassium phosphate, monobasic	007778770	2	03/29/74
Povidone	009003398	11	08/23/83
Procaine	000059461	2	07/01/54
Procaine hydrochloride	000051058	1	11/30/54
Propyl gallate	000121799	1	08/19/71
Propylene glycol	000057556	6	10/26/79
Propylparaben	000094133	38	12/14/87
Saccharin sodium anhydrous	000128449	1	10/13/58
Sesame oil	008008740	49	01/02/87
Sodium acetate	006131904	20	02/29/84
Sodium acetate, anhydrous	000127093	2	11/26/82
Sodium bicarbonate	000144558	1	12/18/74
Sodium bisulfite	007631905	16	02/26/86
Sodium carbonate	000497198	1	11/20/85
Sodium chlorate	007775099	1	06/12/79
Sodium chloride	007647145	66	12/22/87
Sodium citrate	006132043	29	04/03/87
Sodium formaldehyde sulfoxylate	000149440	5	08/02/77
Sodium hydroxide	001310732	89	07/17/87
Sodium metabisulfite	007757746	9	12/22/87
Sodium phosphate	007632055	12	02/27/85
Sodium phosphate, dibasic	007782856	11	03/03/87
Sodium phosphate, dibasic, anhydrous		4	12/04/86
Sodium phosphate, monobasic	007558807	12	12/04/86
Sodium salicylate	000054217	1	08/09/60
Sodium sulfate	007727733	1	01/16/76

Intramuscular (cont)

Sodium sulfite	007757837	2	02/13/74
Sodium tartrate	000868188	1	10/13/58
Sorbitan monopalmitate	001338405	2	12/23/75
Sorbitol	000050704	2	09/12/79
Sorbitol solution	003959433	1	11/01/50
Starch	009005258	1	06/27/52
Sulfuric acid	007664939	5	06/11/79
Sulfurous acid	007782992	1	02/26/86
Thimerosal	000054648	4	08/23/83
Thioglycerol	000096275	4	04/03/73
Tromethamine	000077861	1	01/09/79
Urea	000057136	1	11/01/50
1-tetradecyl-4-picolinium chloride	002748881	6	10/20/82

Intraocular

Calcium chloride	010035048	2	05/21/86
Hydrochloric acid	007647010	2	05/21/86
Magnesium chloride	007791186	2	05/21/86
Potassium chloride	007447407	2	05/21/86
Sodium acetate	006131904	2	05/21/86
Sodium chloride	007647145	2	05/21/86
Sodium citrate	006132043	2	05/21/86
Sodium hydroxide	001310732	2	05/21/86

Intraperitoneal

Benzyl alcohol	000100516	1	09/23/74
Dextrose	005996101	1	09/23/74
Hydrochloric acid	007647010	6	03/26/86
Mannitol	000069658	3	07/07/86
Sodium acetate	006131904	1	09/23/74
Sodium bicarbonate	000144558	1	06/23/78
Sodium bisulfite	007631905	5	01/29/86
Sodium carbonate	000497198	1	02/19/59
Sodium chloride	007647145	4	07/03/86
Sodium citrate	006132043	4	09/30/83
Sodium hydroxide	001310732	5	03/26/86
Sodium metabisulfite	007757746	1	11/05/81
Sulfuric acid	007664939	4	09/30/83

Intrapleural

Benzyl alcohol	000100516	1	09/23/74

Intrapleural (cont)

Citric acid	000077929	2	08/30/68
Dextrose	005996101	1	09/23/74
Hydrochloric acid	007647010	1	09/23/74
Mannitol	000069658	3	07/07/86
Sodium acetate	006131904	1	09/23/74
Sodium carbonate	000497198	1	02/19/59
Sodium chloride	007647145	4	07/03/86
Sodium citrate	006132043	2	08/30/68
Sodium hydroxide	001310732	1	09/23/74

Intraspinal
Dextrose	005996101	2	07/07/82
Hydrochloric acid	007647010	4	04/15/87
Sodium hydroxide	001310732	4	04/15/87

Intrasynovial
Acetic acid, glacial	000064197	5	03/14/79
Benzyl aclohol	000100516	14	02/17/84
Buffer, acetic acid-sodium acetate		1	11/15/77
Carboxymethylcellulose sodium	009004324	8	11/05/81
Citric acid	000077929	1	07/11/62
Creatinine	000060275	3	03/01/77
Edetate disodium	006381926	4	03/01/77
Hydrochloric acid	007647010	7	11/05/81
Isotonic sodium chloride solution	008028771	1	12/06/79
Methylcellulose	009004675	1	12/06/79
Methylparaben	000099763	3	12/06/79
Phenol	000108952	1	08/31/61
Polyethylene glycol 3350		2	09/05/61
Polyethylene glycol 4000		6	03/26/79
Polysorbate 80	009005656	14	02/17/84
Propylparaben	000094133	3	12/06/79
Sodium acetate	006131904	5	03/14/79
Sodium bisulfite	007631905	4	03/01/77
Sodium chloride	007647145	15	11/05/81
Sodium citrate	006132043	3	02/17/84
Sodium hydroxide	001310732	11	11/05/81
Sorbitol	000050704	1	02/17/84
Sorbitol solution	003959533	1	07/25/56

Intrasynovial (cont)

1-tetradecyl-4-picolinium chloride	002748881	3	03/26/79
Intrathecal			
Benzyl aclohol	000100516	3	05/09/86
Citric acid	000077929	2	08/30/68
Edetate calcium disodium	023411349	3	12/31/85
Hydrochloric acid	007647010	13	07/17/87
Pentetate calcium trisodium	012111249	1	03/11/76
Sodium chloride	007647145	9	03/10/87
Sodium citrate	006132043	2	08/30/68
Sodium hydroxide	001310732	15	07/17/87
Tromethamine	000077861	2	12/31/85
Intratracheal			
Benzyl alcohol	000100516	2	07/10/86
Carboxymethlcellulose sodium	009004324	1	05/17/54
Hydrochloric acid	007647010	1	07/10/86
Peanut oil	008002037	1	05/17/54
Sodium chloride	007647145	3	07/10/86
Sodium citrate	006132043	1	05/17/54
Sodium hydroxide	001310732	2	07/10/86
Intratumor			
Benzyl alcohol	000100516	2	05/09/86
Hydrochloric acid	007647010	1	03/31/82
Sodium carbonate	000497198	1	02/19/59
Sodium chloride	007647145	3	05/09/86
Sodium hydroxide	001310732	2	05/09/86
Intrauterine			
Barium sulfate	007727437	1	02/04/76
Crospovidone	009003398	1	04/30/53
Diatrizoic acid	000117964	1	11/19/58
Edetate calcium disodium	023411349	1	04/30/53
Edetate disodium	006381926	1	11/19/58
Ethylene vinyl acetate copolymer		1	02/04/76
Hydrochloric acid	007647010	1	04/08/86
Meglumine	006284408	1	11/19/58
Potassium phosphate, monobasic	007778770	1	04/30/53
Silicon	007440213	1	02/04/76
Sodium citrate	006132043	1	11/19/58

Intrauterine (cont)

Sodium hydroxide	001310732	1	04/08/86
Titanium dioxide	001309633	1	02/04/76

Intravascular

Edetate calcium disodium	023411349	9	12/31/85
Edetate disodium	006381926	3	10/09/80
Hydrochloric acid	007647010	6	12/31/85
Isotonic sodium chloride solution	008028771	1	10/26/76
Potassium hydroxide	001310583	1	10/26/76
Sodium carbonate	000497198	3	07/02/80
Sodium citrate	006132043	3	10/09/80
Sodium hydroxide	001310732	6	12/26/85
Sodium phosphate, monobasic	007558807	1	09/30/63
Sodium phosphate, monobasic, monohydrate	010049215	1	01/26/71
Tromethamine	000077861	2	12/31/85

Intravenous

Acetic acid		8	12/23/87
Acetic acid, glacial	000064197	5	07/20/84
Albumin human	009006535	3	03/25/83
Albumin, aggregated		3	03/20/78
Albumin, colloidal		1	03/25/83
Albumin, microsphere human serum		1	02/23/76
Alcohol		2	01/05/82
Alcohol, dehydrated	000064175	4	05/08/87
Ammonium acetate	000631618	1	02/28/83
Arginine		1	12/31/86
Ascorbic acid	000050817	4	02/23/76
Benzenesulfonic acid solution		1	11/23/83
Benzyl alcohol	000100516	54	05/03/87
Butylated hydroxyanisole	008003245	1	08/08/85
Butylated hydroxytoluene	000128370	1	08/08/85
Calcium gluceptate	017140602	1	01/27/82
Chlorobutanol	000057158	3	02/22/85
Citric acid	000077929	26	12/22/87
Citric acid monohydrate	005949291	1	12/31/85
Citric acid, hydrous	015686654	1	12/20/62
Cysteine hydrochloride	000052891	1	05/29/81
Dextrose	005996101	4	03/05/87

Intravenous (cont)

Dextrose, anhydrous	000050997	1	12/31/85
Diatrizoic acid	000117964	6	09/23/82
Edetate calcium disodium	023411349	12	07/26/85
Edetate disodium	006381926	25	12/22/87
Egg yolk phosphatides		2	08/27/84
Ethylenediamine	000107153	5	05/30/85
Ferrous citrate	022242531	1	12/17/73
Gelatin	009000708	4	08/18/78
Gentisic acid	000490799	1	02/18/81
Gentisic acid ethanolamine	007491352	1	11/06/81
Gluceptate sodium	013007857	1	05/25/78
Glycerin	000056815	2	08/27/84
Guanidine hydrochloride	000050011	2	02/23/76
Hydrochloric acid	007647010	158	12/24/87
Iodamide	000440584	1	07/24/78
Iodohippurate sodium	000133175	1	12/28/84
Iofetamine hydrochloride		1	12/24/87
Ioxaglic acid	059017640	1	07/26/85
Isotonic sodium chloride solution	008028771	4	12/30/77
Lactic acid	008012213	1	07/31/84
Lactose	000063423	3	05/20/85
Lidofenin	059160291	1	10/31/86
Mannitol	000069658	21	07/17/87
Medrofenim		1	01/21/87
Medronate disodium	025681894	3	03/25/83
Medronic acid	001984152	2	02/17/81
Meglumine	006284408	5	07/26/85
Methylparaben	000099763	28	12/22/87
N-2-hydroxyethylpiperazine N'-2'-ethanesulphonic acid		1	12/23/85
Oxidronate sodium		1	02/18/81
Oxyquinoline	000148243	1	12/23/85
Pentetate pentasodium		1	04/15/76
Phenol	000108952	2	08/06/85
Phosphoric acid	007664382	1	10/17/85
Poloxamer 188		2	03/25/83
Polyethylene glycols		1	03/29/63
Polysorbate 20	009005645	3	09/25/86
Polysorbate 80	009005656	2	12/23/85

Intravenous (cont)

Potassium hydroxide	001310583	1	01/25/85
Potassium metabisulfite	004429429	1	05/25/51
Potassium phosphate, dibasic	007758114	1	06/10/74
Potassium phosphate, monobasic	007778770	3	11/06/81
Propylene glycol	000057556	9	05/08/87
Propylparaben	000094133	21	12/22/87
Sodium acetate	006131904	13	12/23/87
Sodium acetate, anhydrous	000127093	1	11/18/76
Sodium ascorbate	000134032	1	09/25/86
Sodium bicarbonate	000144558	9	03/05/87
Sodium bisulfite	007631905	7	10/02/87
Sodium carbonate	000497198	3	11/20/85
Sodium chloride	007647145	131	12/24/87
Sodium citrate	006132043	11	03/18/87
Sodium citrate anhydrous	000068042	1	05/17/76
Sodium dithionite	007775146	2	12/17/86
Sodium hydroxide	001310732	177	12/24/87
Sodium iodide	007681825	1	02/09/59
Sodium metabisulfite	007757746	14	12/22/87
Sodium phosphate	007632055	13	12/24/87
Sodium phosphate, dibasic	007782856	9	04/07/87
Sodium phosphate, dibasic, anhydrous		1	02/23/76
Sodium phosphate, monobasic	00755807	8	09/25/86
Sodium phosphate, monobasic, monohydrate	010049215	3	09/07/76
Sodium pyrophosphate	007722885	3	06/30/87
Sodium sulfite	007757837	3	08/06/85
Sodium thiosulfate	010102177	1	08/18/78
Sodium thiosulfate, anhydrous	007772987	3	04/17/78
Sodium trimetaphosphate	007785844	1	11/19/76
Stannic chloride	007646788	1	04/15/76
Stannous chloride	010025691	16	06/30/87
Stannous fluoride	007783473	3	08/05/82
Stannous tartrate	000815850	1	11/18/76
Sulfuric acid	007664939	8	05/05/87
Tartaric acid, DL-	000133379	1	02/22/85
Thimerosal	000054648	2	01/10/67
Thioglycerol	000096275	11	12/22/87

Irrigation

Acetic acid, glacial	000064197	1	06/08/84
Hydrochloric acid	007647010	6	04/08/86
Methylparaben	000099763	1	06/28/66
Sodium bisulfite	007631905	1	06/11/79
Sodium citrate	006132043	1	06/11/79
Sodium hydroxide	001310732	4	04/08/86
Sulfuric acid	007664939	1	06/11/79

IV-SC

Benzyl alcohol	000100516	27	12/30/87
Calcium hydroxide	001305620	1	12/12/80
Citric acid	000077929	1	07/29/55
Glycerin	000056815	1	08/13/74
Hydrochloric acid	007647010	21	12/30/87
Isotonic sodium chloride solution	008028771	1	02/22/80
Methylparaben	000099763	3	05/20/76
Phenol	000108952	2	08/13/74
Phosphoric acid	007664382	1	08/13/74
Propylparaben	000094133	3	05/20/76
Sodium carbonate	000497198	1	05/07/73
Sodium chloride	007657145	20	04/07/86
Sodium citrate	006132043	1	07/29/55
Sodium hydroxide	001310732	22	12/30/87

IV (infusion)

Acetic acid		8	03/29/85
Acetic acid, glacial	000064197	27	07/23/87
Alcohol		7	12/17/87
Alcohol, dehydrated	000064175	15	04/30/87
Ammonium sulfate	007783202	1	03/11/81
Ascorbic acid	000050817	5	02/13/86
Aspartic acid	000056848	1	11/04/86
Benzenesulfonic acid solution		1	11/23/83
Benzethonium chloride	000121540	1	10/18/78
Benzyl alcohol	000100516	63	12/01/87
Buffer, acetic acid-sodium acetate		1	02/13/74
Butylated hydroxyanisol	008003245	4	08/08/85
Butylated hydroxytoluene	000128370	4	08/08/85

IV (infusion) (cont)

Calcium phosphate, dibasic	007757939	1	12/17/86
Chlorobutanol	000057158	6	03/29/85
Citric acid	000077929	40	02/11/87
Citric acid monohydrate	005949291	2	12/31/85
Citric acid, hydrous	015686654	1	12/03/86
Dextrose	005996101	34	07/02/87
Dextrose, anhydrous	000050997	2	12/31/87
Diatrizoic acid	000117964	2	09/23/82
Dicyclohexyl-carbodiimide		1	03/11/81
Diethanolamine	000111422	6	08/07/87
Diethylamine		1	03/11/81
Disofenin	065717977	1	03/16/82
Edetate calcium disodium	023411349	3	09/23/82
Edetate disodium	006381926	13	10/16/87
Egg yolk phosphatides		8	09/25/84
Ethylenediamine	000107153	6	05/30/85
Gelatin	009000708	1	12/23/87
Gentistic acid ethanolamide		3	10/10/85
Gentisic acid ethanolamine	007491352	1	01/17/83
Glycerin	000056815	10	09/25/84
Hydrochloric acid	007647010	169	12/23/87
Iodamide	000440584	1	07/10/78
Iodipamide	000606177	1	06/27/55
Lactic acid	008012213	6	12/31/87
Lactose	000063423	6	06/08/84
Lactose, hydrous		1	03/28/86
Mannitol	000069658	17	11/04/86
Meglumine	006284408	3	09/23/82
Methylparaben	000099763	27	12/22/87
N,N-dimethylacetamide	000127195	1	03/11/81
Phenol	000108952	4	12/21/77
Phospholipid		2	01/23/81
Phosphoric acid	007664382	4	04/13/87
Polyethylene glycol 300	025322683	2	11/10/83
Polyoxyl castor oil	008047163	1	11/14/83
Polyoxyl 40 castor oil		1	19/04/78
Polysorbate 20	009005645	4	08/08/85
Polysorbate 80	009005656	4	08/08/85
Polyvinyl chloride	009002862	2	02/02/79
Potassium chloride	007447407	1	01/31/85

IV (infusion) (cont)

Potassium hydroxide	001310583	3	01/25/85
Potassium metabisulfite	004429429	9	11/18/85
Propylene glycol	000057556	19	12/17/87
Propylparaben	000094133	20	12/22/87
Saccharin sodium	006155573	2	07/08/87
Saccharin sodium anhydrous	000128449	1	12/23/57
Sodium acetate	006131904	6	12/31/86
Sodium bicarbonate	000144558	10	01/08/87
Sodium bisulfite	007631905	53	12/22/87
Sodium carbonate	000497198	6	07/10/86
Sodium chloride	007647145	72	12/22/87
Sodium citrate	006132043	25	02/11/87
Sodium citrate anhydrous	000068042	1	06/23/70
Sodium desoxycholate		2	04/13/87
Sodium dithionite	007775146	7	10/17/86
Sodium hydroxide	001310732	172	12/31/87
Sodium L-lactate	000867561	3	01/06/76
Sodium metabisulfite	007757746	37	12/17/87
Sodium phosphate	007632055	12	02/27/85
Sodium phosphate, dibasic	007782856	22	07/02/87
Sodium phosphate, dibasic anhydrous		6	04/13/87
Sodium phosphate, monobasic	007558807	20	07/08/87
Sodium phosphate, monobasic, dihydrate		1	03/28/86
Sodium phosphate, monobasic, monohydrate	010049215	3	03/31/78
Sodium sulfite	007757837	1	02/17/84
Sodium tartrate	000868188	3	07/08/87
Stannous chloride	010025691	1	03/16/82
Sulfuric acid	007664939	9	05/05/87
Tartaric acid, DL-	000133379	1	02/22/85
Thiazoximic acid		1	03/11/81
Trithiazoximic acid		1	03/11/81
2-ethyl-hexanoic acid		1	03/11/81
7-amino-cefphalosporic acid		1	03/11/81

Nasal

Acetic acid, glacial	000064197	1	05/18/70
Alcohol		1	08/04/49
Alchol, dehydrated	000064175	1	12/17/65

Nasal (cont)

Benzalkonium chloride	008001545	1	03/18/83
Chlorobutanol	000057158	3	02/21/78
Chondrus extract	008015950	1	05/02/52
Citric acid	000077929	1	03/20/62
Citric acid monohydrate	005949291	1	05/18/70
Cryofluorane	000076142	1	12/17/65
Dichlorodifluoromethane	000075718	1	12/17/65
Edetate disodium	006381926	2	03/18/83
Glycerin	000056815	2	05/18/70
Glycine	000056406	1	05/02/52
Hydrochloric acid	007647010	2	11/30/79
Menthol	000089781	1	03/29/48
Methylparaben	000099763	3	12/11/75
Phenylmercuric acetate	000062384	1	05/02/52
Potassium chloride	007447407	1	12/11/75
Potassium phosphate, monobasic	007778770	1	12/11/75
Propylparaben	000094133	2	05/18/70
Saccharin sodium anhydrous	000128449	1	05/02/52
Sodium acetate	006131904	1	05/18/70
Sodium chloride	007647145	6	11/30/79
Sodium citrate	006132043	1	11/30/79
Sodium phosphate	007632055	2	05/18/70
Sodium phosphate, dibasic	007782856	1	12/11/75
Sorbitol	000050704	2	05/18/70
Tragacanth	009000651	1	05/02/52

Nerve block

Acetic acid, glacial	000064197	1	07/21/77
Acetone sodium bisulfite	000540921	4	11/15/79
Ascorbic acid	000050817	1	10/03/72
Benzyl alcohol	000100516	1	12/08/72
Calcium chloride	010035048	6	12/01/86
Chlorobutanol	000057158	6	11/15/79
Citric acid	000077929	6	10/13/87
Citric acid monohydrate	005949291	1	02/04/80
Edetate calcium disodium	023411349	2	10/03/72
Edetate disodium	006381926	18	01/22/85
Hydrochloric acid	007647010	46	10/13/87
Isotonic sodium chloride solution	008028771	1	02/04/80
Lactic acid	008012213	1	07/29/76

Nerve block (cont)

Methylparaben	000099763	45	10/13/87
Potassium chloride	007447407	7	12/01/86
Potassium metabisulfite	004429429	2	01/22/85
Potassium phosphate, monobasic	007778770	2	07/29/76
Propylparaben	000094133	6	01/30/79
Sodium bisulfite	007631905	14	09/09/80
Sodium carbonate	000497198	1	12/08/72
Sodium chlorate	007775099	1	09/15/72
Sodium chloride	007647145	85	10/13/87
Sodium citrate	006132043	1	03/13/72
Sodium hydroxide	001310732	73	10/13/87
Sodium L-lactate	000867561	1	10/03/72
Sodium metabisulfite	007757746	27	10/13/87
Sodium phosphate	007632055	1	12/03/73
Sodium phosphate, dibasic	007782856	3	12/03/73
Thioglycerol	000096275	1	10/03/72

Ophthalmic

Acetic acid		1	04/02/63
Acetic acid, glacial	000064197	2	04/10/80
Alcohol		1	08/31/82
Alcohol, dehydrated	000064175	1	06/11/87
Alginic acid	009005327	2	07/29/74
Amerchol-CAB	008029047	2	12/03/86
Antipyrine	000060800	1	03/23/51
Benzalkonium chloride	008001545	92	12/31/87
Benzethonium chloride	000121540	2	01/08/87
Benzoyl peroxide	000094360	1	04/30/74
Boric acid	010043353	40	02/09/87
Calcium chloride	010035048	1	06/08/59
Carbomer 940	009007174	1	10/01/84
Cetyl alcohol	000124298	2	09/24/85
Chlorobutanol	000057158	17	05/17/85
Chlorobutanol, anhydrous	001320667	1	09/25/85
Cholesterol	000057885	1	12/09/53
Citric acid	000077929	4	12/17/86
Citric acid monohydrate	005949291	1	12/31/86
Creatinine	000060275	4	07/21/86
Crospovidone	009003398	1	08/02/73
Diethanolamine	000111422	1	01/22/75
Dioctylphthalate		1	07/29/74

Ophthalmic (cont)

Edetate disodium	006381926	76	02/09/87
Edetate sodium	000064028	3	01/10/85
Ethyl acetate	000141786	1	07/29/74
Ethylenl glycol dimethacrylate	000097905	2	04/30/74
Ethylene oxide	000075218	1	12/18/64
Ethylene vinyl acetate copolymer		1	07/29/74
Glycerin	000056815	10	12/17/86
Glyceryl monostearate		2	09/24/85
Hydrocarbon gel, plasticizer	008049658	2	04/02/57
Hydrochloric acid	007647010	40	12/31/87
Hydroxyethyl cellulose	009004620	6	02/11/86
Hydroxypropyl methylcellulose	009004653	18	11/17/86
Hydroxypropyl methylcellulose 2910		2	12/28/82
Isotonic sodium chloride solution	008028771	1	05/02/80
Jelene	008049669	1	12/08/80
Lanolin	008020846	2	05/26/83
Lanolin alcohols	008013341	1	09/04/85
Lanolin nonionic derivatives		1	01/07/75
Lanolin, anhydrous	008006540	13	12/28/82
Magnesium chloride	007791186	1	06/08/59
Mannitol	000069658	3	05/02/80
Methacrylic acid	000079414	1	08/02/73
Methylcellulose	009004675	6	08/24/72
Methylparaben	000099763	21	05/05/87
Mineral oil	008012951	46	12/03/86
Mineral oil, light		3	12/29/60
N,N-dimethyl-P-toluidine	000099978	1	04/30/74
Nitric acid	007697372	1	10/04/63
Nonoxynol	026027383	1	12/17/86
Octylphenol polymethylene		1	11/22/74
Petrolatum	008009038	50	12/03/86
Petrolatum white		4	09/04/85
Phenethyl alcohol	000098851	1	02/24/56
Phenylethyl alcohol	000060128	2	03/13/80
Phenylmercuric acetate	000062384	4	12/03/86
Phenylmercuric nitrate	000055685	4	01/22/75
Poloxamer		5	06/11/87
Polyethylene	009002884	3	12/12/80

Ophthalmic (cont)

Polyethylene glycol 300	025322683	2	07/21/70
Polyethylene glycol 400	009004960	1	12/28/82
Polyethylene glycol 8000		1	03/24/83
Polyethylene glycols		1	08/31/81
Polyoxyl 40 stearate	009004993	6	09/25/85
Polypropylene glycol	009003150	1	09/25/85
Polysorbate 20	009005645	4	11/17/86
Polysorbate 80	009005656	23	07/21/86
Polyvinyl alcohol	009002895	13	12/31/86
Potassium acetate	000127082	1	04/02/63
Potassium chloride	007447407	9	02/09/87
Potassium phosphate, monobasic	007778770	4	12/19/85
Propylene glycol	000057556	12	06/11/87
Propylparaben	000094133	21	05/05/87
Sodium acetate	006131904	5	12/31/87
Sodium bicarbonate	000144558	1	03/31/77
Sodium bisulfate	007681381	1	03/28/83
Sodium bisulfite	007631905	11	07/21/86
Sodium borate	001303964	14	07/21/86
Sodium carbonate	000497198	9	02/09/87
Sodium carbonate hydrate	005968116	1	03/06/74
Sodium chloride	007647145	65	12/31/87
Sodium citrate	006132043	11	12/31/86
Sodium citrate anhydrous	000068042	1	02/18/75
Sodium hydroxide	001310732	49	12/31/87
Sodium metabisulfite	007757746	7	12/19/85
Sodium nitrate	007631994	1	10/04/63
Sodium phosphate	007632055	9	12/17/86
Sodium phosphate, dibasic	007782856	27	01/08/87
Sodium phosphate, dibasic, dihydrate	010028247	1	08/17/78
Sodium phosphate, dried		1	04/02/63
Sodium phosphate, monobasic	007558807	25	05/05/87
Sodium phosphate, monobasic, monohydrate	010049215	7	02/27/86
Sodium sulfate, anhydrous	007757826	2	12/13/84
Sodium sulfite	007757837	4	02/18/75
Sodium thiosulfate	010102177	24	05/05/87
Sorbitan monolaurate	005959897	1	11/26/47
Sulfuric acid	007664939	2	12/13/84

Ophthalmic (cont)

T-butyl peroctoate		1	06/18/76
Thimerosal	000054648	12	06/11/87
Titanium dioxide	001309633	2	07/29/74
Triton 720	000118967	5	01/16/76
Tyloxapol	025301024	4	02/11/86
2-hydroxyethyl methacrylate	000868779	1	08/02/73

Oral

Acacia	009000015	362	10/29/87
Acacia mucilage	008047389	3	08/13/80
Acacia syrup	008047378	1	10/13/82
Acetic acid, glacial	000064197	3	12/16/85
Acetic anhydride	000108247	1	06/25/65
Acetyl tributyl citrate		3	12/22/86
Acetylated monoglycerides		41	12/03/87
Aerosil-200		23	12/16/87
Agar	009002180	2	04/21/72
Alcohol		160	12/21/87
Alcohol, dehydrated	000064175	57	10/16/87
Alcohol, denatured	008024451	14	10/10/86
Alcohol, diluted	008000166	9	03/16/79
Alginic acid	009005327	40	11/27/87
Alpha-tocopherol acetate DL-	000054228	1	06/23/76
Alpha-tocopherol, DL-	000364501	2	08/07/72
Althea		1	04/21/67
Aluminum	007429905	1	03/24/76
Aluminum hydroxide	001302290	3	05/16/73
Aluminum hydroxide gel	012040594	1	07/07/72
Aluminum oxide	001344281	1	05/01/84
Aluminum silicate	014504951	6	04/20/77
Aluminum slicate pentahydrate		1	08/12/77
Amberlite	009002191	8	02/09/87
Amberlite IR-120	009002237	1	09/09/59
Amberlite XE-88	009002340	7	03/07/86
Ammonia	007664417	1	05/22/81
Ammonia solution	008007576	1	06/23/69
Ammonium chloride	012125029	9	06/09/87
Ammonium hydroxide		1	09/07/76
Ammonium phosphate, dibasic	007783280	1	11/02/87
Anethole	012002403	7	01/14/87
Anethole spirit (anise)	000104461	3	06/24/77

Oral (cont)

Anise oil	008007703	7	04/09/87
Anise, star		1	02/10/82
Antifoam	008051089	7	10/10/85
Aquacel 126	008029149	1	04/20/59
Aquacoat ECD		2	12/10/81
Ascorbic acid	000050817	23	12/31/87
Ascorbic palmitate	000137666	2	06/20/75
Attapulgite, activated	001337764	6	12/03/82
Avicel CL 611		2	02/13/87
Beeswax		40	09/02/87
Bentonite	001302789	7	06/15/81
Benzoic acid	000065850	28	10/10/86
Benzoin	009000059	1	06/13/73
Benzyl alcohol	000100516	22	12/30/87
Benzyl benzoate	000120514	1	12/22/69
Beta-naphthol	000135193	4	01/13/76
Betose		2	11/08/63
Bismuth subcarbonate	005892104	3	07/11/74
Butyl aclohol	000071363	10	06/08/84
Butylated hydroxyanisole	008003245	8	03/31/87
Butylated hydroxytoluene	000128370	11	12/11/87
Butylparaben	000094268	31	07/13/87
Calcium acetate	000062544	1	05/08/72
Caclium ascorbate	005743271	1	10/26/72
Calcium carbonate, precipitated	000471341	137	09/10/87
Calcium carrageenan		1	08/04/78
Calcium chloride	010035048	3	04/27/83
Calcium citrate	000813945	2	06/11/79
Calcium hydroxide	001305620	3	04/12/84
Calcium phosphate	010103465	27	06/18/87
Calcium phosphate, dibasic	007757939	317	12/30/87
Calcium phosphate, dibasic, dihydrate	007789777	50	06/18/87
Calcium phosphate, tribasic	012167747	34	10/13/87
Calcium pyrophosphate	007790763	5	03/22/78
Calcium salicylate	000824351	1	10/22/81
Calcium silicate	010101390	7	03/23/87
Calcium stearate	001592230	192	11/27/87
Calcium sulfate	007778189	116	11/06/87
Calcium sulfate dihydrate	010101414	32	05/24/82

Oral (cont)

Calcium sulfate hemihydrate	010034761	1	06/23/76
Calcium sulfate, anrydrous		3	01/26/84
Candelilla wax		5	08/20/86
Capsicum oleoresin	008023776	1	01/14/87
Caramel	008028895	16	03/02/87
Carbomber		2	08/12/81
Carbomer 934	009007163	7	01/24/83
Carboxymethyl starch	009057061	6	05/20/83
Carboxymethyl starch sodium salt	009063381	813	12/31/87
Carboxymethylcellulose	009000117	3	11/23/87
Carboxymethylcellulose sodium	009004324	70	12/17/87
Carboxypolymethylene	009007209	2	03/20/75
Cardamom		1	01/08/75
Carmellose calcium	009050048	4	09/28/87
Carmine	008022933	1	06/10/69
Carmine solution	008001807	2	09/23/74
Carnauba wax	008015869	268	12/08/87
Carrageenan	009000071	3	09/19/79
Castor oil	008001794	32	10/29/87
Castor oil, hydrogenated	008001783	14	01/22/87
Cellulose		129	10/19/87
Cellulose acetate phthalate	009004380	20	07/16/87
Cellulose microcrystalline/ carboxymethylcellulose sodium		2	02/02/87
Cellulose microcrystalline, aqueous		20	01/02/87
Cellulose, microcrystalline	009004346	1,687	12/31/87
Cellulose, oxidized		16	07/25/77
Cellulosic polymers		1	04/09/68
Cetearyl alcohol		4	05/29/87
Cetyl alcohol	000124298	6	06/25/86
Cetyl esters wax	001190632	1	05/07/68
Cetylpyridinium chloride	000123035	10	05/24/85
Cherry		1	09/29/77
Cherry juice	008012995	1	11/25/81
Chlorothen	000148652	1	09/06/79
Cinnamaldehyde	000104552	2	07/14/82
Cinnamon		1	01/08/75
Cinnamon oil	008007805	16	04/09/87

Oral (cont)

Citric acid	000077929	235	12/22/87
Citric acid monohydrate	005949291	3	06/10/87
Citric acid, hydrous	015686654	4	03/25/83
Clove oil	008000348	12	06/11/85
Cocoa bean		1	12/13/72
Cocoa butter		1	04/20/59
Coconut oil	008001318	1	06/20/75
Coffee		1	04/20/59
Coloring suspension		1	11/10/54
Confectioner's glaze		1	03/18/85
Coriander oil	008008524	12	06/11/85
Corn oil	008001307	37	02/28/86
Corn syrup		12	07/01/86
Cottonseed oil, hydrogenated		64	08/14/87
Croscarmellose sodium		437	12/28/87
Crospovidone	009003398	308	11/25/87
Cyclohexane	000110827	1	06/25/65
Cyclomethicone		1	04/07/86
Cysteine hydrochloride	000052891	1	08/20/71
Decaglycerol tetralinoleate		1	10/26/72
Dextrates		1	09/06/72
Dextrin	009004539	6	04/02/79
Dextrose	005996101	22	11/25/87
Dextrose, anhydrous	000050997	1	05/06/59
Di-pac (97% sucrose–3% modified dextrins		23	98/10/81
Diacetylated monoglycerides	008029923	64	11/06/87
Dibutyl phthalate	000084742	2	12/11/79
Dibutyl sebacate		5	12/15/87
Dichlorofluoromethane	000075434	1	04/20/65
Dimethicone	009006659	3	09/02/87
Dioctylphthalate		1	06/30/69
DIPAC (Diisopropylbenzothiazyl-2-sulfenamide)		5	11/10/82
Docusate sodium	000577117	46	09/10/87
Docusate sodium/sodium benzoate		13	07/16/87
Dry flo		1	11/13/84
Dusting powder		6	10/03/83
Dye beige P-1437		1	04/14/83

Oral (cont)

Dye black			04/14/83
Dye black lake blend (LB9972)		2	03/19/87
Dye black (LB442)		1	07/30/85
Dye blue		5	09/10/80
Dye blue #1 (LB4451)		2	07/30/85
Dye blue lakolene		2	05/14/75
Dye brown		4	06/24/81
Dye brown lake		1	10/15/86
Dye brown (LB 292)		1	09/26/85
Dye brown (LB464)		1	07/30/85
Dye burnt sienna	012000576	2	09/10/87
Dye caramel		10	01/14/87
Dye caramel acid proof 100		1	10/31/84
Dye DC blue #2 lake	000130201	4	08/07/87
Dye DC blue #6	000482893	4	09/21/77
Dye DC green #3 lake		2	06/17/77
Dye DC green #5	004403901	5	08/30/78
Dye DC red #17	000085869	1	01/25/62
Dye DC red #19	000081889	1	12/18/85
Dye DC red #21	015086949	1	08/07/61
Dye DC red #21 lake		1	03/26/64
Dye DC red #22	000548265	8	05/10/85
Dye DC red#27	002134158	3	12/20/85
Dye DC red #27 aluminum lake		3	07/14/87
Dye DC red #28	004618239	28	12/08/87
Dye DC red #3 lake		5	01/15/87
Dye DC red #30	002379740	18	10/01/86
Dye DC red #30 aluminum lake		13	09/09/87
Dye DC red #30 lake		7	07/07/87
Dye DC red #33	003567666	66	09/18/87
Dye DC red #33 lake		4	11/17/86
Dye DC red #36		4	09/07/77
Dye DC red #4 lake		1	01/14/60
Dye DC red #40 lake		4	05/11/84
Dye DC red #6	005858811	1	01/26/84
Dye DC red #7	005281049	7	03/20/86
Dye DC red #7 calcium lake		9	07/14/87
Dye DC red #7 lake		6	11/03/86
Dye DC red lake		1	11/17/86
Dye DC violet #2 lake		1	01/15/74
Dye DC yellow		1	06/08/84

Oral (cont)

Dye DC yellow #10	008004920	247	12/31/87
Dye DC yellow #10 aluminum lake		64	10/07/87
Dye DC yellow #10 HT lake		3	09/24/87
Dye DC yellow #10 lake		133	12/31/87
Dye DC yellow #11	008003223	1	01/25/62
Dye DC yellow #5 lake		24	02/07/85
Dye DC yellow #6		3	03/19/87
Dye DC yellow #6 lake		28	11/02/87
Dye FDC black (LB260)		1	08/10/84
Dye FDC blue #1	002650182	312	12/08/87
Dye FDC blue #1 aluminum lake		199	12/31/87
Dye FDC blue #1 HT aluminum lake		9	09/24/87
Dye FDC blue #1 lake		26	10/14/87
Dye FDC blue #2	000860220	62	10/26/87
Dye FDC blue #2 aluminum lake	012227859	81	12/16/87
Dye FDC green #3	002353459	40	10/19/87
Dye FDC green (LB3323)		1	08/25/81
Dye FDC green LB 9583		1	12/06/83
Dye FDC (LB 483)		1	03/20/86
Dye FDC purple LB 588		1	03/20/86
Dye FDC red #3	016423680	186	12/08/87
Dye FDC red #3 lake		8	07/17/87
Dye FDC red #3 aluminum lake	012227780	105	12/18/87
Dye FDC red #33		1	03/06/87
Dye FDC red #40		188	12/08/87
Dye FDC red #40 lake		55	12/24/87
Dye FDC red #7 aluminum lake		4	12/22/87
Dye FDC yellow #10		18	09/04/87
Dye FDC yellow #10 lake		35	12/18/87
Dye FDC yellow #5 aluminum lake	012227699	102	08/19/86
Dye FDC yellow #6	002783940	491	12/31/87
Dye FDC yellow #6 HT lake		2	09/19/86
Dye FDC yellow #6 aluminum lake	012227600	303	12/18/87
Dye FDC yellow #7		1	07/13/79

Oral (cont)

Dye FDC yellow (LB 282)		1	07/15/87
Dye green		11	10/15/82
Dye green (emerald lake blend)		1	12/06/83
Dye green (emerald lake 9207)		1	09/10/85
Dye green dispersion AS 9204		1	05/22/87
Dye green lake blend (LB 482)		1	09/26/85
Dye green PMS-579		1	10/30/86
Dye green PR-1333		1	04/14/83
Dye hercules lemon yellow		1	01/30/85
Dye lakolene yellow #5		1	11/06/74
Dye lavender		1	09/01/78
Dye mint green		3	02/11/76
Dye ochre 3506		1	06/15/79
Dye orange		9	10/15/82
Dye pink		3	07/25/77
Dye purple blend lake		1	11/15/76
Dye purple LB 562 lake blend		1	07/30/85
Dye red		7	12/17/82
Dye red #3 lake HT		1	12/01/78
Dye red cotolene-P		1	08/29/85
Dye rich yellow 062		1	09/10/80
Dye white cotolene-P		2	07/15/86
Dye white TC-1032		1	04/14/83
Dye yellow		3	03/21/85
Dye yellow LB 104		1	03/17/83
Dye yellow LB 9706		4	03/19/87
Dye yellow ochre	001345262	3	08/22/85
Edetate calcium disodium	023411349	15	11/25/86
Edetate disodium	006381926	77	11/06/87
Edetate sodium	000064028	3	04/15/86
Elm		1	01/19/67
Ethyl acetate	000141786	3	09/10/87
Ethyl maltol	004940118	1	11/22/85
Ethyl phthalate	000084662	21	10/30/85
Ethyl vanillin	000121324	18	07/02/87
Ethylcellulose	009004573	250	12/31/87
Ethylenediamine	000107153	3	08/19/83
Ethylparaben	000120478	1	04/07/86
Ethylparaben sodium		2	12/30/86
Eucalyptus oil	008000484	1	01/14/87

Oral (cont)

Eudragit E 30 D		2	04/07/86
Eudragit L 100	052932726	1	07/25/85
Eugenol	000097530	1	09/22/77
Fatty acid esters, saturated		1	05/22/81
Feculose		1	08/19/66
Ferric oxide		8	07/10/86
Ferric oxide, red	001309371	26	12/31/87
Ferrosoferric oxide	001317619	17	04/29/87
Film coating solution, aqueous IM-163		3	03/02/87
Firmenich 51.226/T		1	07/19/82
Flavor		35	10/15/84
Flavor abbatisle		1	07/07/72
Flavor anise		2	07/31/84
Flavor apple	008047914	3	03/06/87
Flavor apricot		3	11/23/82
Flavor apricot peach		2	11/22/85
Flavor apricot with other natural flavors		1	07/19/82
Flavor apricot 24829		1	08/19/83
Flavor banana	000123922	7	09/11/84
Flavor banana FMC 23406		1	11/19/87
Flavor banana mint		1	09/12/85
Flavor banana SA84		1	02/02/87
Flavor berry citrus blend 9756		1	03/26/79
Flavor berry cream		1	08/15/80
Flavor bitterness modifier 15555		1	04/03/87
Flavor black cherry	008010433	1	05/23/75
Flavor black currant		5	04/18/84
Flavor blueberry		1	11/09/87
Flavor bubble gum		1	09/19/79
Flavor buttercaramel		1	12/05/56
Flavor buttermint toffee		1	08/29/78
Flavor buttermint 24020		2	12/16/85
Flavor butterscotch		6	11/09/87
Flavor butterscotch F-1785		3	03/06/87
Flavor butterscotch 61005-U		1	11/27/87
Flavor caramel		1	12/30/71
Flavor cheri-beri PFC-8573		2	08/06/87
Flavor cheri-beri PFC-8580		1	03/25/83

Oral (cont)

Flavor cherry	50	06/22/87
Flavor cherry burgundy 11650	1	09/01/83
Flavor cherry cream	2	11/07/86
Flavor cherry E.P. modified 151	1	12/28/79
Flavor cherry F-232	1	12/16/82
Flavor cherry FMC 22872	1	10/25/84
Flavor cherry FMC 8513	3	10/12/84
Flavor cherry H&R pharma 004	1	01/16/85
Flavor cherry L-1233	1	07/11/73
Flavor cherry N-2755	1	03/03/83
Flavor cherry R-6556	2	02/13/87
Flavor cherry raspberry	1	03/29/84
Flavor cherry vanilla compound A77487	1	11/20/81
Flavor cherry wild NV-101-1489	2	02/13/87
Flavor cherry wild PFC 14783	1	02/04/86
Flavor cherry WL-1093	1	06/28/85
Flavor cherry WL-18022	1	06/16/87
Flavor cherry 18.612	1	02/02/87
Flavor cherry 3321	1	09/20/85
Flavor cherry 338614	1	12/17/87
Flavor cherry 349	1	10/10/86
Flavor cherry 50091OU	1	05/31/75
Flavor cherry-anise PFC 9758	2	03/01/82
Flavor cherry, wild	16	06/18/87
Flavor chocolate	6	03/25/83
Flavor chocolate cream	2	06/13/55
Flavor citrus	1	11/07/80
Flavor citrus-vanilla	1	12/18/87
Flavor cocoa	1	06/20/72
Flavor coconut custard	2	01/26/84
Flavor coconut 41	2	08/01/86
Flavor cola FMC 15740	2	03/02/87
Flavor cough syrup 819	1	04/20/84
Flavor cream	7	07/14/81
Flavor creme de menthe	3	05/15/87
Flavor creme de menthe 14677	2	05/15/87
Flavor currant mint	1	03/05/63
Flavor custard	3	03/25/83
Flavor E-472	1	12/28/79

Oral (cont)

Flavor essence lemon terpeneless		1	08/02/72
Flavor essence orange terpeneless		1	08/02/72
Flavor F-5397A		2	04/27/83
Flavor felton 6-R-9		1	07/23/86
Flavor fig		3	06/20/79
Flavor fritzche tangerine #51465		1	11/08/84
Flavor fritzsche		4	03/22/85
Flavor fritzsche lemon mint #54369		1	10/31/84
Flavor fritzsche peach mint #106109		1	10/31/84
Flavor fritzsche 21028-D		1	03/07/85
Flavor fritzsche 46215		1	01/28/86
Flavor frtizsche 75021		1	03/07/85
Flavor fruit		2	11/23/83
Flavor fruit mint 75588		1	01/08/79
Flavor fruit punch		1	01/08/79
Flavor fruit punch #716		1	12/21/87
Flavor fruit TAK 20008		1	11/23/83
Flavor fruit 84.6422		1	01/13/84
Flavor grape		6	07/03/86
Flavor grape IFF 13549478		1	06/19/87
Flavor grape nectar PFC 8599		1	09/07/82
Flavor grape 13405873		1	02/12/86
Flavor grapefruit		2	02/26/76
Flavor grenadine		1	08/27/62
Flavor guarana		6	11/22/85
Flavor haverstroo ZD 49284		1	01/13/84
Flavor Kola (cola)		1	01/05/78
Flavor lemon	008020197	7	08/96/84
Flavor lemon extract		3	01/18/83
Flavor lemon FMC #10471		1	03/04/83
Flavor lemon lime		1	09/22/77
Flavor lemon vanilla		1	09/02/81
Flavor lemon 812		1	12/12/86
Flavor licorice		2	01/07/83
Flavor lime		3	01/18/83
Flavor mafco-magnasweet 180		1	08/16/77
Flavor maple		1	06/26/78
Flavor maque tree 377(bush)		1	07/05/56
Flavor masking #33321		1	11/22/85
Flavor MCP lemon duramone 4409A		1	07/22/85

Oral (cont)

Flavor MCP lime duramone 6419		1	07/22/85
Flavor mint		5	10/10/85
Flavor mixed fruit		3	10/16/87
Flavor mixed fruit 01-10428		1	11/09/87
Flavor natural and artificial (compound no. 57820/A)		2	12/18/80
Flavor orange	008050326	27	06/10/87
Flavor orange #4168		2	06/12/81
Flavor orange #7679		2	03/23/84
Flavor orange banana WL-18093		1	06/16/87
Flavor orange extract I-1805		1	08/17/79
Flavor orange G 10431		1	03/10/87
Flavor orange P-5614		2	03/15/85
Flavor orange PFH-730016U		1	10/08/82
Flavor orange sour (blood orange)		1	07/19/82
Flavor orange terpeneless		1	09/12/80
Flavor orange 13334		1	06/22/87
Flavor orange-lemon terpeneless		3	12/29/80
Flavor orbit serene 20340		1	04/26/85
Flavor passion fruit		2	04/06/70
Flavor peach		2	08/06/84
Flavor peach F9770		1	06/28/85
Flavor peach mint		1	06/08/82
Flavor peach 13503584		3	06/11/85
Flavor peach-pineapple FMC 14258		1	04/22/87
Flavor peach/pineapple		3	12/31/87
Flavor peppermint		19	11/09/87
Flavor peppermint K373		1	01/16/85
Flavor peppermint stick FMC 16170		2	12/16/85
Flavor peppermint 517		1	02/02/87
Flavor peppermint, natural spraylene		3	07/01/82
Flavor pineapple		11	03/23/87
Flavor pineapple N-2566		2	03/15/85
Flavor pineapple orange imit		1	05/07/68
Flavor pineapple-coconut		1	10/10/85
Flavor punch		1	07/11/73

Oral (cont)

Flavor raspberry		35	12/12/86
Flavor raspberry blend F-1840		1	02/21/85
Flavor raspberry blend PFC 8407		2	12/16/85
Flavor raspberry F-1784		1	12/17/84
Flavor raspberry 1840		1	07/27/83
Flavor refraichissement		1	03/16/82
Flavor root beer		3	09/22/77
Flavor rum and butter		1	07/07/72
Flavor sherry		1	06/25/80
Flavor spearmint		3	07/01/82
Flavor strawberry		25	05/15/87
Flavor strawberry F-5665		1	12/16/85
Flavor strawberry 14953		1	05/15/87
Flavor strawberry 5210(FD&D)		1	12/20/83
Flavor strawberry 55058		1	10/31/84
Flavor tangerine		1	12/03/86
Flavor tetrarome		1	01/05/78
Flavor tutti frutti		4	08/14/80
Flavor tutti frutti P-5400		2	03/15/85
Flavor tutti frutti WL-18481		2	12/22/87
Flavor vanilla		18	11/22/85
Flavor vanilla creme		4	12/03/86
Flavor vanilla P-1160		2	03/15/85
Flavor vanilla-banana		1	04/24/59
Flavor veralock bubble gum		1	01/18/74
Flavor wild cherry K-321		1	11/19/87
Flavor wintergreen		2	08/06/84
Flavor wintergreen PFC 8421		1	04/03/87
Flavor 18317		1	07/11/73
Flour		17	05/14/85
Food glaze		1	08/12/77
Fragrance unspecified		4	09/28/77
Fructose	007660255	8	12/03/86
Fumaric acid	000110178	1	03/23/87
Galactose, D-	000059234	4	06/20/79
Gelatin	009000708	532	12/31/87
Ginger fluidextract		2	01/14/87
Gluconic acid, D-	000133426	1	08/19/68
Gluconolactone, D-	000090802	1	01/21/52

Oral (cont)

Glucose, liquid	008027563	21	04/09/87
Glutamic acid hydrochloride	000138158	2	03/08/83
Gluten	008002800	1	03/14/6x
Glycerin	000056815	237	12/21/8x
Glycerin polymer solution IM-137		3	06/24/85
Glycerin polymer solution, I-137		2	09/06/85
Glycryl distearate	001323837	7	01/06/8x
Glyceryl monostearate		13	06/25/86
Glyceryl oleate	000544763	7	01/26/84
Glyceryl ricinoleate	001323382	1	07/19/56
Glyceryl stearate/PEG stearate		1	03/13/80
Glycine	000056406	8	07/22/85
Glycol, bis(n-methyl-N-(2-chloroethyl)aminoacetate) dihydrochloride	013323574	3	05/04/82
Glycyrrhizin, ammoniated	001407030	2	11/29/79
Grapefruit juice		1	08/27/62
Guar gum	009000300	27	12/01/86
Gum base, chewing		2	11/13/84
Gum rosin	008050100	5	07/13/87
High fructose corn syrup		2	12/31/87
Histidine	000071001	1	12/12/86
Hydrochloric acid	007647010	30	10/16/87
Hydrochloric acid, diluted		1	11/07/85
Hydrochlorothiazide	000053935	1	07/15/87
Hydroxyethyl cellulose	009004620	5	05/29/87
Hydroxypropyl cellulose	009004642	187	11/06/87
Hydroxypropyl methylcellulose	009004653	300	12/30/87
Hydroxypropyl methylcellulose phthalate		6	12/22/86
Hydroxypropyl methylcellulose 100	009004653	1	10/08/86
Hydroxypropyl methylcellulose 2208	009004653	3	07/02/87
Hydroxypropyl methylcellulose 2906	009004653	1	01/19/83

Oral (cont)

Hydroxypropyl methylcellulose 2910		56	11/27/87
Ink black (pharmaceutical)		3	12/31/87
Ink black A-10450		6	05/22/84
Ink black A-10509		3	06/11/87
Ink black A-1057		1	03/23/82
Ink black imprinting FGE-1386		4	01/08/87
Ink blue black		1	08/08/79
Ink blue black A-9371		2	09/21/77
Ink edible		13	05/14/85
Ink edible black		16	01/09/87
Ink edible blue		1	04/02/79
Ink edible brown		4	09/14/81
Ink edible red		1	02/01/60
Ink edible red A-8032		2	07/13/87
Ink edible white		11	12/28/83
Ink fine black 2202C		3	06/14/85
Ink fine black 2212		4	09/25/84
Ink light redwood		1	09/09/86
Ink red A-8032		1	07/03/57
Ink white		1	01/08/87
Ink white A-8154		4	04/15/86
Ink white 21-K		1	02/10/58
Invert sugar	008013170	6	06/07/85
Invert syrup, medium		1	01/14/87
Iron oxide		38	09/02/87
Iron oxide, yellow		8	12/29/87
Isopropanolamine		1	06/12/78
Isopropyl alcohol	000067630	22	11/06/87
Isotonic sodium chloride solution	008028771	4	12/30/77
Kaolin	001332587	40	07/15/86
Karion 83 (D-sorbitol content 19-25%)		1	08/11/82
Lactic acid	008012213	7	01/06/87
Lactose	000063423	2,196	12/31/87
Lactose monohydrate	010039266	25	11/19/87
Lactose, anhydrous		10	05/05/87
Lactose, hydrous		53	10/14/87
Landalgene		1	12/19/75

Oral (cont)

Lauryl sulfate		3	06/18/85
Lecithin	008002435	18	09/02/87
Lecithin, soy bean	008030760	3	12/15/86
Lemon juice		2	12/01/78
Lemon oil	008008568	3	12/30/80
Lime extract terpeneless		1	03/18/82
Lime isolate		1	12/30/80
Lime oil, distilled	008008262	1	08/19/77
Liner oil		1	12/30/80
Lubritab		3	06/21/83
Magnesium	007439954	2	04/02/87
Magnesium aluminum silicate	001327431	46	11/19/87
Magnesium carbonate	000546930	30	04/23/85
Magnesium hydroxide	001309428	2	01/30/76
Magnesium oxide	001309484	11	10/26/87
Magnesium silicate	001343889	14	05/04/77
Magnesium stearate	000557040	2,735	12/31/87
Magnesium sulfate	010034998	11	05/15/86
Magnesium sulfate, anhydrous	007487889	2	08/02/79
Magnesium trisilicate	001343904	6	09/12/85
Maleic acid	000110167	1	04/19/83
Malic acid, DL-		1	04/10/86
Malic acid, L-	000097676	1	01/03/74
Malt extract, powder	008002480	1	05/26/55
Maltol	000118718	4	01/30/85
Mandarin oil, expressed	008008319	1	07/01/83
Mannitol	000069658	58	12/29/87
Mannose, D-	000530267	1	06/21/74
Medical antifoam emulsion C		7	03/18/87
Menthol	000089781	32	01/14/87
Menthol, L-	002216515	1	03/29/84
Methyl acrylate	000096333	1	11/05/82
Methyl alcohol	000067561	9	09/10/87
Methyl hydroxyethyl cellulose		2	09/19/85
Methyl salicylate	000119368	1	12/05/56
Methylated spirits		1	05/19/81
Methylcellulose	009004675	147	09/09/87
Methylcellulose 400		1	08/07/79
Methylene chloride	000075092	2	06/26/78
Methylparaben	000099763	319	12/31/87

Oral (cont)

Methylparaben sodium	005026620	1	02/02/87
Microcrystalline wax	008063089	2	02/04/80
Milk	008049987	1	12/13/72
Mineral oil	008012951	32	05/28/87
Mineral oil, light		22	04/09/87
Mistron spray talc		1	05/18/81
Monochloramine solution		1	07/05/56
Monosodium glutamate	000142472	1	12/05/56
Mullein leaf		1	07/01/76
Muscatel wine		1	02/26/76
Myristyl alcohol	000112721	4	06/25/86
Myvacet type 5-00	008029912	1	02/01/60
Neutral oil		1	06/12/86
Non-pareil seed		101	12/15/87
Nu-tab(combination of sugar, starch, and magnesium stearate)		1	03/24/77
Nutmeg oil, expressed	008007123	1	01/08/75
Oleic acid	000112801	15	07/13/87
Opacoat HA2203		1	05/15/79
Opacoat HA4108 (blue)		2	09/18/78
Opacoat HA4711 (lavender)		1	09/18/78
Opacoat HA7013 (clear)		2	12/03/84
Opacode S-1-3110 (green)		2	06/16/86
Opacode S-1-7077		2	09/18/87
Opacode S-1-8025 (black)		1	07/10/86
Opacode S-1-8081 (black)		4	09/19/86
Opacode S-1-8090 (black)		8	04/29/87
Opacode S-1-8092 (black)		3	04/29/87
Opacode S-1-8095		1	04/16/59
Opacode S-1-8100-HV (black)		1	01/28/87
Opacode S-1-8106 (black)		3	05/22/84
Opacode S-1-8110 (black)		1	12/05/85
Opacode S-1-8115 (black)		1	12/07/67
Opadry		3	10/05/87
Opadry (chartreuse)		3	01/20/87
Opadry (clear)		6	01/20/87
Opadry Y-S-8050 (black)		1	10/16/87
Opadry Y-1-1518 (pink)		1	11/08/83
Opadry Y-1-2132 (yellow)		1	02/20/86
Opadry Y-1-2605 (beige)		1	11/08/83

Oral (cont)

Opadry Y-1-3211 (green)	2	10/22/85
Opadry Y-1-4205 (blue)	1	04/16/59
Opadry Y-1-4234 (blue)	2	04/15/86
Opadry Y-1-7000 (white)	6	02/17/87
Opadry Y-1-7000B (white)	1	09/23/86
Opadry Y-5-1244 (pink)	1	07/14/87
Opadry Y-5-1727 (red)	1	10/16/87
Opadry Y-5-2360 (orange)	1	11/27/87
Opadry Y-5-2450 (orange)	6	07/14/87
Opadry Y-5-2451 (orange)	1	07/14/87
Opadry Y-5-3140 (green)	1	07/14/87
Opadry Y-5-4129 (blue)	2	11/27/87
Opadry Y-5-7058 (white)	3	10/03/77
Opadry Y-5-7068 (white)	4	11/18/87
Opadry Y-5-7411 (purple)	1	07/14/87
Opadry Y-5-9006 (brown)	1	07/14/87
Opadry YPS-7-2127	1	05/24/83
Opadry YS-1-1221 (pink)	1	11/12/86
Opadry YS-1-1510 (pink)	2	03/21/86
Opadry YS-1-1522 (pink)	1	12/21/82
Opadry YS-1-1528 (pink)	1	04/30/84
Opadry YS-1-1847 (red)	1	01/02/87
Opadry YS-1-2122 (yellow)	4	09/23/86
Opadry YS-1-2134 (yellow)	3	12/30/87
Opadry YS-1-2136 (yellow)	1	04/30/84
Opadry YS-1-2167 (yellow)	1	07/22/85
Opadry YS-1-2505 (orange)	2	08/17/87
Opadry YS-1-2465	2	08/01/86
Opadry YS-1-2522 (orange)	1	08/02/85
Opadry YS-1-2526 (orange)	1	05/28/87
Opadry YS-1-2527 (orange)	11	11/12/86
Opadry YS-1-2534	8	11/04/86
Opadry YS-1-2548 (orange)	1	08/28/85
Opadry YS-1-2549 (orange)	1	03/02/87
Opadry YS-1-2558 (orange)	4	10/03/86
Opadry YS-1-2563 (orange)	1	04/30/84
Opadry YS-1-2604 (beige)	3	04/30/84
Opadry YS-1-2612 (beige)	1	06/23/86
Opadry YS-1-2619	3	04/25/86
Opadry YS-1-26123 (brown)	1	11/03/86

Oral (cont)

Opadry YS-1-2635 (tan)	1	03/23/87
Opadry YS-1-2669 (rust)	1	09/19/86
Opadry YS-1-3105 (green)	6	11/12/86
Opadry YS-1-3146 (green)	1	08/05/76
Opadry YS-1-3166 (green)	1	10/05/87
Opadry YS-1-4112 (blue)	2	09/11/86
Opadry YS-1-4221 (blue)	2	12/10/86
Opadry YS-1-4229 (blue)	1	04/30/84
Opadry YS-1-4700 (purple)	3	11/18/86
Opadry YS-1-4702 (violet)	3	02/25/83
Opadry YS-1-4710	3	05/19/86
Opadry YS-1-4812 (lavender)	1	05/29/87
Opadry YS-1-7003 (white)	34	02/03/87
Opadry YS-1-7006 (clear)	37	11/27/87
Opadry YS-1-7027 (white)	2	06/16/86
Opadry YS-1-7552 (grey)	3	03/19/87
Opadry YS-1-89193 (clear)	1	02/12/86
Opadry YS-1-9012 (brown)	2	12/08/87
Opadry YS-2-7013 (clear)	1	08/15/78
Opadry YS-3-7011 (clear)	29	12/08/87
Opadry YS-3-7031 (clear)	6	02/17/87
Opadry YS-5-1260 (pink)	1	01/15/87
Opadry YS-5-3116 (green)	1	08/15/78
Opadry YS-5-7068	4	09/29/87
Opaglos clear	1	05/19/81
Opalux As 1406 (pink)	1	12/05/83
Opalux As 1537 (pink)	1	05/19/81
Opalux As 1589 (pink)	4	11/19/82
Opalux As 1771 (violet)	1	08/05/81
Opalux AS 1841 (red)	1	03/02/82
Opalux AS 2006 (yellow)	1	09/25/84
Opalux AS 2007 (yellow)	1	05/18/81
Opalux AS 2086 (chartreuse)	1	12/29/83
Opalux AS 2087	1	06/17/77
Opalux AS 2094	1	05/26/76
Opalux AS 2167 (yellow)	1	01/22/82
Opalux AS 2236	19	12/14/81
Opalux AS 2269 (yellow)	2	12/20/82
Opalux AS 2336 (orange)	1	07/14/87
Opalux AS 2346 (orange)	3	04/03/84

Oral (cont)

Opalux AS 2413	2	02/15/73
Opalux AS 2433 (orange)	2	07/28/81
Opalux AS 2498 (orange)	5	09/25/84
Opalux AS 2512	1	03/23/82
Opalux AS 2532 (orange)	1	08/13/80
Opalux AS 2553 (orange)	2	03/20/81
Opalux AS 2620-B (tan)	1	12/05/83
Opalux AS 2676 Salmon (Jasper red)	2	10/21/83
Opalux AS 2691	1	09/14/81
Opalux AS 2754	1	01/4/82
Opalux AS 2768	1	09/09/87
Opalux AS 3287	1	10/27/69
Opalux AS 3308 (green)	1	04/20/77
Opalux AS 3348-C (green)	1	01/22/87
Opalux AS 3376	1	10/27/69
Opalux AS 3378-C (green)	1	09/15/82
Opalux AS 3389 (green)	1	03/20/81
Opalux AS 3391 (green)	3	09/25/84
Opalux AS 3910 (maroon)	1	02/09/79
Opalux AS 4025	1	09/09/87
Opalux AS 4151 (blue)	1	10/30/80
Opalux AS 4188 (tan)	1	09/29/76
Opalux AS 4208-A (blue)	1	05/14/84
Opalux AS 4270 (blue)	4	11/19/82
Opalux AS 4800 (lavender)	1	07/22/86
Opalux AS 4854 (lavender)	1	07/22/86
Opalux AS 4855 (purple)	2	07/22/86
Opalux AS 4891	1	09/09/87
Opalux AS 5107	1	09/15/80
Opalux AS 5178 (green)	1	10/29/87
Opalux AS 5203 (green)	1	10/29/87
Opalux AS 5205 (green)	1	12/05/83
Opalux AS 5212 (green)	2	06/20/77
Opalux AS 7000-B	6	06/01/82
Opalux AS 7000-P (white)	6	05/21/85
Opalux AS 7001	1	09/09/87
Opalux AS 7535 (gray)	1	09/10/87
Opalux AS 8010-A (black)	1	06/23/76
Opalux AS 8050-L (black)	2	09/29/87

Oral (cont)

Opalux AS 9010 (brown)	2	07/14/81
Opalux brown	1	07/14/81
Opalux red	2	09/29/87
Opaode S-1-7078	1	12/04/87
Opaque buff 031	1	05/13/86
Opaque green 661	1	05/13/86
Opaque ivory 009	1	05/13/86
Opaque orange	3	12/04/87
Opaque peach	1	12/04/87
Opaque red	1	01/08/87
Opaque white	3	06/24/87
Opaque white 999	1	05/13/86
Opaseal	3	05/24/83
Opaspray	27	12/03/87
Opaspray (coral)	1	08/05/77
Opaspray green	1	08/14/87
Opaspray IM-176	2	09/06/85
Opaspray K-1-1230	1	05/25/77
Opaspray K-1-1279	3	11/13/84
Opaspray K-1-1289 (pink)	1	01/03/86
Opaspray K-1-1413 (pink)	1	09/26/84
Opaspray K-1-1414 (pink)	1	01/23/86
Opaspray K-1-1563 (pink)	1	06/23/82
Opaspray K-1-1573 (lavender)	1	09/26/84
Opaspray K-1-1574	1	05/03/82
Opaspray K-1-1584	1	05/24/83
Opaspray K-1-2013 (yellow)	3	02/07/86
Opaspray K-1-2216-A (yellow)	3	05/03/82
Opaspray K-1-2227 (yellow)	1	05/18/81
Opaspray K-1-2228 (yellow)	3	01/09/87
Opaspray K-1-2240 (yellow)	1	06/29/84
Opaspray K-1-2300 (peach)	1	09/25/84
Opaspray K-1-2301 (peach)	1	10/01/86
Opaspray K-1-2303 (orange)	1	09/11/86
Opasrpay K-1-2304 (orange)	1	08/06/85
Opaspray K-1-2314 (orange)	3	11/13/84
Opaspray K-1-2327 (orange)	1	08/14/87
Opaspray K-1-2330 (orange)	1	03/15/85
Opaspray K-1-2335 (orange)	2	02/02/87
Opaspray K-1-2406 (orange)	2	08/10/82

Oral (cont)

Opaspray K-1-2410 (orange)	2	04/13/82
Opaspray K-1-2430	3	05/11/84
Opaspray K-1-2441 (orange)	3	10/15/85
Opaspray K-1-2473	1	08/30/83
Opaspray K-1-2492	1	07/23/86
Opaspray K-1-2531	1	01/04/82
Opaspray K-1-2533 (orange)	1	04/01/82
Opaspray K-1-2568 (orange)	1	08/06/85
Opaspray K-1-2570 (orange)	1	05/27/82
Opaspray K-1-2588 (orange)	1	06/12/85
Opaspray K-1-2614 (beige)	2	01/04/82
Opaspray K-1-2621 (brown)	1	06/23/82
Opaspray K-1-2626 (orange)	1	01/15/86
Opaspray K-1-2630 (brown)	1	08/31/87
Opaspray K-1-2656 (beige)	2	11/08/82
Opaspray K-1-2670 (tan)	1	11/18/83
Opaspray K-1-2674 (beige)	1	09/11/86
Opaspray K-1-2685	1	04/18/85
Opaspray K-1-3000	2	03/02/84
Opaspray K-1-3142 (green)	2	11/03/84
Opaspray K-1-3144 (green)	1	06/12/86
Opaspray K-1-3147	3	01/23/86
Opaspray K-1-3148 (green)	2	07/29/83
Opaspray K-1-3173 (green)	1	08/05/76
Opaspray K-1-3178 (green)	1	12/10/86
Opaspray K-1-3209 (green)	1	06/12/86
Opaspray K-1-3220 (green)	1	09/26/84
Opaspray K-1-3300-A (green)	1	08/05/76
Opaspray K-1-3300-C	1	08/15/83
Opaspray K-1-4108 (blue)	3	09/17/86
Opaspray K-1-4119	1	03/13/80
Opaspray K-1-4136 (blue)	2	01/04/82
Opaspray K-1-4205 (blue)	1	01/04/82
Opaspray K-1-4210-A	1	09/04/80
Opaspray K-1-4214	1	03/13/80
Opaspray K-1-4234 (blue)	2	04/15/86
Opaspray K-1-4235 (blue)	4	01/29/85
Opaspray K-1-4720	2	06/22/82
Opaspray K-1-4728	3	09/25/84
Opaspray K-1-4730	1	03/20/86

Oral (cont)

Opaspray K-1-4731 (purple)		1	03/20/86
Opaspray K-1-4748 (purple)		1	02/02/87
Opaspray K-1-4786		1	03/13/80
Opaspray K-1-7000 (white)		26	01/02/87
Opaspray K-1-70008 (white)		4	12/05/86
Opaspray K-1-9027 (brown)		2	09/16/83
Opaspray K-1-9039-L (brown)		4	11/26/85
Opaspray K-1-9080 (brown)		2	11/13/84
Opaspray K-1-9112 (brown)		1	10/02/87
Opaspray L-1-3305 (green)		1	12/01/86
Opaspray L-1-3306 (green)		1	12/01/86
Opaspray M-1-3439 B (orange)		2	04/10/87
Opaspray M-1-3459 B (orange)		2	04/10/87
Opaspray M-1-3484 B (orange)		2	04/10/87
Opaspray M-1-4399 (blue)		1	12/28/87
Opaspray M-1-711B (white)		2	06/14/85
Opaspray M-1-7111-B		2	02/22/85
Opaspray M-1-7120 (white)		3	12/28/87
Opaspray WD-1270 (pink)		1	02/27/75
Opaspray WD-2009-B (yellow)		1	03/16/76
Orange juice		2	12/18/80
Orange juice, synthetic		1	07/22/81
Orange natural extract		1	03/14/41
Orange oil	008008579	15	08/07/85
Orange oil, terpeneless		3	01/17/85
Orange peel extract		1	03/18/82
Orange peel, sweet		1	06/09/81
Ozokerite	008021554	2	03/04/77
Palm oil–soybean oil, hydrogenated		1	08/05/86
Parabens		8	01/15/85
Paraffin	008002742	11	10/22/87
Parmacoat 606		1	10/15/86
PD base-1000		1	06/12/86
Peanut oil	008002037	3	07/02/87
Peppermint		1	09/02/60
Peppermint oil	008006904	36	09/17/86
Petrolatum	008009038	3	03/06/86
Pharma-sweet 24052		1	10/21/80
Pharmaceutical glaze		131	12/18/87

Oral (cont)

Phosphate buffer		1	11/16/76
Phosphoric acid	007664382	3	02/23/78
Pineapple extract, artificial (H Kohnstamm & Co)		1	07/25/83
Piperonal	000120570	1	11/22/85
Plasdone-alcohol solution		1	07/01/82
Polacrilin potassium	039393765	35	09/01/87
Polishing solution IM-182		3	03/02/87
Poloxamer		10	12/18/87
Poloxamer 188		1	12/10/57
Poloxamer 331		2	02/13/87
Polyethylene	009002884	12	12/20/85
Polyethylene glycol	025322683	85	12/08/87
Polyethylene glycol 1000		5	04/03/87
Polyethylene glycol 1500		1	05/30/73
Polyethylene glycol 1540		3	07/28/75
Polyethylene glycol 200		1	01/27/81
Polyethylene glycol 3350		18	12/31/87
Polyethylene glycol 3500		4	04/15/86
Polyethylene glycol 400	009004960	24	03/18/87
Polyethylene glycol 4000		31	11/07/86
Polyethylene glycol 600		3	02/07/85
Polyethylene glycol 6000		38	04/15/86
Polyethylene glycol 8000		42	12/30/87
Polyethylene glycol-tert-dodecylthioether		1	05/22/84
Polyethylene glycols		16	04/18/83
Polyox	008050622	1	02/03/69
Polyoxyl 20 stearate		1	11/21/79
Polyoxyl 40 stearate	009004993	22	08/03/87
Polyoxyl 8 stearate	009004993	1	03/03/70
Polypropylene glycol	009003150	1	05/11/84
Polysaccharide		1	03/29/82
Polysorbate		6	11/27/87
Polysorbate 20	009005645	6	12/12/86
Polysorbate 40	009005667	4	05/12/62
Polysorbate 60	009005678	5	03/15/85
Polysorbate 80	009005656	110	12/31/87
Polyvinyl acetate	009003207	3	10/22/87
Polyvinyl alcohol	009002895	3	09/10/87

Oral (cont)

Polyvinyl chloride–polyvinyl acetate copolymer		1	04/19/83
Polyvinylpyrrolidone ethylcellulose		1	03/12/79
Potassium carbonate	000564087	29	12/18/87
Potassium chloride	007447407	19	12/15/87
Potassium citrate	006100056	3	01/03/74
Potassium hydroxide	001310583	2	04/09/87
Potassium metaphosphate	007790536	2	05/12/62
Potassium phosphate, dibasic	007758114	5	11/19/87
Potassium phosphate, monobasic	007778770	9	10/24/85
Potassium sorbate	000590001	14	12/18/87
Povidone	009003398	420	12/31/87
Propionic acid	000079094	1	12/23/53
Propylene glycol	000057556	284	12/31/87
Propylene glycol alginate	009005372	3	08/03/73
Propylparaben	000094133	237	12/31/87
Propylparaben sodium	035285699	4	12/28/87
Protein hydrolysate	009015547	1	08/04/66
QUSO–G 32		1	08/11/80
Rapeseed oil	008002139	1	12/15/86
Rosin	008050097	10	09/13/82
Saccharin	000081072	14	01/19/83
Saccharin calcium	006381915	2	07/23/86
Saccharin sodium	006155373	162	06/10/87
Saccharin sodium anhydrous	000128449	19	06/11/85
Satialgine H		1	11/13/84
Sea spen		1	01/18/74
Sesame oil	008008740	4	04/03/87
Shellac	009000593	135	10/29/87
Shellac P.V.P. solution no. 5		1	11/29/82
Shellac P.V.P. solution no. 4		1	11/29/82
Silica gel	007699414	165	11/03/87
Silica, diatomaceous	007631869	43	07/22/86
Silicon	007440213	1	03/16/76
Silicon dioxide	007631869	1,063	12/31/87
Silicone		18	12/29/87
Silicone emulsion		2	01/04/71
Simethicone	008050815	24	07/02/87
Simethicone (medical adhesive B) MDx4-4036		1	09/09/87

Oral (cont)

Soap		1	07/13/87
Soap, eiderdown		7	05/14/84
Sodium acetate	006131904	3	12/10/85
Sodium acetate, anhydrous	000127093	1	11/18/76
Sodium alginate	009005383	7	12/16/86
Sodium aluminosilicate	001344009	1	10/01/69
Sodium aminobenzoate	000555066	4	02/18/75
Sodium benzoate	000532321	204	12/22/87
Sodium bicarbonate	000144558	46	11/27/87
Sodium bisulfate	007681381	1	04/27/83
Sodium bisulfite	007631905	31	04/16/86
Sodium carbonate	000497198	7	02/27/85
Sodium carragenate		1	03/21/61
Sodium cellulose		2	10/15/80
Sodium chloride	007647145	28	07/17/87
Sodium citrate	006132043	140	12/22/87
Sodium citrate anhydrous	000068042	8	12/08/81
Sodium gluconate	000327071	2	11/22/85
Sodium hydoxide	001310732	43	12/23/87
Sodium lactate	000072173	1	12/12/86
Sodium lauryl sulfate	000151213	412	12/28/87
Sodium metabisulfite	007757746	22	01/15/86
Sodium m-lauroyl sarcosinate	000137166	1	09/26/84
Sodium nitrate	007631994	1	11/10/80
Sodium phosphate	007632055	6	06/28/85
Sodium phosphate, dibasic	007782856	15	05/28/86
Sodium phosphate, dibasic, anhydrous		1	06/18/87
Sodium phosphate, monobasic	007558807	7	05/28/86
Sodium phosphate, monobasic, monohydrate	010049215	3	02/23/78
Sodium phosphate, tribasic	007601549	1	07/16/47
Sodium propionate	000137406	15	11/25/86
Sodium salicylate	000054217	1	10/31/55
Sodium stannate		1	11/08/76
Sodium stearate	000822162	10	10/09/80
Sodium succinate		1	04/03/87
Sodium sulfate	007727733	3	02/10/81
Sodium sulfate, anhydrous	007757826	4	03/09/61
Sodium sulfite	007757837	6	04/27/83
Sodium thiosulfate	010102177	5	11/09/79

Oral (cont)

Sodium thiosulfate, anhydrous	007772987	5	10/14/82
Sorbic acid	000110441	21	12/21/87
Sorbitan monolaurate	005959897	6	08/07/85
Sorbitan monooleate	005938385	7	08/12/82
Sorbitan monostearate	001338416	1	07/16/62
Sorbitan solution		1	02/12/86
Sorbitan trioleate	005960065	3	12/09/75
Sorbitol	000050704	79	12/30/86
Sorbitol solution	003959533	93	12/21/87
Soybean oil	008001227	16	09/04/86
Soybean oil, hydrogenated	008016704	5	01/21/87
Spearmint oil	008008795	3	04/12/82
Stanofil		6	05/15/81
Starch	009005258	1,721	12/31/87
Starch 1500		119	12/17/87
Starch 1551		10	09/29/87
Starch, corn		446	12/29/87
Starch, potato		27	04/02/87
Starch, pregelatinized		286	12/29/87
Starch, pregelatinized corn		28	05/08/87
Starch, rice		1	05/01/62
Stear-o-wet C		1	01/29/82
Stear-o-wet M		49	12/03/87
Stearic acid	000057114	1,210	12/30/87
Stearyl alcohol	000112925	3	09/09/87
Succinic acid	000110156	1	04/03/87
Sucrose	000057501	772	12/31/87
Sucrose syrup		2	01/28/86
Sugar compressible		4	09/04/87
Sugar confectioners		23	12/08/87
Sugar fruit fine		4	02/13/87
Sugar liquid		10	01/04/85
Sugar non-pareil seeds		3	08/23/84
Sugar/starch insert granules		2	12/16/82
Sugars (unidentified)		24	01/10/86
Sulfuiric acid	007664939	2	09/07/76
Syloid 244 FP		15	06/18/87
Synasol		1	04/02/79
Synchron oral carrier		7	04/03/85
Syrup	008027472	21	09/29/87

Oral (cont)

Talc	014807966	699	12/31/87
Talc triturate		1	09/09/87
Tamarin fantaisie		1	03/14/41
Tartaric acid	000087694	3	06/12/79
Tartaric acid, DL-	000133379	14	03/25/86
Tartrazine	001934210	219	07/20/87
Tellurium	010028167	1	03/24/76
Terpene resin	009003741	2	06/13/73
Timing solution clear N-7		1	09/01/82
Titanium	007550450	1	06/23/87
Titanium dioxide	001309633	461	12/31/87
Tolu	068916336	1	11/22/76
Tragacanth	009000651	20	10/10/85
Triacetin	000102761	45	09/02/87
Trichloroethane	000102761	1	03/23/77
Trichloromonofluorethane		1	04/20/65
Triethyl citrate	000077930	4	01/02/87
Triglyceride, synthetic		1	08/17/78
Trimyristin		1	10/18/85
Tristearin	000555431	1	08/21/58
Tromethamine	000077861	2	08/05/81
Unspecified ingredient(s)		83	10/28/86
Urea	000057136	1	11/08/73
USA base #8		1	09/17/54
Vanillin	000121335	38	07/10/87
Vegetable oil	008008897	10	12/31/87
Vegetable oils, hydrogenated		39	12/28/87
Vegetable shortening		1	05/18/73
Vegetable stearine		2	12/01/78
Velvetine black powder		1	05/16/74
Vinyl acetate–crotonic acid copolymer		1	02/23/82
Vinyl chloride	000075014	1	10/21/83
Viscarin	008047254	1	06/20/72
Vitamin E	000059029	2	11/24/82
Vythene	001299894	1	03/02/82
Wax blend		2	01/06/81
Wax, candelilla		3	09/08/81
Wax, carnauba yellow		11	04/03/84
Wax, concord		2	08/04/77

Oral (cont)

Wax, dehydag SX	008023403	1	09/10/87
Wax, white	008006404	138	09/10/87
Wax, yellow	008012893	34	12/08/87
Wheat meal		1	07/09/74
Xanthan gum		25	12/31/87
Zein	009010666	22	07/13/87
Zinc stearate	000557051	24	06/23/87
Zinc sulfate	007446200	1	04/06/84
1,1,1-trichloroethane	000071556	13	07/14/87
2-hydroxy-n-cyclopropylmethyl morphinan hydrochloride		1	11/27/59
2-hydroxynicotinic acid		1	01/21/74
2-naptholene sulfonate sodium salt		2	09/09/71

Oral birth control products

Acacia	009000015	12	10/01/76
Amberlite	009002191	1	07/26/79
Calcium acetate	000062544	6	12/30/81
Calcium carbonate, precipitated	000471341	2	11/01/84
Calcium phosphate	010103465	3	12/30/81
Calcium phosphate, dibasic	007757939	6	07/05/78
Carboxymethyl starch	009057061	1	04/30/73
Carboxymethyl starch sodium salt	009063381	4	07/05/78
Castor oil, hydrogenated	008001783	6	12/30/81
Cellulose		7	11/01/84
Cellulose, microcrystalline	009004346	8	01/29/87
Crospovidone	009003398	6	04/04/84
Dye DC green #5	004403901	6	07/18/86
Dye DC yellow #10	008004920	11	12/14/87
Dye DC yellow #10 aluminum lake		8	01/29/87
Dye FDC blue #1	002650182	5	11/01/84
Dye FDC blue #1 aluminum lake		1	03/29/76
Dye FDC blue #1 lake		1	10/02/67
Dye FDC blue #2 aluminum lake	012227859	1	04/04/84

Oral birth control products (cont)

Dye FDC red #3	016425680	6	07/21/82
Dye FDC yellow #10		1	12/14/87
Dye FDC yellow #10 lake		1	04/04/84
Dye FDC yellow #6	002783940	12	12/14/87
Dye FDC yellow #6-aluminum lake	012227600	4	07/05/78
Dye peach		1	01/11/82
Dye red		2	05/15/70
Glycerin	000056815	2	11/01/84
Iron oxide		2	11/01/84
Lactose	000063423	55	12/14/87
Magnesium silicate	001343880	1	10/01/76
Magnesium stearate	000557040	60	12/14/87
Methylparaben	000099763	2	11/01/84
Polacrilin potassium	039393765	10	01/29/87
Polyethylene glycol 8000		2	11/01/84
Povidone	009003398	29	12/14/87
Propylparaben	000094133	2	11/01/84
Sodium benzoate	000532321	2	11/01/84
Sodium lauryl sulfate	000151213	1	07/18/86
Sodium phosphate	007632005	2	10/10/78
Sodium phosphate, dibasic	007782856	1	02/22/64
Sodium phosphate, monobasic	007558807	2	10/10/72
Sodium sulfate	007727733	1	02/22/64
Sodium sulfate, anhydrous	007757826	1	10/10/72
Starch	009005258	36	07/18/86
Starch, corn		9	12/14/87
Starch, pregelatinized		11	07/18/86
Sucrose	000057501	14	11/01/84
Talc	014807966	12	11/01/84
Tartrazine	001934210	2	10/01/76
Titanium dioxide	001309633	2	11/01/84

Otic

Acetic acid		1	09/18/85
Acetic acid, glacial	000064197	3	11/06/85
Aluminum sulfate	010043013	1	08/21/85
Benzlakonium chloride	008001545	6	09/18/85
Benzethonium chloride	000121540	4	03/04/85

Otic (cont)

Boric acid	010043353	1	08/21/85
Calcium carbonate, precipitated	000471341	2	08/21/85
Cetearyl alcohol		1	09/29/87
Cetyl alcohol	000124298	5	11/06/85
Chlorobutanol	000057158	1	02/16/60
Chloroxylenol	000088040	4	03/03/80
Citric acid	000077929	5	03/04/85
Creatinine	000060275	1	09/23/59
Cupric sulfate, anhydrous	007758987	1	11/15/75
Edetate disodium	006381926	3	12/01/81
Edetic acid	000060004	1	12/14/66
Glycerin	000056815	5	09/29/82
Glyceryl monostearate		2	09/29/87
Hydrochloric acid	007647010	6	11/18/82
Hydroxyethyl cellulose	009004620	1	06/29/76
Isopropyl myristate	000110270	1	12/14/66
Lanolin, anhydrous	008006540	1	12/29/60
Methylparaben	000099763	1	12/14/66
Mineral oil	008012951	3	09/29/87
Mineral oil, light		1	12/29/60
Petrolatum	008009038	3	10/23/73
Phenylethyl alcohol	000060128	1	09/23/59
Polyoxyl 40 stearate	009004993	3	09/29/87
Polysorbate 80	009005656	7	11/06/85
Potassium metabisulfite	004429429	3	09/29/82
Potassium phosphate, monobasic	007778770	1	06/29/76
Propylene glycol	000057556	20	09/29/87
Propylene glycol diacetate	000623847	6	03/04/85

Topical

Propylparaben	000094133	1	12/14/66
Sodium acetate	006131904	13	09/10/85
Sodium disulfite	007631905	3	12/01/81
Sodium borate	001303964	1	09/23/59
Sodium chloride	007647145	1	06/29/76
Sodium citrate	006132045	1	09/23/59
Sodium hydroxide	001310732	3	08/21/85
Sodium phosphate, dibasic	007782856	1	06/29/76
Sodium sulfite	007757837	1	12/01/81
Thimerosal	000054648	5	09/29/87

Percutaneous

Aerotex resin 3730		1	12/10/85
Alcohol		1	09/10/86
Aluminum polyester		1	12/31/79
Crospovidone	009003398	5	08/25/82
Cyclomethicone		2	10/19/81
Di-2-ethylhexyl adipate	000103231	1	06/15/87
Dimethicone copolyol	064345237	2	10/19/81
Dioctylphthalate		2	04/10/86
Dow corning elastomer		3	01/08/86
Ethylene vinyl acetate copolymer		3	09/10/86
Glycerin	000056815	5	08/25/82
Hydroabietyl alcohol	001333897	2	05/06/86
Hydrocarbon gel, plasticized	008049658	1	05/06/86
Hydroxypropyl cellulose	009004642	1	09/10/86
Isopropyl palmitate	000142916	6	06/15/87
Lactose	000063423	8	05/06/86
Lactose, hydrous		1	01/08/86
Medical fluid 360		2	10/19/81
Miglyol		2	05/06/86
Mineral oil	008012951	5	09/10/86
Mineral oil, light		2	09/10/86
Polyalcadiene (C4-C5)		1	05/06/86
Polyester		2	10/19/81
Polyethylene glycol 400	009004960	3	01/08/86
Polyisobutylene	009003274	5	09/10/86
Polypropylene	009003070	2	10/10/84
Polyvinyl alcohol	009002895	5	08/25/82
Polyvinyl chloride-polyvinyl acetate copolymer		3	06/15/87
RA-2397		1	12/10/85
RA-3011		1	12/10/85
Silicon dioxide	007631869	11	06/15/87
Silicone		3	10/19/81
Silicone/polyester film strip		1	12/31/79
Sodium citrate	006132043	5	08/25/82
Union 76 amsco-res 6038		1	12/10/85
2,6-Di-T-butyl P-cresol		1	05/06/86

Perfusion/biliary

Glycerin	000056815	1	10/29/85

Topical (cont)

Sodium borate	001303964	1	09/23/59
Sodium chloride	007647145	1	06/29/76
Sodium citrate	006132045	1	09/23/59
Sodium hydroxide	001310732	3	08/21/85
Sodium phosphate, dibasic	007782856	1	06/29/76
Sodium sulfite	007757837	1	12/01/81
Thimerosal	000054648	5	09/29/87

Percutaneous

Aerotex resin 3730		1	12/10/85
Alcohol		1	09/10/86
Aluminum polyester		1	12/31/79
Crospovidone	009003398	5	08/25/82
Cyclomethicone		2	10/19/81
Di-2-ethylhexyl adipate	000103231	1	06/15/87
Dimethicone copolyol	064345237	2	10/19/81
Dioctylphthalate		2	04/10/86
Dow corning elastomer		3	01/08/86
Ethylene vinyl acetate copolymer		3	09/10/86
Glycerin	000056815	5	08/25/82
Hydroabietyl alcohol	001333897	2	05/06/86
Hydrocarbon gel, plasticized	008049658	1	05/06/86
Hydroxypropyl cellulose	009004642	1	09/10/86
Isopropyl palmitate	000142916	6	06/15/87
Lactose	000063423	8	05/06/86
Lactose, hydrous		1	01/08/86
Medical fluid 360		2	10/19/81
Miglyol		2	05/06/86
Mineral oil	008012951	5	09/10/86
Mineral oil, light		2	09/10/86
Polyalcadiene (c4-c5)		1	05/06/86
Polyester		2	10/19/81
Polyethylene glycol 400	009004960	3	01/08/86
Polyisobutylene	009003274	5	09/10/86
Polypropylene	009003070	2	10/10/84
Polyvinyl alcohol	009002895	5	08/25/82
Polyvinyl chloride-polyvinyl acetate copolymer		3	06/15/87
RA-2397		1	12/10/85
RA-3011		1	12/10/85

Percutaneous (cont)

Silicon dioxide	007631869	11	06/15/87
Silicone		3	10/19/81
Silicone/polyester film strip		1	12/31/79
Sodium citrate	006132043	5	08/25/82
Union 76 amsco-res 6038		1	12/10/85
2,6-Di-t-butyl p-cresol		1	05/06/86

Perfusion/biliary

Glycerin	000056815	1	10/29/85

Perfusion/cardiac

Hydrochloric acid	007647010	1	02/26/82
Sodium hydroxide	001310732	1	02/26/82

Periarticular

Diatrizoic acid	000117964	1	08/21/69
Edetate calcium disodium	023411349	1	08/21/69
Meglumine	006284408	1	08/21/69

Peridural

Citric acid	000077929	1	08/30/76
Dextrose	005996101	1	01/23/74
Hydrochloric acid	007647010	2	08/30/76
Methylparaben	000099763	3	08/30/76
Sodium chloride	007647145	4	03/14/77
Sodium hydroxide	001310732	3	03/14/77
Sodium metabisulfite	007757746	1	08/30/76

Rectal

Alcohol		3	11/17/86
Aluminum diacetate	000142030	1	03/06/64
Anise oil	008007703	1	09/23/82
Ascorbic acid	000050817	1	10/05/81
Ascorbyl palmitate	000137666	5	08/14/87
Benzocaine	000094097	1	07/15/74
Benzoic acid	000065850	1	09/11/84
Bismuth subgallate	012263400	1	03/06/64
Butylated hydroxyanisole	008003245	4	08/26/87
Butylated hydroxytoluene	000128370	4	08/26/87
Butylparaben	000094268	1	12/19/77
Calcium stearate	001592230	1	02/19/48
Caramel	008028895	1	06/13/60
Carbomer 934	009007163	1	12/24/87
Carboxypolymethylene	009007209	1	01/12/66

Rectal (cont)

Cerasynt-SE	001319955	1	05/26/76
Cetyl alcohol	000124298	2	02/10/82
Cocoa butter		6	10/04/83
Cocoa butter (Pond's type 520A)		1	09/02/77
Coconut oil, hydrogenated		2	04/30/73
Cryofluorane	000076142	1	02/10/82
Dichlorodifluoromethane	000075718	1	02/10/82
Dimethyldioctadecylammonium bentonite		1	05/13/59
Dye blue		1	10/05/81
Dye DC yellow #10	008004920	1	11/07/68
Dye FDC green #3	002353459	1	11/07/68
Edetate disodium	006381926	4	12/24/87
Edetic acid	000060004	1	08/13/84
Ethylenediamine	000107153	1	04/02/82
Fat, edible		1	09/27/78
Fatty acids, saturated		1	04/30/73
Flavor		1	12/26/73
Flavor banana	000123922	1	09/11/84
Flavor cherry		1	09/11/84
Flavor cherry, wild		2	11/17/86
Flavor lemon vanilla		1	09/02/81
Fluorochlorohydrocarbons		1	07/26/78
Glycerin	000056815	3	08/13/84
Glyceryl monostearate		6	05/12/87
Glyceryl palmitate	001330730	2	04/30/73
Glyceryl stearate/PEG-40 stearate		1	08/26/87
Glycine	000056406	1	09/02/81
Lactose	000063423	1	11/30/48
Lecithin	008002435	2	05/12/87
Magnesium aluminum silicate	001327431	3	11/17/86
Methylparaben	000099763	7	11/17/86
Mineral oil, light		1	05/13/59
Palm kernel oil	008023798	1	02/09/59
Peruvian balsam	008007009	1	03/06/64
Polyethylene glycol 1000		3	10/05/81
Polyethylene glycol 1540		1	11/07/68
Polyethylene glycol 3350		2	08/13/84

Rectal (cont)

Polyethylene glycol 400	009004960	1	11/07/68
Polyethylene glycol 4000		2	10/05/81
Polyethylene glycol 6000		1	11/07/68
Polyethylene glycol 8000		1	08/13/84
Polysorbate		1	08/14/87
Polysorbate 60	009005678	1	11/07/68
Polysorbate 80	009005656	11	08/26/87
Potassium acetate	000127082	1	12/24/87
Potassium metabisulfite	004429429	1	12/24/87
Propylene glycol	000057556	5	11/17/86
Propylene glycol monostearate	001323393	1	07/15/74
Propylparaben	000094133	6	11/17/86
Saccharin	000081072	1	11/30/48
Saccharin sodium	006155573	5	11/17/86
Saccharin sodium anhydrous	000128449	1	12/19/77
Silicon dioxide	007631869	2	09/02/77
Simethicone	008050815	1	12/26/73
Sodium benzoate	000532321	1	12/24/87
Sodium carbonate	000497198	1	05/13/59
Sodium chloride	007647145	3	08/13/84
Sodium citrate	006132043	2	09/02/81
Sodium hydroxide	001310732	1	09/23/82
Sorbitol	000050704	2	09/11/84
Sorbitol solution	003959533	3	11/17/86
Starch	009005258	1	11/30/48
Steareth-10		2	02/10/82
Sucrose	000057501	1	12/19/77
Talc	014807966	1	11/30/48
Tannic acid	001401554	1	08/13/62
Tartaric acid, DL-	000133379	2	10/04/83
Trolamine	000102716	1	02/10/82
Vegetable oils, hydrogenated		8	08/26/87
Wax, emulsifying	008014388	1	02/10/82
Wax, white	008006404	4	07/09/81
Witepsol W-35		2	08/14/87
Xanthan gum		1	12/24/87
Zinc oxide	001314132	1	03/06/64

Retrobulbar

Sodium hydroxide	001310732	1	05/07/59

Retrobulbar (cont)

Route not given
Sodium citrate	006132043	1	10/31/86

Soft tissue
Acetic acid, glacial	000064197	1	03/14/79
Benzyl alcohol	000100516	7	01/25/84
Carboxymethylcellulose sodium	009004324	4	05/24/82
Citric acid	000077929	4	01/25/84
Creatinine	000060275	2	06/19/80
Edetate disodium	006381926	4	05/24/82
Hydrochloric acid	007647010	6	06/19/80
Isotonic sodium chloride solution	008028771	1	12/06/79
Methylcellulose	009004675	1	12/06/79
Methylparaben	000099763	3	06/19/80
Phenol	000108952	2	01/30/79
Phosphoric acid	007664382	2	05/29/81
Polyethylene glycol 3350		2	09/09/75
Polyethylene glycol 4000		4	03/26/79
Polysorbate 80	009005656	5	05/24/82
Propylparaben	000094133	3	06/19/80
Sodium acetate	006131904	1	03/14/79
Sodium bisulfite	007631905	5	05/24/82
Sodium chloride	007647145	9	05/24/82
Sodium citrate	006132043	4	01/25/84
Sodium citrate anhydrous	000068042	1	07/15/75
Sodium hydroxide	001310732	13	01/25/84
Sodium metabisulfite	007757746	1	05/29/81
Sodium phosphate	007632055	3	02/27/79
Sodium phosphate, dibasic	007782856	1	12/31/74
Sodium sulfite	007757837	2	01/25/84
1-tetradecyl-4-picolinium chloride	002748881	4	03/26/79

Subarachnoid
Sodium hydroxide	001310732	1	05/04/84

Subcutaneous
Acetic acid		1	04/09/85
Acetic acid, glacial	000064197	1	08/01/77
Ammonium hydroxide		1	07/26/74
Ascorbic acid	000050817	1	06/08/51
Benzyl alcohol	000100516	4	02/18/86

Subcutaneous (cont)

Calcium chloride	010035048	1	03/22/50
Carboxymethylcellulose sodium	009004324	1	01/04/60
Chlorobutanol	000057158	1	08/01/77
Cresol	008026946	3	01/16/80
Cresol, M-	000108394	10	07/11/86
Diatrizoic acid	000117964	1	09/23/82
Edetate calcium disodium	023411349	2	11/30/84
Edetate disodium	006381926	2	02/18/86
Glycerin	000056815	20	07/11/86
Hydrochloric acid	007647010	21	08/24/87
Isotonic sodium chloride solution	008028771	3	03/17/80
Lactose	000063423	2	09/30/82
Methanesulfonic acid	000075752	1	11/30/84
Methylparaben	000099763	10	09/30/85
Phenol	000108952	12	07/11/86
Phenol, liquified		3	05/30/86
Polysorbate 80	009005656	1	01/04/60
Potassium phosphate, dibasic	007758114	1	07/29/81
Propylene glycol	000057556	1	11/30/84
Propylparaben	000094133	2	05/06/82
Protamine sulfate	009009658	7	10/28/82
Sodium acetate	006131904	6	08/30/83
Sodium acetate, anhydrous	000127093	3	09/30/85
Sodium bisulfite	007631905	1	08/01/77
Sodium chloride	007647145	13	09/30/85
Sodium hydroxide	001310732	22	08/24/87
Sodium phosphate	007632055	12	05/30/86
Sodium phosphate, dihydrate		2	07/11/86
Sodium phosphate, dibasic	007782856	1	04/28/86
Sodium phosphate, monobasic	007558807	1	07/29/81
Sodium thioglycolate	000367511	1	06/08/51
Thimerosal	000054648	1	03/06/51
Zinc acetate	000557346	4	08/30/83
Zinc chloride	007646857	5	08/30/83
Zinc oxide	001314132	6	09/30/85

Sublingual

Butylated hydroxyanisole	008003245	3	04/16/81
Calcium stearate	001592230	5	08/02/79
Carboxymethyl starch sodium salt	009063381	14	02/10/83

Sublingual (cont)

Castor oil	008001794	1	04/16/81
Castor oil, hydrogenated	008001783	1	04/16/81
Cellulose		1	02/13/80
Cellulose, microcrystalline	009004346	27	09/23/86
Corn oil	008001307	1	12/28/76
Cottonseed oil, hydrogenated		2	12/28/77
Croscarmellose sodium		5	09/18/86
Crospovidone	009003398	6	12/08/81
Dextrose	005996101	3	07/29/82
Dye DC yellow #10	008004920	3	03/09/83
Dye DC yellow #10 lake		4	09/18/86
Dye FDC blue #1	002650182	1	02/24/83
Dye FDC blue #1 aluminum lake		1	05/08/84
Dye FDC red #3 lake		1	09/18/86
Dye FDC red #3-aluminum lake	012227780	6	12/08/81
Dye FDC yellow #10 lake		1	11/20/81
Dye FDC yellow #5-aluminum lake	012227699	4	12/08/81
Dye FDC yellow #6	002783940	3	03/09/83
Dye FDC yellow #6-aluminum lake	012227600	3	09/18/86
Flavor orange	008050326	1	07/29/82
Flavor peppermint		2	06/08/84
Gelatin	009000708	2	01/15/81
Hydroxypropyl cellulose	009004642	1	06/08/84
Isopropyl alcohol	000067630	2	12/11/79
Lactose	000063423	37	09/23/86
Magnesium stearate	000557040	36	09/23/86
Mannitol	000069658	12	06/08/84
Peppermint oil	008006904	1	02/24/83
Plusweet		1	07/29/82
Polyethylene glycol 4000		2	04/16/81
Polysorbate 80	009005656	2	04/16/81
Povidone	009003398	4	02/10/83
Saccharin	000081072	2	06/08/84
Saccharin sodium	006155573	2	06/08/84
Silica gel	007699414	1	07/29/82
Silicon dioxide	007631869	16	09/18/86
Sodium bisulfite	007631905	2	08/11/81
Sodium lauryl sulfate	000151213	4	08/02/79

Sublingual (cont)

Sorbic acid	000110441	2	04/16/81
Sorbitol	000050704	2	01/08/81
Starch	009005258	24	03/09/83
Starch, corn		3	06/08/84
Starch, pregelatinized		1	12/03/81
Stearic acid	000057114	13	02/10/83
Sucrose	000057501	2	07/07/80
Talc	014807966	5	04/16/81
Tartaric acid, dl-	000133379	3	07/29/82

Topical

Alcohol		18	10/23/87
Alcohol, dehydrated	000064175	11	10/21/87
Alcohol, denatured	008024451	14	07/23/87
Alcohol, diluted	008000166	2	08/12/77
Alkyl ammonium sulfonic acid betaine (sulfobetaine DEH)		1	07/08/76
Alkyl aryl sodium sulfonate		1	05/17/51
Allantoin	000097596	2	01/07/87
Almond oil sweet	008007690	1	07/27/61
Aluminum acetate	000139128	2	06/07/82
Aluminum chlorhydroxy allantoinate	017175870	1	02/24/56
Aluminum hydroxide	001302290	1	05/15/85
Aluminum hydroxide gel	012040594	3	09/20/85
Aluminum hydroxide gel F 500		4	07/30/86
Aluminum hydroxide gel F 5000		4	07/30/86
Aluminum silicate	014504951	1	05/14/75
Aluminum starch octenylsuc- cinate		1	05/06/87
Aluminum stearate	007047849	1	09/30/83
Aluminum sulfate	010043013	9	05/20/87
Amerchol C	008035301	1	12/18/74
Amerchol L101		1	11/09/84
Amerchol-CAB	008029047	1	09/22/71
Ammonium hydroxide		1	04/24/85
Ammonium nonoxynol 4 sulfate		2	01/07/87
Ammonium salt of C-12-C-15 linear primary alcohol ethoxylate		1	07/08/76

Topical (cont)

Ammonyx		3	12/24/84
Amphoteric-2		2	09/01/83
Amphoteric-9		1	03/17/78
Antifoam	008051089	2	07/16/74
Aquaphor	008029150	3	09/06/85
Arlacel	008029229	2	02/13/75
Asafetida	009000048	1	01/30/74
Avocado oil	008007725	1	07/27/61
Balsam oregon		1	03/31/86
Beeswax		4	12/14/84
Bentonite	001302789	6	09/01/83
Bentonite magma		1	08/25/44
Benzalkonium chloride	008001543	4	04/11/74
Benzoic acid	000065850	6	03/28/85
Benzyl alcohol	000100516	35	12/16/86
Boric acid	010043353	1	12/18/74
Butane	000106978	2	09/02/82
Butyl stearate	000123955	10	05/29/87
Butylated hydroxyanisole	008003245	8	08/30/85
Butylated hydroxytoluene	000128370	13	12/01/78
Butylparaben	000094268	16	07/05/84
Calcium acetate	000062544	9	05/29/87
Calcium hydroxide	001305620	1	04/26/78
Calcium stearate	001592230	1	04/16/69
Candelilla wax		1	08/02/66
Caprylic/capric triglyceride		3	01/24/85
Caramel	008028895	2	09/20/85
Carbitol		1	06/04/48
Carbomer 934	009007163	17	02/03/87
Carbomer 940	009007174	17	08/10/87
Carbomer 941		1	12/16/81
Carboxy vinyl copolymer		1	10/26/84
Carboxymethylcellulose sodium	009004324	6	07/24/86
Carboxypolymethylene	009007209	2	11/12/74
Carnauba wax	008015869	1	01/15/52
Carrageenan	009000071	2	12/17/81
Carrageenan salt		1	12/19/74
Castor oil	008001794	4	05/23/80
Castor oil, hydrogenated	008001783	1	01/20/78
Cellulose, microcrystalline	009004346	1	03/27/58

Topical (cont)

Dextrin	009004539	9	08/02/84
Dichlorodifluoromethane	000075718	4	03/04/61
Diethyl sebacate	000110407	2	08/06/71
Diisopropanolamine	000110974	1	04/02/73
Diisopropyladipate		3	04/06/84
Dimethicone	009006659	1	08/26/59
Dimethicone 350	009006659	2	01/24/80
DMDM hydantoin		2	21/26/85
Docusate sodium	000577117	3	10/26/84
Dye black		1	07/12/60
Dye DC green #5	004403901	7	03/27/79
Dye DC green #6	000128803	1	07/27/61
Dye DC red #19	000081889	4	11/30/84
Dye DC red #36		2	02/07/66
Dye DC red #39	006371557	1	07/16/74
Dye DC yellow #10	008004920	4	09/01/83
Dye FDC blue #1	002650182	6	03/10/86
Dye FDC blue #1 aluminum lake		1	09/25/72
Dye FDC green #3	002353459	3	03/27/79
Dye FDC red #40		2	08/27/81
Dye FDC yellow #6	002783940	3	03/27/87
Dye green		1	07/12/60
Dye red		1	03/10/76
Dye yellow ochre	001345262	1	07/12/60
Edetate disodium	006381926	17	06/06/84
Edetate sodium	000064028	6	10/03/83
Edetate trisodium	000150389	1	07/27/61
Edetic acid	000060004	2	02/03/78
Entsufon		2	08/01/77
Entsufon sodium	002917944	2	05/28/81
Ethomeen C-25	008051523	1	07/08/76
Ethyl acetate	000141786	1	07/15/53
Ethylcellulose	009004573	1	04/09/52
Ethylene glycol	000107211	1	05/17/51
Ethylene oxide	000075218	2	09/24/68
Ethylenediamine	000107153	3	10/08/85
Ethylenediamine dihydro-chloride	000333186	1	07/30/86
Ethylhexanediol	001321342	1	07/22/86

Topical (cont)

Cerasynt-SE	001319955	2	12,
Ceteareth-15		4	08,
Ceteareth-20		8	05,
Ceteareth-30		3	04,
Cetearyl alcohol		21	06,
Ceteth-2		1	03,
Ceteth-20		13	06,
Cetrimonium chloride		1	03,
Cetyl alcohol	000124298	110	10,
Cetyl esters wax	001190632	8	02,
Cetyl palmitate	000540103	1	03,
Chlorobutanol	000057158	1	06,
Chlorocresol	000059507	21	08,
Chloroxylenol	000088040	1	06,
Cholesterol	000057885	5	01/
Choleth-24		1	02/
Cis-n-(3-chloroallyl) hexaminium-chloride		3	11/
Citric acid	000077929	71	07/
Citric acid monohydrate	005949291	4	12/
Citric acid, anhydrous		1	06/
Citric acid, hydrous	015686654	1	06/
Cocamide diethanolamine		7	07/
Cocamide mercaptoethyl amine		1	03/
Cocoa butter (Pond's type 520A)		1	08/
Cocomonoethaholamide	000142789	1	02/
Coconut fatty acid	008037147	2	03/
Coconut mono-ethanolamide		1	07/
Coconut oil	008001318	2	01/
Coconut oil soap, aqueous		1	01/
Cocoyl sodium isethionate		1	03/
Copper phthalocyanine blue	000147148	1	04/
Corn oil	008001307	2	07/
Cream base		2	05/
Creatinine	000060275	1	08/
Crospovidone	009003398	4	08/1
Cryofluorane	000076142	1	04/2
Cyclomethicone		1	04/2
Dehydroacetic acid	000520456	3	11/2
Dehymuls E		1	09/3

Topical (cont)

Ethylparaben	000120478	2	08/12/69
Fatty acid pentaerythriol ester		1	09/30/83
Fatty acids	009013187	1	01/26/78
Fatty alcohol citrate		1	09/30/83
Ferric oxide		1	07/03/85
Ferric oxide, red	001309371	1	07/12/60
Flavor fruit		1	01/18/77
Flavor rhodia pharmaceutical #RF 451		1	03/11/64
Flavor spearmint		2	08/17/81
Flavor vanilla		1	03/06/73
Formaldehyde	000050000	1	02/03/78
Fragrance (RBD-9819)		9	12/03/82
Fragrance bouquet rel essence 9200		1	12/17/79
Fragrance CS-28197		1	10/08/85
Fragrance felton 066M		1	07/22/86
Fragrance florien plus		1	03/10/86
Fragrance H-6540		1	04/24/85
Fragrance meridian		1	03/10/86
Fragrance P O FL-147		4	12/24/84
Fragrance PA 52805		2	07/23/87
Fragrance pera derm D		1	07/03/85
Fragrance soap		2	09/22/49
Fragrance spicy metholated eugenol		1	12/16/81
Fragrance ungerer honeysuckle K 2771		1	04/08/83
Fragrance ungerer N5195		1	11/25/85
Fragrance unspecified		3	06/03/80
Gelatin	009000708	1	03/06/73
Gluconolactone, D-	000090802	4	12/24/84
Glycerides of tallow		4	11/30/84
Glycerin	000056815	68	05/29/87
Glyceryl monostearate		62	05/29/87
Glyceryl oleate/propylene glycol		1	04/27/87
Glyceryl palmitate	001330730	2	09/01/83
Glyceryl ricinoleate	001323382	4	11/04/81
Glyceryl stearate SE		1	03/10/86

Topical (cont)

Glyceryl stearate/PEG-100 stearate		3	12/27/85
Glycol stearate	000111604	5	09/01/83
Herbacol	006365839	2	08/27/81
Hexachlorophene	000070304	1	07/12/60
Hexylene glycol	000107415	3	05/06/87
Hydrocarbon gel, plasticized	008049658	7	10/29/82
Hydrocarbon 40	008041632	1	02/03/78
Hydrochloric acid	007647010	18	10/08/85
Hydrochloric acid, diluted		1	03/06/80
Hydrogen peroxide	007722841	2	01/07/87
Hydroxyethyl cellulose	009004620	3	07/22/86
Hydrooxypropyl cellulose	009004642	7	10/21/87
Hydrooxypropyl methyl-cellulose	009004653	3	03/27/79
Imidazolidinyl urea		1	03/31/86
Irish moss extract		2	08/16/84
Iron oxide		1	04/09/52
Isobutane	000075285	6	09/22/86
Isooctylacrylate		1	07/29/69
Isopropyl alcohol	000067630	36	12/17/87
Isopropyl myristate	000110270	45	10/22/87
Isopropyl palmitate	000142916	46	12/16/86
Isopropyl stearate		1	12/13/74
Jelene	008049669	1	04/01/64
Kathon CG		1	03/10/86
Lactate	000050215	2	11/26/85
Lactic acid	008012213	27	12/16/86
Lactic acid, DL-	000598823	1	08/25/44
Lactose	000063423	9	03/01/85
Laneth	008051965	1	03/10/76
Lanolin	008020846	23	05/29/87
Lanolin alcohols	008013341	5	03/28/80
Lanolin alcohols, acetylated	008028986	1	07/08/76
Lanolin cholesterols		1	05/28/81
Lanolin, anhydrous	008006540	6	12/19/74
Lanolin, hydrogenated	008031445	4	12/23/87
Lanosterol	000079630	1	07/27/61
Lauramine oxide		1	06/22/86
Laureth sulfate		1	10/10/78

Topical (cont)

Laureth 23		3	11/30/84
Laureth 4	009002920	5	04/24/85
Lauric diethanolamide	000120401	7	09/01/83
Lauric myristic diethanolamide		2	05/28/81
Lauric myristic monoethanol-amide		1	04/30/71
Lavender		2	07/30/86
Lecithin	008002435	1	02/03/78
Lemon oil	008008568	1	10/26/84
Limonene	000138863	1	08/02/82
Linear alcohol ethylene oxide adduct		1	11/25/85
Linear tridecyl benzene sulfonate		1	09/25/72
Magnesium aluminum silicate	001327431	8	04/24/85
Medical antifoam emulsion C		1	09/20/85
Menthol	000089781	3	04/29/82
Methyl salicylate	000119368	1	10/26/84
Methyl stearate	000112618	1	10/16/78
Methylcellulose	009004675	8	04/24/85
Methylparaben	000099763	119	01/07/87
Methylphenylpolysiloxane		1	05/20/66
Microcrystalline wax	008063089	2	08/02/66
Mineral oil	008012951	128	08/10/87
Mineral oil, light		35	12/23/87
Monostearic hydrazide		1	09/25/72
Multisterol extract		6	09/11/85
Myristyl alcohol	000112721	1	12/30/82
Myristyl lactate		1	11/25/85
Myristyl stearate	008016771	1	11/27/74
N-decyl-methyl sulfoxide		1	08/12/77
N,N-dimethyl lauramine oxide		4	07/24/86
Nitric acid	007697372	1	08/30/85
Nonoxynol	026027383	1	05/09/58
Nonoxynol iodine		1	01/15/64
Octoxynol	009010439	1	11/02/78
Octoxynol-1	009036195	1	12/01/80
Octoxynol-9	009002931	3	01/07/87
Octyldodecanol	005333426	3	02/17/84
Oleic acid	000112801	3	02/03/78
Oleth 20	009004982	1	01/20/78

Topical (cont)

Oleyl alcohol	000143282	1	06/21/60
Oleyl oleate		1	01/10/85
Olive oil	008001250	1	02/03/78
Orvus K liquid		2	11/30/84
Paraffin	008002742	9	12/16/86
Pectin	009000695	1	03/06/73
Peglicol-5-oleate		2	12/23/82
Pegoxol 7 stearate		2	12/23/82
Pentosanpolysulphate sodium	001300727	1	02/03/78
Pentylamine	000110587	1	05/17/66
Perfume B-8412		1	03/07/49
Perfume compound bouquet 10328		2	12/17/81
Perfume E-1991		1	05/15/85
Perfume GD 6504		2	10/08/85
Perfume oil, gardenia		1	01/10/85
Perfume 3949-5		1	11/04/81
Perfume 520A		1	09/01/83
Perfume 91-122		2	05/14/75
Perfumes		9	12/01/80
Petrolatum	008009038	153	05/29/87
Petrolatum, white		40	12/23/87
Phenylethyl alcohol	000060128	1	10/16/78
Phosphoric acid	007664382	24	08/10/87
Pine needle oil		1	08/02/82
Plastibase-50W		3	06/28/85
Poloxamer		3	08/30/85
Polyethylene	009002884	11	10/09/85
Polyethylene glycol	025322683	2	01/07/87
Polyethylene glycol 1000		4	05/14/85
Polyethylene glycol 1500		2	05/17/51
Polyethylene glycol 1540		5	07/22/81
Polyethylene glycol 200		2	06/03/77
Polyethylene glycol 300	025322683	7	07/22/81
Polyethylene glycol 3350		5	12/31/87
Polyethylene glycol 400	009004960	20	12/31/87
Polyethylene glycol 4000		12	05/11/81
Polyethylene glycol 6000		1	06/26/84
Polyethylene glycol 8000		2	10/17/75
Polyethylene glycol 900		1	10/04/45

Topical (cont)

Polyethylene glycols		7	04/19/82
Polyox	008050622	2	10/19/76
Polyoxyethylene alcohols		7	10/08/85
Polyoxyethylene propylene		1	07/16/74
Polyoxyethylene sorbitan monoisostearate		1	04/08/83
Polyoxyethylene 25 propylene glycol stearate			
Polyoxyl distearate			
Polyxoyl stearate	009009409	2	10/22/81
Polyoxyl 150 distearate	009005087	2	11/22/78
Polyoxyl 2 stearate		5	04/24/85
Polyoxyl 4 dilaurate		1	06/22/86
Polyoxyl 40 stearate		1	12/19/79
Polyoxyl 50 stearate		1	12/03/82
Polyoxyl 75 lanolin	009004993	49	12/16/86
Polyoxyl 8 stearate		1	06/06/85
Polyoxypropylene 15 stearyl ether		2	07/22/86
Polyoxypropylene 26 oleate	009004993	6	10/08/85
Polypropylene		1	03/01/78
Polypropylene glycol		1	01/12/73
Polysorbate	009003070	1	02/22/77
Polysorbate 20	009003150	1	03/24/61
Polysorbate 40		2	06/23/81
Polysorbate 60	009005645	20	05/29/87
Polysorbate 80	009005667	10	07/05/84
Polyvinyl alcohol	009005678	66	10/22/87
Potassium carbonate	009005656	14	10/22/87
Potassium hydroxide	009002895	1	05/29/87
Potassium sorbate	000584087	1	02/03/78
Povidone	009003398	2	02/25/87
Product HAT		2	11/30/84
Promalgen type g		1	03/28/73
Promulgen D		1	12/16/81
Promulgen G	009009614	4	11/26/85
Propane	000074986	2	09/02/82
Propionic acid	000079094	1	06/04/48
Propyl alcohol, N	000071238	2	06/04/48
Propyl gallate	000121799	4	05/30/80
Propylene carbonate	000108327	1	09/22/71

Topical (cont)

Propylene glycol	000057556	197	10/23/87
Propylene glycol monolaurate	001322878	1	08/02/66
Propylene glycol monostearate	001323393	23	05/06/87
Propylene oxide	000075569	1	07/24/78
Propylparaben	000094133	92	07/30/86
Protein hydrolysate	009015547	1	03/31/86
Pyrithione zinc	003590236	1	07/24/67
Pyrithyldione	000077043	1	07/24/67
Quaternium-15		4	04/24/85
Saccharin	000081072	5	06/03/77
Sesame oil	008008740	1	07/27/61
Silicon	007440213	4	08/19/78
Silicone		2	01/21/74
Silicone emulsion		2	04/03/85
Simethicone	008050815	20	08/14/86
Sipon L-20	008024304	1	02/13/75
Soap, castile	008029387	1	09/25/72
Soap, potassium		1	04/14/78
Sodium acetate, anhydrous	000127093	1	12/13/74
Sodium alkyl sulfate	008036542	1	01/21/74
Sodium benzoate	000532321	3	05/28/81
Sodium bisulfite	007631905	4	09/25/87
Sodium chloride	007647145	7	03/10/86
Sodium citrate	006132043	7	02/25/87
Sodium dodecylbenzene-sulfonate	012068212	1	05/14/75
Sodium formaldehyde sulfoxylate	000149440	1	05/30/80
Sodium glyceryl alkyl ether sulfonate alkyl		1	09/24/68
Sodium hydroxide	001310732	67	08/10/87
Sodium iodide	007681825	1	05/09/58
Sodium laureth sulfate		1	01/12/73
Sodium lauryl sulfate	000151213	34	06/06/84
Sodium lauryl sulfoacetate	001847581	1	10/19/76
Sodium N-lauroyl sarcosinate	000137166	1	09/24/68
Sodium N-methyl-N-coco-oil acid taurate		1	03/20/72
Sodium phosphate	007632055	7	02/17/84
Sodium phosphate, dibasic	007782856	10	01/07/87

Topical (cont)

Sodium phosphate, dibasic, anhydrous		1	05/03/65
Sodium phosphate, dried		1	03/17/78
Sodium phosphate, monobasic	007558807	19	08/10/87
Sodium phosphate, monobasic, monohydrate	010049215	5	07/10/84
Sodium pyrrolidone carboxylate		2	11/26/85
Sodium stearate	000822162	1	04/30/71
Sodium sulfate	007727733	1	09/25/72
Sodium sulfite	007757837	2	10/22/87
Sodium sulfosuccinated undecylcenic monoalkyloamide		1	12/03/82
Sodium tallowate		1	01/06/71
Sodium xylenesulfonate		1	04/14/78
Solulan	008042511	2	12/24/84
Sorbic acid	000110441	49	07/30/86
Sorbitan monooleate	005938385	16	12/23/85
Sorbitan monopalmitate	001338405	7	08/14/86
Sorbitan monostearate	001338416	59	10/22/87
Sorbitan sesquioleate	008007430	6	12/27/85
Sorbitan solution		1	07/30/86
Sorbitan trioleate	005960065	1	07/27/61
Sorbitol	000050704	11	03/28/85
Sorbitol solution	003959533	31	04/27/87
Soybean flour		1	02/13/75
Soybean oil	008001227	2	02/03/78
Spermaceti	008002231	15	11/30/77
Squalane	000111013	2	08/16/74
Squalene	000111024	1	06/21/60
Starch	009005258	4	04/06/79
Stearalkonium chloride	000122190	2	03/31/86
Stearalkonium hectorate		1	09/02/82
Steareth	009005009	4	02/03/78
Steareth-10		1	08/08/83
Steareth-2		1	03/10/86
Steareth-21		1	03/10/86
Stearic acid	000057114	54	12/14/84
Steartrimonium hydrolized animal protein		1	03/10/86
Stearyl alcohol	000112925	75	10/22/87

Topical (cont)

Sucrose	000057501	1	04/01/64
Sucrose polyesters		1	08/12/77
T-butyl hydroperoxide	000075912	1	01/26/78
Talc	014807966	9	07/03/85
Tall oil	008002264	1	12/01/80
Tartrazine	001934210	3	05/14/75
Tenox		6	10/05/84
Terpineol, alpha	000098555	1	08/02/82
Thimerosal	000054648	3	02/01/79
Titanium dioxide	001309633	24	05/06/87
Tocopheryl acetate, D-alpha	000058957	1	06/21/60
Trichloromonofluoromethane		4	05/04/61
Trideceth 10		2	12/24/84
Triglycerides, unspecified length		1	01/20/78
Trihydroxy stearin	010248745	1	05/30/80
Trilaneth-4 phosphate		1	01/10/85
Trilaureth 4 phosphate		1	01/10/85
Trisodium hedta	000139899	1	03/10/76
Triton x-200 sodium salt of alkylauryl polyether sulfonate		2	10/19/76
Trolamine	000102716	21	08/16/84
Trolamine alkyl sulfate		2	02/15/73
Trolamine lauryl sulfate		7	09/18/84
Tromethamine	000077861	1	07/29/70
Vanillin	000121335	1	01/15/52
Vegetable oil	008008897	1	04/14/78
Viscarin	008047254	1	12/17/79
Vitamin E	000059029	1	07/27/61
Wax, dehydro SX	008023403	7	05/29/87
Wax, emulsifying	008014388	22	12/14/84
Wax, white	008006404	17	05/06/87
Wax, yellow	008012893	2	08/02/66
Xanthan gum		3	07/19/74
Zinc acetate	000557346	2	07/03/85
1-(3-chloroallyl)-3,5,7-triaza-1-azoniaadamantane chloride	004080313	2	11/30/77
1-0-tolylbiguanide	000093696	1	03/10/76
1,2,6-hexanetriol	000106694	2	06/26/84
2-amino-2-methyl-1-propanol	000124685	5	08/16/84

Topical (cont)

6-methoxy-2-(4-styryl-3-sulfo-phenol)-2-H-benzotriazole	001333659	1	09/25/72
Transmucosal			
Cryofluorane	000076142	1	10/31/85
Dichlorodifluoromethane	000075718	1	10/31/85
Ether	000060297	1	10/31/85
Menthol	000089781	1	10/31/85
Neutral oil		1	10/31/85
Peppermint oil	008006904	1	10/31/85
Ureteral			
Benzyl alcohol	000100516	1	04/07/59
Diatrizoic acid	000117964	2	09/23/82
Edetate calcium disodium	023411349	3	09/23/82
Edetate disodium	006381926	1	02/19/57
Hydrochloric acid	007647010	1	04/07/59
Meglumine	006284408	2	09/23/82
Methylparaben	000099763	1	02/19/57
Propylparaben	000094133	1	02/19/57
Sodium citrate	006132043	1	02/19/57
Sodium hydroxide	001310732	1	04/07/59
Urethral			
Diatrizoic acid	000117964	1	04/01/77
Edetate calcium disodium	023411349	2	04/01/77
Edetate disodium	006381926	1	08/02/55
Hydrochloric acid	007647010	1	04/01/77
Meglumine	006284408	1	04/01/77
Sodium phosphate, monobasic	007558807	1	08/25/76
Sodium phosphate, monobasic, monohydrate	010049215	1	04/12/72
Vaginal			
Acetic acid, glacial	000064197	2	12/30/65
Allantoin	000097596	1	01/27/87
Alum, potassium	007784249	1	01/18/77
Asafetida	009000048	1	01/30/74
Benionite	001302789	1	01/18/77
Benzoic acid	000065850	5	04/01/83
Benzyl alcohol	000100516	2	02/16/79
Butylated hydroxyanisole	008003245	4	12/31/87

Vaginal (cont)

Butylated hydroxytoluene	000128370	2	06/09/86
Calcium lactate	000814802	1	04/19/85
Carboxymethylcellulose sodium	009004324	2	12/30/65
Cellulose, microcrystalline	009004346	3	10/17/85
Cetearyl alcohol		1	11/08/78
Cetyl alcohol	000124298	14	12/31/87
Cetyl esters wax	001190632	3	02/16/79
Cholesterol	000057885	3	06/09/86
Choleth		3	11/09/87
Cis-N-(3-chloroallyl) hexaminium-chloride		1	06/03/77
Citric acid	000077929	3	04/01/83
Citric acid monohydrate	005949291	1	05/26/47
Crospovidone	009003398	4	04/19/85
Cryofluorane	000076142	2	12/10/63
Dichlorodifluoromethane	000075718	2	12/10/63
Diethylaminoethyl stearamide phosphate	007490882	1	12/10/63
Diethylaminoethyl stearate	003179815	1	12/30/65
Diglycol stearate	000106116	1	01/27/87
Edetate disodium	006381926	1	01/31/84
Ethylcellulose	009004573	6	10/17/85
Fragrance (RBD-9819)		1	12/30/65
Gelatin	009000708	2	11/02/78
Glutamic acid, DL-	000617652	1	05/26/47
Glycerin	000056815	10	01/27/87
Glyceryl monostearate		12	11/09/87
Glyceryl stearate/PEG stearate		1	11/25/85
Guar gum	009000300	1	09/12/45
Hydroxypropyl methylcellulose	009004653	1	04/19/85
Isopropyl myristate	000110270	1	12/31/87
Lactic acid	008012213	6	01/27/87
Lactic acid, DL-	000598823	1	01/27/87
Lactose	000063423	14	01/27/87
Lactose, hydrous		1	01/27/87
Lanolin	008020846	3	06/09/86
Lanolin, anhydrous	008006540	1	09/01/82
Lecithin	008002435	6	11/09/87
Lecithin, soy bean	008030760	1	09/12/45
Magnesium aluminum silicate	001327431	1	12/30/86

Vaginal (cont)

Magnesium stearate	000557040	4	04/19/85
Methyl salicylate	000119368	1	02/11/59
Methyl stearate	000112618	1	10/16/78
Methylcellulose	009004675	1	01/31/84
Methylparaben	000099763	16	11/09/87
Mineral oil	008012951	4	11/25/85
Myristic acid	000544638	1	07/12/63
Nonoxynol	026027383	1	02/11/59
Octyldodecanol	005333426	2	02/16/79
Peanut oil	008002037	8	11/09/87
Perfumes		1	12/10/63
Phenylethyl aclohol	000060128	1	10/16/78
Phosphoric acid	007664328	7	11/09/87
Polyethylene	009002884	1	01/18/77
Polyethylene glycol 1000		1	11/28/78
Polyethylene glycol 3350		1	01/27/87
Polyethylene glycol 400	009004960	2	01/27/87
Polyethylene glycol 4000		2	11/15/82
Polyethylene glycol 6000		1	02/11/80
Polyethylene glycol 8000		1	10/17/85
Polyethylene glycols		1	07/12/63
Polyoxyl palmitate	009004948	1	11/28/78
Polyoxyl stearate		1	12/30/65
Polyoxyl 100 stearate		1	11/25/85
Polysorbate 20	009005645	3	02/02/77
Polysorbate 60	009005678	4	12/31/87
Polysorbate 80	609002895	2	12/30/65
Polyvinyl alcohol	009002895	2	12/30/65
Promulgen D		1	06/03/77
Propylene glycol	000057556	16	12/31/87
Propylene glycol monostearate	001323393	1	10/16/78
Propylparaben	000094133	13	11/09/87
Silicon dioxide	007631869	1	04/19/85
Sodium citrate	006132043	1	04/01/83
Sodium hdyroxide	001310732	1	05/26/47
Sodium iodide	007681825	1	02/11/59
Sodium lauryl sulfate	000151213	4	09/19/85
Sodium metabisulfite	007757746	1	04/01/83
Sodium phosphate, dibasic	007782856	1	02/11/59
Sodium phosphate, monobasic	007558807	1	06/03/77
Sodium phosphate, monobasic,			

Vaginal (cont)

monohydrate	010049215	1	06/03/77
Sorbic acid	000110441	1	04/01/83
Sorbitan monostearate	001338416	3	11/25/85
Starch	009005258	6	04/03/84
Starch, corn		4	10/17/85
Stearamidoethyl diethylamine		3	11/09/87
Stearic acid	000057114	19	11/09/87
Stearyl alcohol	000112925	3	12/31/87
Suppocire	008043150	1	08/23/77
Tartaric acid, DL-	000133379	1	01/18/77
Tartrazine	001934210	1	11/02/78
Trolamine	000102716	4	01/27/87
Vegetable oils, hydrogenated		2	08/15/84
Wax, white	008006404	1	10/16/78
Wecobee FS		1	03/15/82
Witepsol E-85		1	11/25/85
Witepsol S-55		1	11/25/85

Index

A

Acacia, 123,175,294
Accidental poisonings, 147
Acesulfame, 140
Acetate buffers, 171
Acid alcohols, 111
Acidic polymers for tablet coating, 124
Acrylate adhesives, 350
Acrylic monomers, 287
ACTH, 20
Actinic reticuloid, 246
Activation of complement, 348
Acute laryngeal edema, 303
Adhesive tape, 349
Adipic acid, 287,352
Adjuvant, 350
Adverse effects of excipients by class of excipient, 88
  bulk, 89,201
  coloring agents, 159,253
  coatings, 123,223
  flavoring agents, 133,231
  other products, 167,287
Adverse first-use responses, 347
Aflatoxin, 177
Agar, 287
Airway resistance, 329
Albumin, 127,227,228
Albuminuria, 233
Alcohols, (See also specific alcohols), 20,98,106,143,202, 211,212,310
Aldehyde sensitivity, 147
Aldehydes, 143,238

Alginates, 229,287
Allergen, 35,40,43,61
Allergic antibody, 61
Allergic contact dermatitis, 53
Allergic purpura, 268,272
Allergic reactions, 23
  bulk materials, 201
  coatings, 223
  flavoring agents, 231
  coloring agents, 253
  other addition products, 287
Allergy, 18,23,225
Alpha-tocopherol, 312,313
Alternate pathway of complement, 24
Aluminum monostearate, 113
Aluminum oxide, 352
Aluminum silicate, 105
Amaranth, 163,274
Amino acid buffers, 171
Ammonia, 92,101
Amphoteric emulsifiers, 290
Amyl butyrate, 153
Anaphylactic reactions, 291
Anaphylactic shock, 239
Anaphylactoid reactions, 20,205, 215,217,268,297
Anaphylatoxins, 21,46
  C3a and C5a, 32
Anaphylaxis, 23,202,204,236,245, 272,274,315,317
Anethole, 151
Angioedema, 249
Animal studies, 13
Animal toxic effects, 346
Anionic agents, 173,289,290

449

Anise, oil of, 151,152
Anthraquinones, 254
Anti-cholinergiclike effects, 174
Antiidiotypic antibodies, 33
Antibodies, 25,306
Antibody dependent cell cytotoxicity, 30
Antifoaming agents, 123
Antigen-induced lymphocyte transformation (proliferation), 76, 77
Antigens, 24
Antimicrobials, 177,178,296
Antinuclear antibody (ANA), 72
Antioxidants, 177,181,312
Appendix-Inactive Ingredient Guide, 359
Aqueous formulations, 211
Arlacel, 290
Aromatic acohols, 238
Aromatic oils, 146
Arthritis, 225
Arthus phenomenon, 50
Artificial excipients, 2
Artificial sweeteners, 137
Aspartame, 137,139,233
Aspirin intolerance, 150,268
Asthma (See also Bronchoconstriction), 163,188,189,203,228, 229,248,268,273,276,287, 348
Atopic dermatitis, 236
Atopy, 39,40
Autoantibodies, 45,46,72
Autoimmune diseases, 49
Autooxidation, 315
Azelaic acid, 352
Azo colors (dyes), 254,257

B

B cell factors, 31
B cells, 27

B lymphocytes, 24
Balsam of Peru, 238,239,241
Balsams, 238,241
Bananas, 153
Barbiturate buffers, 172
Basophilic hypersensitivity, 52
Basophils, 44,45
Beeswax, 105,210,211
Benefit-risk ratio, 14
Bentonite (soap clay), 105
Benzaldehyde, 153
Benzalkonium chloride, 292,293, 353
Benzoic acid, 180,239,308,309,310
Benzyl alcohol, 179,310
Benzyl benzoate, 112,308
Benzylkonium chloride, 174
BHA, 312,313,314
BHT, 313,314
Bicarbonate salts, 95
Bile salts, 95
Bioerodible ocular devices, 344
Biocidals, 20
BNPD (2-bromo-2-nitropropane-1, 3-diol), 305,306
Bone cement, 344
Borate buffers, 170
Bovine collagen, 344,350,351
Bradycardia, 351
Bronchial challenge test, 62,79
Bronchial obstruction, 214
Bronchoconstriction, 293,318,319
Bronchospasm, 226,247
Bronopol (BNDP), 181
Buffers, 169,289
Bulk fillers, 89,201
Burning sensation, 248
Butane, 189,190
Butanetriols, 100
Butylated hydroxyanisol (BHA), 312, 313, 314
Butylated hydroxytoluene (BHT), 181, 313, 314
Butylene glycol, 104

C

C3b receptors, 32
C5a, 46
Calciphylaxis, 94
Calcium, 171
Calcium metabolism, 170
Calcium oxalate, 101
Calcium phosphate, 93
Calcium sulfate, 93
Camphor poisoning, 148
Cancers in rats, 163
Canthaxanthin, 254,278
Capsules, 121,223
Caramel, 136,278
Caraway oil, 149
Carbomer, 123,124,227
Carbon dioxide, 92
Carbopol, 124,125
Carbowax, 101
Carboxymethylcellulose, 97,287,288
Carboxyvinyl polymers (carbomer)
   122,125
Carcinogenesis, 161
Carcinogenic potential, 138,160
Cardiac arrhythmias, 186,188,189
Cardiac sensitization, 188
Cardiotoxic properties, 328
Carmine, 163,278
Carnaubawax, 125
Carrier protein, 24
Carriers, 89
Casein, 287
Cassia oil, 238
Castor bean, 108
Castor oil, 108
Catgut, 348
Cationic agents, 174,292
Celery, 235
Celiac disease, 124,225
Cell-mediated immunity, 19,50,53,
   73
Cell-mediated responses, 225

Cellacephate, 125
Cellular sensitization, 19
Cellulose, 97
Cement, 128
Central nervous system depression,
   186
Certified drug colorants, 253
Cetalkonium chloride, 292
Cethexonium bromide, 292
Cetrimide, 174,292
Cetrimonium bromide, 292
Cheilitis, 148,245
Chelating agents, 177,183,323
Chemical polymers, 343
Chemotactic factors, 44,66
Chest tightness, 248
Chloracetamide, 312
Chloramine, 178
Chloramine-T, 310,328
Chlorbutanol, 179
Chlorhexidine, 353
Chloride, 96
Chlormethylsilane, 123
Chlorobutanol, 310,353
Chlorocresol, 178,296,297
Chloroform, 153,187
Chocolate, 237
Cholesterol, 128
Cholinergic urticaria, 351
Chromic catgut, 348
Chromium, 352
Chromosomal changes, 184
Cinnamaldehyde, 246,247
Cinnamic alcohol, 238
Cinnamic aldehyde, 147, 149, 238
Cinnamon oil, 238,241
Citrate buffers, 171
Citric acid, 94
Citronella oil, 349
Class I MHZ antigens, 24
Class II MHZ antigens, 24
Classification of adverse reactions,
   17

Clonidine patches, 349
Closed patch test, 74
Clq-binding assay, 69
Cluster differentiation (CD) anti-
    gens, 27
CMC (carboxymethylcellulose), 287
Coatings, 121,223,230
Cobalt, 352
Cochlear potentials, 124
Cocoa, 145
Cocoa alkaloids, 145
Cocobetaine, 290
Coconut diethanolamine, 290
Coconut oil, 102,107
Collagen, 122
Colloid volume substitutes, 217
Colorants (coloring agents), 159,
    253,345
Colostomy devices, 349
Complement, 32,48
Complement receptor 1 (CR1), 32
Complement-dependent cytotoxic
    antibodies, 67
Compliance, 15
Composition of coloring agents,
    161
Compressed CO_2, 186
Condoms, 347,350
Conglutinin-binding assay, 69
Conjunctival challenge tests, 78
Connective tissue, 45
Contact allergy, 304
Contact cheilitis, 227
Contact dermatitis, 19,36,51,73,
    207,208,209,210,211,212,
    213,214,224,228,229,236,
    246,268,287,288,292,293,
    294,297,298,299,306,308,
    310,313,317,318,321,322,
    323,325,327,346,347,348,
    349,351
  acrylic adhesives, 350
  adhesive tape, 349
  alcohols, 212,310
  alginates, 229
  anionic surfactants, 290
  beeswax, 211

[Contact dermatitis]
  benzalkonium chloride, 293
  benzoic acid, 310
  boric acid, 308
  2-bromo-2-nitropropane-1,3-diol
      (BNPD), 306, 307
  butylated hydroxyanisole, 313
  butylated hydroxytoluene (BHT)
      313
  carboxymethylcellulose, 288
  chlorocresol, 297
  cinnamaldehyde, 246
  colostomy devices, 349
  essential oils, 246
  ethylenediamine, 321,322
  ethylenediaminetetracetic acid
      (EDTA), 323
  ethylene oxide, 325
  food flavors, 236
  formaldehyde, 306
  glutaraldehyde, 327
  glycerin, 214
  hearing devices, 349
  isopropyl myristate, 210
  lanolin, 209
  methylmethacrylate, 228,287
  needles, 348
  nitroglycerin patches, 349
  nordihydroguaiaretic acid
      (NDGA), 313
  olive oil, 213
  pacemakers, 349
  parabens, 298,299
  petrolatum, 207
  polyethylene glycol, 208
  propolis, 211
  propylene glycol, 208
  quaternium-15, 307
  quinoline dyes, 277
  rubber antioxidants, 346,347
  sesame oil, 213
  siloxane, 224
  skeletal system appliances, 351
  sorbic acid, 308
  sulfites, 317,319
  tartrazine, 268

[Contact dermatitis]
  tragacanth, 294
  triethanolamine, 292
Contact lenses, 126,128
Contact mucositis, 246
Contact sensitivity, 81,235,241,
    290,296
Contact sensitization, 211,272,277
Contact urticaria, 204,208,212,
    215,239,245,247,297,298,
    309,312,347,349
  adhesive pads, 349
  alcohol, 204,212
  balsam of Peru, 239,245
  benzoic acid, 239,309
  butylated hydroxyanisole (BHA),
    312
  butylated hydroxytoluene (BHT),
    312
  cassia oil, 239, 245
  chlorocresol, 297
  cinnamic acid, 247
  cinnamic aldehyde, 239,245,247
  cornstarch, 347
  dimethylsulfoxide (DMSO), 215
  ethyl vanillin, 239,245
  methyl salicylate, 247
  parabens, 298
  polyethylene glycols, 298
  propylene glycols, 208
  rubber latex, 347
  sodium benzoate, 309
  sorbic acid, 239,247,309
  zinc diethyldithiocarbonate,
    347
Contact-type eruptions, 232
Containers, 126
Contraceptive diaphragms, 350
Controlled release, 97,103,121
Controlled release binding agents,
    167,283
Copper, 172
Copper-containing intrauterine
    devices, 351
Corn oil (maize oil), 107
Cornstarch, 201,206,295

Cornstarch surgical glove powder,
    347
Corticosteroid formulations with
    parabens, 300
Corticosteroid formulations with
    sorbic acid, 308
Cotton linters, 348
Cottonseed oil, 107,112,113
CR1 receptors, 48
CR2 receptor, 33
CR3 receptor, 33
CR4 receptor, 33
Cremophor EL, 112,290,291
Cross intolerance, 150
Cross-reactions, 321
Cross-sensitivity, 346
Cryoglobulins, 69
Cuprammonium cellulose, 127,347
Cuprophan dialyzers, 348
Cutaneous flushing, 203
Cyclamates, 137,138,139,140,233,
    234
Cytokines, 31
Cytotoxicity, 18,29
Cytotoxic antibodies, 68
Cytotoxic hypersensitivity reac-
    tions, 35
Cytotoxic T cells, 27,30

                    D

D&C colors, 253
Deaths due to asthma, 188
DEHP (Dihexylethylphthalate),
    346
Delaney Amendment, 162
Delayed hypersensitivity, 32,36,50,
    76
Delayed-hypersensitivity T cells,
    29,50
Delisting of colors, 163
Dental amalgams, 300
Dental caries, 99
Dermatitis herpetiformis, 124
Detergents, 113,290

Device materials, 350
Devices, 343
Dextran, 216,288
Dextrates, 96
Dextrim (starch gum), 96
Dextrose, 96
Diabetics, 99
Diacids, 111
Diagnostic procedures for
    human hypersensitivity,
    59
Dialysis membranes, 127
Dialyzer devices, 347
Dialyzer-associated adverse events,
    348
Diarrhea, 162,202,226
Dichlormethylsilane, 123
Dicrolenes, 112
Digestive tract, 345
Digitalis, 96
Dihexylethylphthalate (DEHP), 227
Dill oil, 148
Dimethicone, 123
Dimethylsulfoxide (DMSO), 109,
    215,350
Direct patch test, 73
Direct skin test reactions, 320
Direct skin tests, 60
Direct toxicity, 148
Disaccharide, 201
Dispensers, 345
Disposable hollow-fiber dialyzers,
    328
Disulfiram, 99
DMSO (Dimethylsulfoxide), 109,
    216
Dose-response curve, 13
Double-blind oral challenge tests,
    78
Draize tests, 75
Drug delivery systems, 344
Dumping syndrome, 96
Dusting powders, 103
Dyes (See also colors), 161

E

Effector T cells, 27
Effervescent formulations, 95
Effervescent tablets, 90
Egg albumin, 227,287
Elixirs, 99,101
Emollient, 105,108
Emulsifiers, 172,189,290
Emulsions, 106
Enteric coatings, 125,168
Enteric film formers, 227
Enzyme-Linked Immunosorbent
    Test (ELISA), 63
Eosin, 163
Eosinophils, 44,225
Epileptogenic, 139
Epoxidized soybean oil, 288
Epoxy resins, 349
Erodible drug dispensers, 345
Erythromycin, 227
Erythrosine, 163,276
Esophagus, 122
Essential oils (See also oils), 238,
    239,146,147,148
    synthetic derivatives, 237
Esters, 143
Ethanol (See also Alcohols), 98,99,
    143,202,203,204
Ethanolamine, 350
Ethers, 143
Ethyl alcohol (See Ethanol)
Ethyl Oleate, 112
Ethylene glycol, 101,111
Ethylene oxide, 184, 324, 325, 326
Ethylenediamine, 182,289,320,
    321,322
Ethylenediamine tetraacetic acid
    (EDTA), 183, 321, 323
Eugenol, 147,238,239,241,245
Exercise-induced anaphylaxis, 235
Experimental contact hypersensiti-
    vity, 81

Experimental respiratory sensitiza-
    tion, 82
External use dyes (EXT D&C),
    254
Extractable nuclear antigens, 73
Eye appliances, 352

F

Fat embolism, 112,113,128
Fatal reactions, 151
Fatality rate, 188
Fatty alcohols, 176,296
FD&C dyes, 253
    Blue no. 2 (Brilliant Blue), 277
    Red dye no. 4 (Ponceau SX), 274
    Green no. 3 (Fast Green), 277
    Red dye no. 17, 275
    Red no. 36, 275
    Yellow no. 10, 277
    Yellow no. 11, 277
    Yellow no. 6, 274
FDA certification-exempt dyes,
    278
Fillers, 89,90
Fixed oils, 112
Flatulence, 123,202
Flavoring agents, 246
Fluoran dyes, 275,276
Fluorocarbon propellants, 186,187,
    188,189,328
Fluorohydrocarbons, 329
Food allergies, 236
Food anaphylaxis, 234
Food hypersensitivity, 234
Food immune complexes, 235
Formaldehyde, 181,305,306,327,
    348,351,352
Formaldehyde antibodies, 306,328
Formaldehyde-releasing agents, 305
Formalin (See Formaldehyde)
Formic acid, 110
Forty-eight/eighty (48/80), 20
Fructose, 99,100,135
Fructose-1-P-aldolase, 99

Fruit flavors, 141
Furfural, 110

G

Galactose, 93
Gallic acid esters, 312
Gastrointestinal disturbances, 215,
    236
Gastrointestinal symptoms, 247,
    274
Gelatin, 122,168,216,223,344
Gelatin capsules, 122
General skin test hyerresponsive-
    ness, 40
Germall, 180,305
Giant papillary conjunctivitis
    syndrome, 352
Ginger, 145
Ginger jake paralysis, 107
Gingilli oil, 107
Glass, 127
Glucose, 93,96,135,231
Gluten, 123,124,225,226
Gluteraldehyde, 326,344
Glycerin (glycerol), 99,100,108,
    111,122,135,204,214
Glycine, 171
Glycols, 101,104,111,204,207
Glycosuria, 100
Glycosylation-enhancing factor
    (GEF), 42
Glycosylation-inhibitory factor
    (GIF), 42
Glycyrrhetinic acid, 237
Granule-associated mediators,
    43
Granulomatous mastitis, 123
Granulomatous panniculitis, 139,
    233
Granulomatous reactions, 224
GRAS, 161
Gum arabic, 294
Gum guar, 294
Gums, 124
Gynecologic appliances, 345

H

Hair sprays, 123
Halothane-induced hepatitis, 328
Haptenic reaction, 24
Hard paraffin, 104
Hard plastic lenses, 344
Headache, 215,139
Hearing devices, 349
Hemagglutination techniques, 67
Hemodialysis, 306
Hemodialysis reactions—Types A &
    B, 324,347
Hemolysis, 110,184
Hepatic dysfunction, 186
Hepatotoxic, 150
Hereditary factors, 39
High affinity receptors ($F_{c\ell}$ R1), 43
Higher alcohols, 143
Histamine, 44,65,237
Histamine-releasing agents, 229,247
Histamine-releasing properties, 216,
    227
HLA–DR4 class II antigen, 350
Human hypersensitivity, 34
Human leukocyte antigens (HLA), 24
Human serum albumin, 172,216
Humectants, 108
Humoral antibodies, 24
Hydantoin, 94
Hydrogen gas, 92
Hydrogenated lanolin, 209
Hydrogenated vegetable oil, 176
Hydrous wool fat, 105
Hydroxyethyl starch, 216
Hydroxylamine, 172
5-Hydroxymethyl furfural, 110
Hydroxysulfonate adduct, 315
Hyperaldosteronism, 237
Hypereosinophilia, 348
Hyperkinesis, 268,273
Hypertonic hyperosmolar solutions,
    110,211
Hypoglycemia, 99
Hypotension, 351

Hypotonic Solutions, 110
Hypromellose, 97

I

Idiosyncrasy, 19
Idiotypic network, 33
IgA antibodies, 306
IgD antibodies, 270,271
IgE antibodies, 19,31,35,62,225,
    270
IgE receptors, 43
IgE-binding factors, 42
IgE-mediated reactions, 31
IgG antibody, 45,47
IgM antibodies, 306
Imidazolidinyl urea, 305
Imitation flavors, 141
Immediate hypersensitivity, 18,35,
    39
Immediate hypersensitivity reac-
    tions, 35
Immune complexes, 19,35,46,47,
    48,49,50,68,72
Immune response genes, 40
Immunopathogenesis of human
    hypersensitivity, 39
Immunotoxicological surveys, 79
Immunotoxicology, 18
Implantable lenses, 344
Impurities, 15
India gum, 294
Indigo carmine, 277
Indigoids, 254,277
Inorganic agents, 300
Inorganic salts, 140
Insomnia, 145
Insulin, 110
Interferon, 24
Interleukin 4, 31,42
Intolerance, 19,209,212,225,226
Intracutaneous skin tests, 60,73
Intradermal implants, 350
Intradermal tests, 60,73

Intramuscular route, 110
Intrauterine devices, 345,351
Ionic agents, 173
Ionic/nonionic equilibrium, 169
Irritant contact dermatitis, 210
Isobutane, 189,328
Isocyanates, 348
Isoeugenol, 238
Isopropyl alcohol, 98
Isopropyl myristate, 108,112,123, 210
Isopropyl palmitate, 108
Isoproterenol, 188

K

K cells, 30
K_1 oxide, 112
Karaya gum, 294,349
Kernicterus, 180
Ketosis, 100

L

Lactase, 92
Lactase deficiency, 136,202
Lactic acid, 92
Lactose, 92,136,202
Lactulose, 92,101
Lakes, 161
Langerhans epidermal cells, 30,52
Lanolin, 105,209,210
Lanolin alcohol, 105
Late cutaneous reactions, 61
Late phase response, 50
Lavender oil, 151
Leaching, 98
Leaching of nickel, 348
Lecithin, 168
Lemon oil, 151
Lens cleaning solutions, 353
Leukocyte inhibitory factor, 52,77
Leukotriene, 44,46

Levulinic acid, 110
Licorice, 145,237
Limited compatibility, 140
Limonene, 151
Lincomycin, 139
Linoleic acid, 108
Lipids, 128
Lipoid granulomata, 104
Lipoid pneumonia, 104
Liquid formulations, 97,202
Liquid paraffin, 104
Liquid petrolatum, 104
Liquids, (lotions, emulsions, suspensions), 106,211
Listed colorants, 253
Local irritation, 122
Locust gum, 294
Lotions, 106
Low affinity IgE receptors $(F_{c\varrho} R2)$, 43
Lozenges, 99
Lubricants, 123,175,176,295
Lymphadenopathy, 224
Lymphokines, 24,52

M

Macrogol, 101
Macrophages-inhibiting factor, 52, 77
Macrophage, 30
Maize oil, 107
Mannitol, 101,205,216,217
Maple syrup, 136
Mast cells, 44,45
Mediators of allergic reaction, 64
Medical appliances, 343
Medical Device Amend. 1976/ Federal FD&C Act, 343
Medical devices, 344
Medical plastic appliances, 346
Membrane attack complex (C5b6789), 33,46

Membrane lipid-derived mediators, 44
Menthol, 153,238,239,241
Mercaptobenzothiazole, 347
Mercurialentis, 179
Mercury amalgam, 301
Mercury compounds, 300,303
Methacrylate monomers, 351
Methanol (methyl alcohol), 98,143
Methemoglobinemia, 182
Methyl alcohol (methanol), 98,143
Methyl salicylate, 149,150,239
Methylcellulose, 175,202,288,295
Methylenediphenyldiisocyanate MDI, 348
Methylmethacrylate, 128,228,349, 351
MHC Class I antigens, 24
MHC Class II antigens, 24
MHC Class III antigens, 32
Microemboli, 224
Microencapsulation, 121,123,127, 168,227,228,229
Microscopic implantable spheres, 344
Migraine headaches, 233
Mineral hydrocarbons, 103
Mineral oil, 104,106
Miscarriage, 184
Mono (2-ethylhexyl) phthalate (MEHP), 346
Monoclonal rheumatoid factor assay, 70
Monosaccharides, 101,201
Monosodium glutamate (MSG), 248,249
Mortality rate, 189
Mouth preparations, 218
Mucilages, 124
Musk ambrette, 241,243

N

N blood group antigen, 328
Nasal challenge test, 62,78
Natural dyes, 161
Natural flavors, 141,142,143,234

Natural killer cells (NK), 24,30
Necrotizing vasculitis, 241
Needles and sutures, 348
Neomycin, 124
Neurotoxicity, 179
Neutrophil chemotactic factor of anaphylaxis, 66
Neutrophils, 225
Nickel salts, 347,352
Nickel-sensitive persons, 348
Nitrogen gas, 186
Nitroglycerin patches, 349
Nonaqueous solvents, 112
Nonbiodegradable materials, 228
Noncertifable colorants, 254
Nonhuman albumin, 227
Nonimmunologic basophilic histamine release, 247
Nonimmunologic contact urticaria (NICU), 247,310
Nonionic surfactants, 173,174,179, 290
Nonspecific irritant reactions, 203, 214,215
Nordihydroguaiaetic acid (NDGA), 181,312
Nose drops, 104
Nutmeg oil, 151

O

O-Acetylsalicylic anhydride, 287
Occlusive dressings, 102
Ocular inserts, 344
Oils
  essential oils
    anise, 151
    camphor, 148
    caraway, 149
    cinnamon, 149
    cloves, 149,238
    dill, 148
    eucalyptus, 150
    lavender, 151
    lemon, 151

[Oils]
  [essential oils]
    nutmeg, 151
    orange, 151
    peppermint, 149,241
    persic, 108
    rose, 150
    spearmint, 149,241
    wintergreen, 149
  vegetable oils
    coconut, 102,107
    cottonseed, 107,112,113
    corn, 107
    olive, 107,212,213
    peanut, 206
    poppyseed, 108
    rapeseed, 108
    safflower, 108
    sesame, 107,212,213
    soybean, 206
Olive oil, 107,212,213
Open patch tests, 73
Ophthalmic medical devices, 344
Ophthalmic solutions, 106
Ophthalmologic topical preparations, 103
Oral formulations, 201
Oral challenge, 270
Orange oil, 151
Organ challenge tests, 61,77
Organic acids and their salts, 308
Organic mercury, 300
Orofacial granulomatosis, 246
Oxidation, 102

P

Pacemaker devices, 349
Papain, 353
Parabens, 180,298,299,353
Paraffin, 104,123,125,175
Paraffinomas, 104
Paregoric, 99
Paraplegia, 179
Parenteral formulations, 109,216

Parenteral nutrition, 112
Paresthesia, 351
Passive transfer tests, 61
Patch testing, 103
Peanut oil, 206
Pectin, 288
PEG (See Polyethylene Glycol)
Penetration of skin, 102
Penicillin, 287
Peppermint, 238
Peppermint oil, 149,241
Percutaneous drug delivery, 103
Perfumes, 147
Periorbital edema, 224
Persic oil, 108
Pessaries, 350
Petrolatum, 103,104,206
pH, 106,169,170
Phagocytes, 24
Pharmagel, 122
Phenol, 178,238,296
Phenylacetaldehyde, 238
Phenylalanine, 139
Phenylethylamine, 237
Phenylmercuric nitrate/acetate, 179,353
Phenylmercuric proprionate, 303
Phenylmercuric salts, 303
Phosphate buffers, 170
Phospholipid dispersions, 344
Photosensitivity dermatitis, 146, 233,322
Photosensitization, 232,241,276
Phototoxicity, 161,163
Phthalate plasticizers, 227,288, 348
Phthalic acid, 125
Phthalic acid anhydride, 288, 346
Pigments, 161
Pimelic acid, 352
Piperonal, 143
Pitkin menstruum, 112
Plain collagen sutures, 348
Plaster of paris, 93,111
Plasticizers, 125,126,344
Plastics, 126

Platelet-activating factor (PAF), 44, 66
Pleuripotential stem cells, 26
Pneumonitis, 225
Poly-l-lysine, 124,227
Polyacrylate, 349
Polyanhydride polymers, 352
Polyethoxylated castor oil, 112
Polyethylene, 126
Polyethylene glycols (PEG), 101, 104,208
Polymers, 227,349
Polymers (acidic, basic), 124
Polymethyl methacrylate (PMMA), 128,351,352
Polymyxin B, 20
Polyneuropathy, 107
Polyols, 122
Polypropylene, 126
Polystyrene, 126
Polyvinyl chloride (PVC), 126,288, 346
Polyvinylpyrrolidone (PVP), 168, 169,229,288
Pompholyx, 304
Poppyseed oil, 108
Potassium bicarbonate, 95
Potassium bisulfite, 314
Potassium chloride, 140
Potassium metabisulfite, 314
Povidone, 168
Powders, 90
Preservative-free diet, 274
Preservatives, 176,296
Prick tests, 60
Primary irritants, 102,308
Propellants, 184,328
Prophetic patch tests, 75
Propolis, 210,211
Propyl gallate, 182
Propylene glycol, 100,101,104, 204,208,209
Propylgallate, 313
Prostaglandins, 44,66
Proteoglycans, 44
Provisional colorants, 253

Pseudoallergic reactions, 20,59,77, 237,247,272,309,314,329
Pulmonary leukostasis, 348
PVC (See Polyvinyl chloride)
PVP (See Polyvinyl pyrrolidone)

Q

Quaternium-15, 305
Quinoline dyes, 254,277

R

Radioallergosorbent tests, 63
Raji cell assay, 71
Rancidity, 102
Rapeseed oil, 108
Reactions to specific dyes, 162
Recall antigens test battery, 76
Red blood cells, 328
Red cell "ghosts", 128
Reflex mediated reactions, 329
Regenerated cellulose membranes, 347
Regulation of coloring agents, 161
Regulatory cells, 27
Renal perfusion, 124
Renal tubular acidosis, 234
Repeat open application skin tests, 78
Reproductive system, 163
Resins, 123
Rose oil, 150
Rubber appliances, 346,349
Rubber stoppers, 123
Rubber tree extracts, 347
Rubbing alcohol, 106

S

Saccharin, 137,138,231,232,233
Safflower oil, 108

Safrole, 150
Salicylism, 150
Saline, 110
Salts, 234
Sarcomas, 161
Scleroderma, 215,225
Serum albumin, 216,344
Serum sickness, 47,49
Serum IgE, 62
Sesame oil, 107,212,213
Shellac, 123,226,289
Silicates, 105,210
Silicon dioxide, 168
Silicone, 123,223,224,225
Silicone teflon sponge, 352
Siloxanes, 350
Simethacone, 123
Skeletal system appliances, 351
Skin adhesive devices, 349
Sodium benzoate, 180,308,309
Sodium bicarbonate, 95
Sodium bisulfite, 314
Sodium chloride, 140
Sodium fluorescein, 275
Sodium lauryl sulfate, 173,290
Sodium metabisulfite, 314
Sodium sulfite, 314
Sodium-restricted diet, 140
Soft plastic lenses, 344
Solid formulations, 201
Solids (gels, ointments, creams),
    103,206
Sorbic acid, 179,247,308,309,353
Sorbic acid reactors, 309
Sorbitan esters, 174,290
Sorbitans, 174
Sorbitol, 101,122,136,205
Sorbitol intolerance, 205
Soybean oil, 206
Spans, 290
Spearmint oil, 149,241
Stabilizers, 320
Starch, 91
Stasis dermatitis, 210
Stearic acid, 123
Sterilizing agents, 324

Stiffening agents, 172,289
Subcutaneous route, 110
Substituted catechols, 238
Sucrase, 100
Sucrose, 99,135,231
Sugar alcohols (See Alcohols), 205
Sugars, 135,201,231
Sulfidopeptide leukotrienes, 44, 66
Sulfite aerosols, 318
Sulfite oxidase deficiency, 319
Sulfite oxidation, 319
Sulfite reactivity, 315,318,319
Sulfites, 182,314,315,317
Sulfur dioxide, 122,318,319
Sunset yellow, 274
Suppositories, 113,217
Surfactants, 101,172,173
Suspending, emulsifying, and stiff-
    ening agents, 172,289
Suspensions, 106
Sweetening agents, 135,231
Sympathomimetic reactions, 145
Synovitis, 224
Synthetic dyes, 161
Synthetic flavoring agents, 152,154
Synthetic phospholipids, 168
Synthetic sweeteners, 231
Synthetic vanillin, 239
Syrups, 99

T

T-cell receptor, 27
T-cells, 24,27
    T-helper cells, 30
    T-suppressor cells, 30
    $T_D CD4$ cells, 36
Tablet coatings, 123,223
Tachycardia, 145
Talc, 176,295
Tantalum, 349
Tartrazine, 162,257,268,270,271,
    272,273
Terpenes, 238
Tetramethylthiuram, 347

Thimerosal, 179,303,304,353
Throat preparations, 218
Thromboangiitis obliterans, 350
Thrombophlebitis, 110
Thymol, 178,296
Tier I assays, 80
Tier II assays, 80
Tinctures, 99
    tincture of orange, 248
Titanium, 349,352
Titanium oxide, 278
Tonicity, 110
Tooth enamel, 171
Topical drug delivery, 102
Topical ophthalmic preparations,
    218
Topical otic preparations, 218
Toxic effects, 163
Toxic potential, 13
Toxicity, 17
Tragacanth gum, 174,175,294
Transdermal delivery systems, 349
Transfer factor, 52
Transient gluten intolerance, 225,
    226
Transitional medical devices, 343
Triethanolamine, 292
Triethanolamine stearate, 290,291
Triethylenetetramine, 289
Trioses, 92
Trioxylmethylene, 305,306
Triphenylmethane dyes, 277
Triphenylmethanes, 254
Tris buffers, 172
Trivial risks, 162
Tryptase, 44,66
Tuberculin-like intradermal tests,
    76
Tuberculin-type delayed hypersen-
    sitivity, 304
Tweens, 290
Two-tiered system of immune
    function testing, 80
Type I hypersensitivity, 18,306
Type II hypersensitivity, 19,45,66

Type III hypersensitivity, 19,47
Type IV hypersensitivity, 36, 50

U

Unabsorbable complex, 139
United States National Toxicology
    program, 80
Urticaria, 202,204,205,208,226,
    232,233,236,245,268,272,
    274,276,294,297,349,350

V

Vaginal devices, 350
Vaginal products, 218
Vaginitis, 350
Vanillin, 145,153,238,247
Vanishing creams, 102
Vaseline, 104
Vegetable gums, 293 294,351
Vegetable oils (See Oils)
Vehicle tray for patch testing, 102
Ventricular tachycardia, 328
Vertigo, 205
Vials, 123
Vinyl chloride, 288
Vinyl chloride monomer, 346
Vinyl chloride toxicity, 189
Vitamin B_{12}, 319
Vitamins, 112
Vomiting, 319
Vulvitis, 350

W

Water, 98,106,109
Waxes, 125,168
Wheezing (See also Asthma, Bron-
    choconstriction), 236
White petrolatum, 206
Wine, 99

Wool alcohols, 105,209
Wool grease, 105

X

Xanthene dyes, 254,275
Xenobiotics, 79
Xylitol, 101,136,205

Y

Yellow petrolatum, 206,207

Z

Zinc dithiocarbamate, 289,347
Zinc-deficient diets, 183

About the Authors

Murray Weiner is Acting Director of the Division of Clinical Pharmacology and Toxicology, and Clinical Professor of Medicine, at the University of Cincinnati in Cincinnati, Ohio, where he has taught since 1972. From 1957 through 1971 he held various research and management positions with Geigy Pharmaceuticals, a division of Ciba-Geigy, serving finally as Vice President and Director of Biologic Research. From 1971 to 1981 he was Vice President, Research and Scientific Affairs, Merrell Research Center. The author or coauthor of some 200 articles and book chapters, he has published several books, including *Nicotinic Acid* (with J. van Eys) and *Drug Interaction Compendium* (both titles, Marcel Dekker, Inc.). He served on several editorial boards, including the journal *Immunopharmacology* and is editor of Marcel Dekker, Inc.'s Clinical Pharmacology Series. A Fellow of the American College of Physicians and New York Academy of Sciences, he is a member of numerous professional societies, including the American Society for Clinical Research and the American Society of Pharmacology and Experimental Therapeutics. Dr. Weiner received the B.S. degree (1939) from the College of the City of New York, M.S. degree in biochemistry and M.D. degree (both in 1943) from New York University College of Medicine.

I. Leonard Bernstein is Clinical Professor of Medicine and Environmental Health Sciences and Co-Director of the Allergy Research Laboratory and the Allergy Training Program at the University of Cincinnati Medical School in Cincinnati, Ohio. The author or coauthor of more than 200 articles, book chapters, and proceedings papers, he currently serves as a director of the American Board of Allergy Immunology, as a governor of the American Board of Internal Medicine, and as a chairman of the Food and Drug Administration's Pulmonary-Allergy Drug Advisory Committee. He is a Fellow and Past President of the American Academy of Allergy, Fellow of the American College of Physicians, and a member of the American Thoracic Society, American Society for Clinical Research, American Association of Immunologists AOA, and Sigma Xi. He has been and currently serves as a consultant for over a dozen peer-reviewed journals in allergy and chest disease as well as the *Journal of the American*

Medical Association, New England Journal of Medicine, and *Journal of Laboratory and Clinical Medicine.* Dr. Bernstein received the M.D. degree (1949) from the University of Cincinnati Medical School.